CUSPID

Volume 1

JOHN LASZLO

CUSPID

Clinically

Useful

Safety

Procedures

In

Dentistry

JOHN LASZLO

To order additional copies of this book, contact:
Xlibris
800-056-3182
www.Xlibrispublishing.co.uk
Orders@Xlibrispublishing.co.uk
714120

PREFACE TO CUSPID

The purpose of these two volumes is to provide a foundation enabling you to learn, revise and then test your knowledge of clinically useful safety procedures in dentistry and by doing so; you will be practising safely and in accordance with the latest evidence based clinical guidelines.

By reading the 5 chapters in these two books, a significant proportion of the requirements for Enhanced Continuing Professional Development (ECPD) that will maintain your registration with the General Dental Council (GDC) can be readily and easily achieved.

Whether you are already in practise, or returning to work after a career break, studying for an examination to register with the UK GDC, or another dental regulator, or to achieve your membership of one of the Royal College of Surgeons Dental Faculties (the MFDS or MJDF examinations), the clinically oriented information in this textbook, together with the essential skills and the clinical experience you have already gained during your training will be of benefit for yourself and for your patients.

Much of the work in a dental practice is based on the technical subjects learned at dental school which are often combined with and modified by the latest information provided by the dental trades' manufacturing and supply companies. While your clinical decisions are supported by such learning, we must not forget that dentistry, despite being corporatized and monetized is neither a trade nor is it a business, it is a health care profession. At the very heart of this profession lies your knowledge of anatomy, physiology, biochemistry, pathology and pharmacology.

It is the medical problems which your patients bring with them and not the surgical ones created in the dental clinic that are the most likely to cause havoc with a patient's health and compromise that delicate balance in the stable environment of safety you and your dental team operate within.

Dentistry and the manner in which it is delivered can and does influence the fine balance between the state of wellness and the state of illness being continually played out in your patient's bodies and in their minds. If this equilibrium isn't fully appreciated or respected, there are dental patients whose health can with some subtlety and a remarkable ease almost imperceptibly drift towards a state of morbidity and if such a change is not immediately recognized, the further descent towards mortality could follow at a rate which can be alarming.

Thankfully such incidences are rare, in fact they are extremely rare, but they do occur and when they do, the loss of one's professional standing or the end of a career standing before the GDC, even though catastrophic, is nothing compared to the loss of a patient's life, even more so if the loss is from a set of circumstances that could have been foreseen and thus prevented.

The work of your colleagues in the nursing, medical and surgical disciplines in secondary care can also be influenced by the actions and inactions of those in primary care. It is therefore of fundamental importance in dentistry, firstly with respect to the patient and secondly with respect to all of your colleagues that an awareness of the scope and the extent of your dental treatment and its relationship to any additional care is understood and maintained. This awareness begins with obtaining and then: <u>maintaining</u> consent all the way to the conclusion of treatment, whether this treatment is by your own hands or by those of the specialist to whom you refer your patient.

Effective communication between dentists, doctors and nurses working in primary and secondary care is essential. The inability to communicate either among or between: dental, medical and nursing professionals have so often been the underlying cause of misunderstandings and mistrust that have led to an unintended conflict that ultimately compromised both patient care and clinical safety.

Undoubtedly with further clinical experience, postgraduate training and specialization to keep up with progress in the profession or other clinical or regulatory developments, the focus of one's dental knowledge deepens, but as it deepens, so often its breadth narrows and so a paradox presents itself in clinical practise: The less qualified but more experienced member of the dental team may be better positioned to identify problems as they begin to unfold than the highly qualified specialist who has, overall; far less clinical experience!

There have been occasions in surgery when a nudge matronizingly and attentively delivered from the dental nurse has moved a newly qualified dentist's hand (the one holding the forceps) from a child's fifth premolar to their fourth premolar, may be from the left to the right side of the mouth or even from the upper to the lower arch and by doing so, disaster was swiftly averted for the patient and disgrace was elegantly (but still) narrowly avoided for the dentist. In this example and with deference, the altruism of team work and the honesty of reflection are the bedrock upon which respect is earned and solid careers are built, not only in dentistry but for any professional in any discipline.

Whether you are working in a general practice, a sedation centre, or a specialist clinic with patients at the extremes of age and health or not, the monitoring and recognition of trends and changes in the patient's vital signs are everyone's responsibility. This is essential, but what is arguably more important than this, or a mastery of the latest developments in clinical practise, is the ability to listen, to work with and to respect the experiences and understand the proficiencies of your colleagues and....to know your own limitations before they remind you of them with more than just a nudge.

The importance for each and every one of your dental team members to participate in your ECPD while you work through this book must be emphasized, not least of all because all members of the dental team can use these two volumes to complete their CPD and their Personal Development Portfolios too.

With today's reliance on electronic media and the stride of clinical research from beginnings *in-silico,* sidestepping the *in-vitro* and *in-vivo* stages, to stamp an authority *in-clinico* is being achieved at a pace that is incredible as it is startling. For sure there is a risk of floundering in an illustrious wake of digital progress, but perhaps what is more important than marching along to the latest developments in dentistry (and often paying for the privilege), is the ability and the need to build a solid foundation of clinical knowledge upon which these latest developments can be understood. While the enchantment of electronic media will continue evolving with ever more accessible but complex and delicate forms, a text book that can be picked up, passed around, dropped, have coffee spilled on and then be written in, that needs no renewal or subscription fee and can be easily replaced if lost will still have a place in clinical learning.

These two books were written for everyone working in dentistry and they were written so you can read, study and learn from these books and do so together with your colleagues. Team work should begin with your Enhanced CPD and the lessons learned by studying together can then be put into practise in the clinic where you will be working together.

In the first volume, in Chapter 1, medical emergencies and the steps required to deal with the most commonly occurring of these are presented together with the 2015 algorithms from the UK Resuscitation Council. In Chapter 2, the mechanisms of how drugs work; their actions, reactions and the potential for adverse interactions that could compromise clinical safety are explored. Although the GDC have not made medicine and drug safety a core topic for Enhanced CPD from 2018, this is an area of clinical practice that is so safety critical it cannot be ignored.

In the second volume, the technical considerations of infection control are covered in Chapter 3, while in Chapter 4, the latest IRR 17 and IR (ME) R 18 regulations for X-ray and radiation safety are presented. While those chapters should prove to be a useful source of revision for the dentist, it is hoped they will be read by the members of the dental team who routinely and in some dental practices almost exclusively deal with these two essential and safety critical activities, without which a dental practice simply cannot function.

In Chapter 5, the subject of oral cancer is presented and we should acknowledge the GDC's quite correct decision to recognise the importance of oral cancer by making it a core component of Enhanced CPD. This chapter concludes with a small section on palliative end of life care; an important but often overlooked area of clinical dental practise that is becoming increasingly prevalent as more of our patients achieve old age. Undoubtedly you will have treated and looked after many patients from their days of health, through various stages of their life's journey and to its end.

While palliative care is not yet part of the GDC's core of Enhanced CPD, nevertheless, it is our duty to recognize and if possible to remedy not only the dental needs, but the clinical needs of our patients living with many illnesses at the end of their lives.

With advances in clinical care, we will attend to patients living with and suffering with illnesses, from which only a few years ago they would have succumbed... passing-on at a younger age and an earlier stage of the disease process. But despite the life-giving and life-extending benefits of modern medicine, the end of life is an outcome that awaits all of us and so it remains our duty to provide the best care for every one of our patients regardless of either, their age, or their time of life; or the time that remains in their life.

Our care has to be given with kindness; it has to be given with compassion and as Carl Rogers urged: It has to be given with an unconditional positive regard. Not only must we care, we must care enough to share our knowledge with our medical and nursing colleagues to support their work in caring for our patients.

While we cannot prolong life, our aim should be to preserve its quality and I hope these two volumes will in some small way help you to achieve that aim and you will be doing so safely for all of your patients all of the time.

An Appreciation

In the past four years many of you will have read and studied from Clinical Problems in Dentistry. With several thousand copies sold, I wish to thank you all for the part you played in that unexpected success and for your feedback that was positive and your feedback that was constructive. In a quote attributed to Jonas Salk and then to Tom Sachs, it is stated the reward for hard work is the opportunity to do more and so an invitation to write another book arrived some two years after that book was published. In truth it was hard to sit down and to begin the process of writing all over again, but I would recommend that you all give it a go, it is painful, it is difficult and I hope this book makes it worth the effort.

My intention was to write a book to pass on the lessons I have learned. Foremost; so you don't make the same mistakes I have, secondly; so you can be a better dentist than I have been and finally; to make dentistry a safer place for you and for your patients, a safer place than it has been for me and my patients. Yes I have made mistakes and apologised to my patients, but none so serious that I haven't been forgiven and I haven't stopped learning from those mistakes and from the kindness and the humanity of my patients. So this book is for our patients and our profession.

The influence of the following individuals, who are no longer with us, whose example and inspiration will remain long after their passing, should be remembered and this book is also for them.

Professor Crispian Scully, one word from me would be too much but a thousand words from the dental profession too few; for his encouragement and his words of advice given to so many including myself, his contribution to our profession was and will be beyond measure.

Professor Robert Yemm and Professor David Stirrups whose capabilities and patience, their kindness and understanding were tested by my inexperience and enthusiasm as a dental student, whose lessons and wisdom now form a significant part of the dentistry that I and we all practise.

Lt Col Mike Argue MC MBE whose drive and determination to succeed in the face of adversity and overwhelming odds set an example for all of us who had that rare privilege to serve under him.

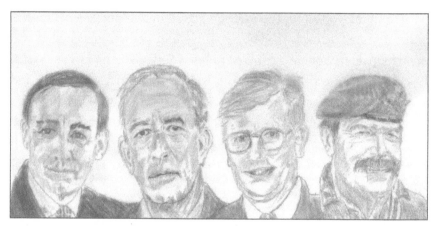

Ad unum omnes

This book was written for you to learn from my mistakes, to make you a better dentist and to make dentistry safer for you and for your patients. I hope that at least something of the essence these great men will have passed into this work. While that bar they set was high...very very high, with the words of Alfred, Lord Tennyson they have now crossed the bar.

It is with a sense of personal and professional regret that they didn't live to see a return of their efforts and investment in me but from this book and with time I hope their investment will become your reward.

An Acknowledgment

Without the support and guidance of Mr Roger Farbey MBE and the staff of the BDA library: Helen Nield, Damyanti Raghvani, Amy Grinnell and Janet Laws, this book could not have been written and I am grateful for their encouragement and their help to complete this work. I have been fortunate to have the help of many, among the many, the support of a few should be recognized:

Dr Derek Keilloh suggested why this book needs to be written. Mr William Fyfe-Jones provided advice and guidance on nursing practice in the NHS. Mr James Badenoch QC of 1 Crown Office Row shared his own experiences of anaesthesia and advised on patient consent.

Professor Mervyn Singer, University College London advised on COPD and palliative care.

Professor Aly Rashid NHS England Responsible Officer made several professional recommendations.

His Honour John Hillen, Blackfriar's Crown Court, Recorder Rajiv Thacker of Garden Court Chambers, Mr Neil Baki of 25 Bedford Row Chambers and Mr Nev Niyazi of McKenzies all provided a valuable legal input to ensure this work would be completed.

Some two decades ago... without the work of Mr Alan Jenkins, (6 Pump Court) now of Serjeant's Inn Chambers, none of this would have happened...nothing... at all....

But because it has, I now wish to express my gratitude to Miss Marianne Lehmann for her administration, support and attention to detail. Dr Adrien Bercu Ph. D Friebourg Switzerland for his directions in this project.

Dr Nikki Davey for sharing her thoughts and experiences of providing dentistry and care at the end of life.

The staff of X-Libris: Emman Villaran, Francine Diola, Charles del Mar and Dion Seller for their work, Mr Brian Westbury of Dental Protection for adding yet another dimension to the legal issues.

Mr Adam Stanley and colleagues of the BDIA.

Mr Chirag Patel BSc Hons CDT RCS (Eng), Sheetal, Ankur, Suryakant, Anandiben and family for their fellowship and friendship.

Claire Daley, editor and her colleagues of the Royal College of Physicians, for their work with the NEWS charts. Sue Hampshire and colleagues in the UK Resuscitation Council, for their medical emergency algorithms.

For feedback and content evaluation, we wish to thank Dr. Edward M. Mills, Dental Surgeon and Roupa Gokal, Dental Student.

Down all these years and long after we served: Dave Stevenson, Ian Millar and Brian Harmer for sticking to our principles, setting the standard and holding the bar that carries us onwards and carries us upwards.

A Dedication

And now when it's all said and it's all done and there's no more to write, for the sacrifices and her love, waiting for me to finish, this book is for my mother...This book is for all our mothers.

Marianne Laszlo
1st January 1931 – 26th March 2017

MHDSRIP.

INTRODUCTION TO CUSPID VOLUME 1

Using this book will help you to complete your requirements for Enhanced CPD.

The GDC inform us that:

Continuing Professional Development (CPD) for dental professionals can be defined as: lectures, seminars, courses, **individual study and other activities** that can be included in your CPD record if they can be <u>reasonably expected</u> to advance your professional development either as a dentist or as a dental care professional and such activities are relevant to your practise or your intended practise of dentistry[1].

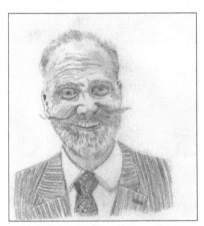

The GDC go on to recommend: CPD is a valuable source of support for dentists and dental care professionals to maintain and update their clinical skills, knowledge and professional behaviours[1,2].

All registered dental professionals have a legal duty to maintain and develop their working knowledge and clinical skills so the dental treatment and oral care provided is <u>safe</u> and of the very best standard. To maintain registration with the GDC, specific CPD requirements must be met.

Participating in CPD is therefore a compulsory part of your registration with the GDC and the evidence that you are doing so needs to be retained. The CPD scheme has made an important contribution to patient safety and the previous requirements in place for nearly a decade have now been replaced with a new set of requirements entitled: Enhanced CPD. This is effective from the start of 2018 for dentists and from August 2018 for all other dental care professionals registered with the GDC.

There are a minimum number of hours that must be completed during your five year CPD cycle and these can include contributions from:

I. Lectures.
II. Seminars.
III. Courses.
IV. **Individual study.**
V. **Other activities.**

Almost anything can be included in your CPD record, however as underlined above and repeated again; such activity has to be <u>reasonably expected</u> to advance your professional development as a dentist or as a dental care professional and it must be <u>relevant to your practise of dentistry</u>. Examples of these can include:

I. Courses and lectures.
II. **Training sessions.**
III. **Peer Review and Clinical Audit.**
IV. **Reading journals and text books.**
V. Attendance at conferences and E-learning activity.

By working your way through this textbook you can undertake all of those activities highlighted in the above boxes *e.g:* Individual study, or with your colleagues; you can participate in: Other activities, such as: Training sessions, Peer Review and Clinical Audit and together with reading journals or other professional publications, this text book can provide you not only with a foundation for your 5 year program of Enhanced CPD, but also a framework that you can use to support the plans for your personal and professional development which the GDC require you to undertake from 2018 onwards.

As a reminder: In your 5 year CPD cycle there will be a minimum number of CPD hours you must complete. These minimums are determined by your registration status; whether you are registered as a dentist or a dental care professional (DCP). From January 2018 for dentists and from August 2018 for dental care professionals, the following changes to CPD came into effect:

I.   There is an increase in the number of verifiable hours you must complete.

II. There is now a requirement to spread these hours evenly across 5 years.

III. Due to the requirement for non-verifiable CPD being removed, there will be an overall reduction in the CPD hours for all dental professionals.

IV. There will be a need to make a mandatory annual declaration of the CPD hours you have completed and that you are meeting the requirements for the specific subject or core areas.

V.   As noted above: There is now a requirement for a Personal Development Plan to be completed.

The verifiable hours required over a five year CPD cycle will be:

I.	Dentists and Specialists: **100 Hours.**
II.	Dental Therapists and Hygienists: **75 Hours.**
III.	Orthodontic Therapists: **75 Hours.**
IV.	Clinical Dental Technicians: **75 Hours.**
V.	Dental Nurses and Technicians: **50 Hours.**

Furthermore under these new requirements, you will need to keep a CPD record including:

I. A **Professional** and/or a **Personal Development Plan**.
II. Details of the CPD you have undertaken and the CPD you plan to undertake.
III. The learning outcomes which may evolve throughout your 5 year CPD cycle.
IV. A log of completed CPD, including: date, number of hours and outcomes achieved.
V. Evidence such as a certificate for each CPD activity you have completed.

The GDC have also stated:

You may find it helpful to carry out CPD with other people, particularly other members of the dental team. This may be particularly helpful if you are a sole practitioner. In some circumstances, it will be useful for a dental team to carry out training together – for example, training to handle medical emergencies in the practice[1]. Therefore the five chapters in this two volume text book can be used to undertake those activities outlined from the GDC's recommended list of CPD sources and these can be:

I. **Individual study.**

II. **Other activities.**

III. **Training sessions.**

IV. **Peer review and Clinical Audit.**

V. **Reading journals and text books.**

By participating in these activities and using this first volume, the following two subject areas in your 5 Year cycle of Enhanced CPD can be completed:

> **I.   Medical Emergencies.**
>
> **II.   Medicine and Drug Safety *.**

* Despite the GDC not including Medicine and Drug Safety in your core CPD, given the safety critical nature of this subject, it is recommended as an essential part of your Enhanced CPD.

From the second volume, the following topics in your 5 Year Enhanced CPD cycle can be completed:

> **III.   Disinfection and Decontamination.**
> **IV.   Radiography and Radiation Protection.**
> **V.   Oral Cancer Early Detection.**

If you are a dentist or a DCP completing your CPD under the transitional arrangements available until you fully participate in the Enhanced CPD scheme, by reading the chapters in this book and recording the dates and times in the logs provided, there is sufficient material for you to claim general CPD to a level that is well in excess of the minimum requirements laid down by the GDC under both the previous and the present guidelines. If you are in the transitional phase of your CPD, the GDC "Enhanced CPD Transition Tool" is available from: https://gdc.onlinesurveys.ac.uk/ecpdtool. Using this together with this book will greatly assist you in completing your CPD requirements.

To claim Enhanced CPD you will need to read and revise the subjects within the chapters and then answer questions relevant to the sections you have selected. Your CPD can then be verified by recording the dates and duration for such activity in the CPD logs and signing the certificates provided at the end of each chapter.

A counter signature from one of your GDC, GMC or NMC registered colleagues or your dental practice manager can attest to this activity being verifiable and thus your participation in such CPD qualifies for Enhanced Continuing Professional Development.

For such activity to be carried out as Enhanced CPD, as a guide:

> **It should take 1 hour to read, revise and review the material for some 10 multiple choice questions. However, some of you may take longer and more of you may take less than this. Your feedback on your individual study speeds would be most welcome!**

In the two volumes there are a total of 650 multiple choice questions. Some questions have single answers, many questions have multiple answers and a few questions have a range of answers. By taking one hour for every 10 questions (you can choose the subject, the questions and the time taken to discuss the results), a total of 65 hours of Enhanced CPD can be recorded just by studying for and then answering the multiple choice questions.

If these are completed in five years, this is neither an onerous nor an intensive exercise and by the end of your CPD cycle, a considerable amount of your Verifiable, Core and Enhanced CPD can be covered and completed in the company of your colleagues, either as a part of your dental practice team-training or as Peer Review Exercises. This activity can be easily accomplished during your working hours, comfortably exceeding the GDC minimum rate to participate in Enhanced CPD which is:

> **10 Hours every 2 Years.**

Following from this approach to your CPD, if you are a dentist you will be left with 35 hours to allocate for those courses with mandatory attendance, such as: First Aid, Immediate Life Support and Paediatric Life Support. Even though your attendance on such courses is mandatory, by reading the material in this textbook, you will firstly be able to revise and secondly you will be able to reflect on your attendance on these courses. By doing so, you can with a measure of confidence gain so much more from your attendance than if no background reading or study were undertaken beforehand.

If you are a clinical dental technician, an orthodontic therapist or a hygienist, you could complete 65 out of your 75 hours, while nurses and technicians could participate with their senior colleagues to complete or possibly even exceed the Enhanced CPD requirements just by reading these two books then answering the multiple choice questions at the end of each chapter.

We shouldn't overlook the opportunity to participate in Peer Review Exercises and that such activity can count towards Enhanced CPD! If you choose to select and focus on topics from within the 5 chapters, it would not be unreasonable of the GDC to expect that some 3 Hours +/- 1 Hour from each of the 5 chapters could be (or should be) set aside for Peer Review of those subjects. Therefore another 15 to 20 Hours of CPD could be reasonably claimed in a 5 Year CPD Cycle just by using the data in these books both for Peer Review and for your Personal and Professional Development Portfolio thus:

> **80 Hours to 85 Hours of Verifiable Enhanced CPD can be achieved from these text books.**

In essence: For DCP registrants using these books, the Enhanced CPD requirements to maintain GDC registration can be met and for dentists using this book; setting aside another 20 hours across a 5 Year CPD cycle for further verifiable CPD is no longer an inaccessible pinnacle or an insurmountable obstacle to contemplate on your professional journey while ensuring your continued registration!

For some time now, verifiable CPD has been defined by the GDC as requiring the documentary evidence that the dentist or the dental care professional has actually undertaken the CPD and further documentary evidence is required to prove that the CPD you undertake will have the following:

> I. **Concise educational aims and objectives**
> II. **Clear anticipated outcomes**
> III. **Quality controls.**

If you are using this book as a basis for your Enhanced CPD, then the GDC state you must keep a record of this for up to 5 years <u>after</u> the end of your CPD cycle. In order to meet the GDC requirements, your CPD record must include the documentary evidence attesting to the verifiable nature of the CPD. This can be achieved by completing and signing the: log sheets, the certificates and the feedback forms found at the end of each chapter after the answers for the multiple choice questions.

Please don't forget to collect counter signatures from your registered colleagues who also participate in your CPD. Without these, the GDC could reasonably question whether or not the CPD activity is verifiable. Adding to this, the GDC have stipulated for CPD to be verifiable at least one of the following learning outcomes must be demonstrated for each activity you complete[2]:

> I. **Effective communication** with patients, the dental team and others, including obtaining consent, dealing with complaints and raising concerns.
> II. **Effective management** of yourself and effective management of others or effective work with others in the dental team; in the interests of patients at all times.
> III. **Providing constructive leadership where appropriate**.
> IV. **Maintaining and developing knowledge and skills** within your field of practice.
> V. **Maintaining skills, behaviours and attitudes** which maintain patient confidence in you and the dental profession while putting the patients' interests first.

Given the broad scope of these learning outcomes, if you study each of the five chapters and answer the questions at the end of each chapter, then you can demonstrate that you have maintained and developed the knowledge and skills within your field of practise. (Outcome IV). With your participation, appraisal and reflection, the other outcomes from the above list can also be achieved.

All verifiable CPD must be quality controlled.
While the GDC do not quality assure CPD activity, from April 2013, the GDC did expect that some form of quality assurance must be in place. The educational content of this textbook when used for verifiable CPD has been effectively quality controlled by the following means at the relevant stages[3,5] :

1. Quality controls in place before CPD:

I.	Each chapter has numbered citations with references for further reading. The chapter on medical emergencies comprehensively covers this GDC core CPD subject.
II.	The publisher and their editorial board have content evaluated this work.
III.	The chapters and questions are evidence based on the professional standards not only for dentistry but for those professionals who are allied to dentistry.
IV.	Any policies and procedures referred to have no commercial bias; this text book was written for educational purposes only and is published on a not-for-profit-basis.
V.	Your feedback will be incorporated in subsequent editions and amendments to this work will be made as our knowledge in the subject areas continues to grow.

2. Quality controls during the CPD activity:

I.   Confirmation of your participation and the length of study time can be achieved by signing the log sheets and whenever necessary, a counter signature can attest to the verifiable nature of any CPD activity that you are claiming.

II.   The delivery of educational standards can be evaluated through feedback and by making reflective notes as you progress through your 5 year CPD cycle using this book as a framework for your professional development portfolio.

III.   In accordance with the GDC's principles for CPD: The aims, objectives and anticipated learning outcomes are clearly set out at the beginning of each chapter.

IV.   During dental team training and group exercises, there will be opportunities for reflection from all participants.

V.   The questions at the end of each chapter provide an opportunity to assess whether the learning outcomes and educational objectives have been reached.

3. Quality control after completion of the CPD:

I.   Those who take part in Enhanced CPD can record their participation in the log sheets.

II.   There should be post-delivery evaluation that can be noted in the feedback forms.

III.   Should any questions or doubts arise from using this text book for CPD, the author, the editors and the publisher can be notified of such concerns.

IV.   All contributions improving this CPD resource will be acknowledged.

V.   There is an opportunity to provide feedback both offline and online.

CUSPID Volume 1 Clinically Useful
Safety Procedures in Dentistry.
Annual Record of Accumulated Verifiable CPD

Name: .... **GDC Number:** ....
CPD Start date..................

I. Know your compulsory CPD start date.
II. Be certain of how many hours of CPD the GDC required you to complete.
III. Plan your CPD activities to meet your requirement for registration.
IV. Record your CPD.
V. Every year: submit proof of your completed CPD hours to the GDC.

Dentists needs to complete 100 hours of Verifiable CPD in a 5-year cycle.

Therapists Hygienists and Clinical Dental Technicians need to complete 75 hours.

Dental nurses need to complete 50 hours of verifiable CPD in a 5-year cycle.

Dental Technicians need to complete 50 hours of verifiable CPD in a 5-year cycle

As a reminder: Using CUSPID should count towards your Enhanced CPD activity given that:

I. The educational aims and objectives are listed at the start of each chapter.

II. Clear goals are set out in the introduction to each chapter.

III. At the end of each chapter, the opportunity to give feedback is provided.

IV. A record of the duration in CPD hours can be recorded in the log sheets; these can be accumulated over the 5 year CPD cycle.

V. On completing each chapter or parts of a chapter, the total can be entered in the certificate of participation attesting to your total hours of verifiable CPD.

Please retain and copy your recorded totals every year for the GDC CUSPID Volume 1

Chapter 1 of 5 Medical Emergencies	Total: 80 MCQs 8 Hours	MCQs Completed:	Hours Claimed:	Signed and dated:
				Countersigned
Chapter 2 of 5 Medicine and Drug Safety	Total: 165 MCQs 16.5 Hours	MCQs Completed:	Hours Claimed:	Signed and dated:
				Countersigned:

Please copy as necessary and place in your portfolio or submit to the GDC.

CUSPID Log sheet for verifiable CPD

Date and venue	Method eg: self study or training sessions	Topic(s) Covered	Pages studied:	MCQs used:	Reflection and areas for improvement? If so what?	CPD Hours	Signed

(Copy as necessary to add further CPD).

Total hours this page:

CUSPID
Clinically Useful Safety Procedures In Dentistry

Main CPD Topic:

Focused subject:

Verifiable CPD Record and Certificate for:

Name:

GDC Number:

Professional Role:

Pages accessed:

For the CPD Period:

MCQ Questions answered:

Verifiable CPD hours claimed:

Signed:
Date:

Counter signed:
Date:

Name + GDC number:

(Copy as necessary to document and record additional CPD).

References to Introduction Volume 1.

1. General Dental Council. Continuing Professional Development for Dental Professionals.
   Available online from:
   file:///C:/Users/Owner/Downloads/Continuing%20Professional%20Development%20for%20Dental%20Professionals.pdf
   Accessed June 2017.
2. General Dental Council. Enhanced CPD.
   Available online from:
   https://www.gdc-uk.org/professionals/cpd/enhanced-cpd
   Accessed June 2017.
3. General Dental Council. Quality Controls for Verifiable CPD.
   Available online from:
   file:///C:/Users/Owner/Downloads/Quality%20Controls%20for%20Verifiable%20CPD%20advice%20sheet%20(3).pdf
   Accessed June 2017.
4. European Commission for Education, Audiovisual and Culture Executive Agency (EACEA). Harmonisation & Standardisation of European Dental Schools. Programmes of Continuing Professional Development for Graduate Dentists – Dent CPD: Lifelong Learning Erasmus programme (#509961-LLP-1- 2010-1-UK-ERASMUS-EMHE).
   Available online from:
   http://www.dentcpd.org/workpackages/WP4/CPD_activity_evaluation_toolkit_for_dental_educators.pdf
   Accessed June 2017.

CHAPTER ONE

Medical Emergencies

CONTENTS

INTRODUCTION

In this first chapter, we will look at the more common medical emergencies occurring in your patients. The specific ways in which you and your dental team will need to manage them will be explained. As a reminder, the GDC recommend that in your Verifiable CPD: 10 hours of Medical Emergency training must be undertaken and logged in every 5-year cycle.

The GDC, the Surgical Royal Colleges, and the Post Graduate Dental Deaneries in the UK also recommend that training in this core subject is undertaken on a regular basis as there is firm evidence demonstrating that after completing a practical course in CPR, (Cardiopulmonary Resuscitation) your skills diminish quite rapidly (in a number of weeks) without regular refresher training.[1][2][3.]

The reason for this less than optimal skill retention is that in the UK, medical emergencies are relatively rare occurrences in dental practices. So thankfully, you do not get to use your skills for real, that often; if at all, hence the need to keep practicing them regularly.

In order to keep your clinical skills at an optimum level with respect to medical emergency training, Professor St. John Crean's advice, in line with the Faculty of Dental Surgery, Royal College Surgeons, England, is to do three things on a regular basis:

> I. Practise
> II. Practise
> III. Practise.

On reflection, specifically for medical emergencies, if you feel the need to improve your skills in this safety critical core area, there are many training courses and training venues available where you can indeed: Practise, Practise and Practise.

In addition to that, in our digital age, there are many mobile phone applications, some of them freely available with which you can refresh your practical knowledge and run through your procedural skills, doing so at a suitable time when (or if) you have a few moments free in your dental practice to practise, practise, practise.

You get the point and your trainers in medical emergency training will no doubt stress this point too.

The dental clinic where you work will be compliant with either the CQC the Care Quality Commission (in England), the Care and Social Services Inspectorate (in Wales), the Regulation and Quality Improvement Inspectorate (in Northern Ireland) or the Care Inspectorate (in Scotland). If you work in a hospital, for a dental corporate body or the uniformed or armed services, there will be clearly defined training schedules to ensure you and other members of your dental team will undergo regular training in CPR (Cardio Pulmonary Resuscitation), basic airway management and the use of an AED (Automatic External Defibrillator). Working within such a framework will mean you will be compliant with the most up to date guidance or standards for the jurisdiction in which you are currently working[4].

Wherever you are working, three safety driven principles to remember are:

I. **Medical emergencies in the dental practice can be life-threatening.**
II. **All equipment and emergency drugs should be immediately available.**
III. **There must be regular training so you can effectively deal with medical emergencies.**

The Educational Aims and Objectives of this chapter:

I.   Remind, Revise and Renew your active working knowledge of the common medical emergencies you were trained to deal with while studying for your qualifications.

II. To keep you updated with the latest information on medical emergencies, so you can efficiently deal with any patient or member of the public who presents with any of the medical emergencies we will look at in this chapter.

III. To enable you and your dental team to work effectively together to achieve the best outcome for anyone who needs your help in a medical emergency.

The expected outcomes from this chapter:

I.   Actively read this chapter, making notes and revisions to your knowledge where necessary.

II. To be aware of the latest guidelines on medical emergencies from the GDC, the Resuscitation Council UK, your professional associations and the post graduate dental faculties in the UK and Irish Royal Surgical College's Dental Faculties.

III. Where and when necessary; anticipate and prevent a medical emergency from occurring.

IV. Should a medical emergency occur: You will be trained to treat the patient to ensure the best outcome for all those involved.

V.   Demonstrate your participation in regular group training exercises, with other members of your dental team to demonstrate your knowledge and practical skills are maintained to an appropriate level.

VI. Correctly answer the multiple choice questions at the end of this chapter to demonstrate that you have read and understood the principles of dealing with medical emergencies.

Quality Control

If the questions you answer are marked by a third party, with your regular CPR exercises being logged and the results from your performance in these exercises being audited, together with documented training by an appropriately qualified resuscitation officer in CPR and the other medical emergencies, then working through this chapter will count towards your enhanced CPD in this core subject. The information in this chapter should be discussed in your regular dental practice meetings. By doing so and with your personal background reading, this chapter should count towards your enhanced CPD in this core subject and this can be used for your Personal Development Plan.

You must be prepared to deal with medical emergencies

With very good reason, your patients, your colleagues and your professional regulator, will demand as a dental professional that you are adequately prepared and able to deal with medical emergencies while at work. One suggested reason to be prepared is there seems to be an increase in the number of medical emergencies occurring in dental practices.[5] Although no precise reasons for such an upward trend have been identified, one factor may be the increasing age of the dental patient population with an increased risk of age related co-morbidities.[5,6] Should you happen upon a medical emergency while in a public place or at any occasion while outside of work, you would be expected to deal with such an event until the arrival of a first aider or an emergency responder. I think you will agree, those are reasonable things to be expected of any health care professional.

With all medical emergencies, prevention has to be better than intervention and correction. So the patient's medical history and history of their medication has to be up to date, not only that; but all members of your dental team need to be aware of data in a patient's history that can positively contribute to the way you deal with their care.

If a medical emergency occurs, then you have to act in a way that prevents further harm from occurring. The first task is to ensure both the safety of your patient and yourself. In extreme, but thankfully rare cases, you will have to focus your efforts on the patient, keeping them alive until help arrives and they can be transferred from your care into the care of an expert nursing or medical facility.

Timing is critical. Your intervention to assist the patient and alerting of the emergency services has to be both immediate and effective.

Following your intervention and alerting of the emergency services, you then need to stop any further deterioration in the patient's medical condition. As a member of a dental team, it is reasonable to expect that you and your colleagues should be able to recognize the more common life threatening conditions that might appear in a dental patient and to act accordingly in the event of a medical emergency

These conditions might be:

I.   A Myocardial Infarct.
II. A Cardiac Arrest.
III. An Anaphylaxis.

Furthermore, you will need to identify those conditions, that although not immediately life threatening may quickly develop into life threatening ones.

These conditions might be:

I.   Asthma
II. Epilepsy
III. Diabetes
IV. Choking

In any of the above conditions and with many of the other medical emergencies, you will need to act alone or as an integral part of your dental team to maintain the patient's Airway, carry out basic life support procedures to assist <u>Breathing</u>, deliver oxygen and administer emergency drugs to maintain the patient's <u>Circulation</u>.

Essentially this is the A B C you will already be familiar with.

Where necessary, you may need to apply and use an Automatic External Defibrillator (AED) and contact the emergency services, co-ordinating their arrival and handing over your dental patient into their medical care.

So that such vital procedures can be carried out wherever and whenever they are needed, there has to be a program of regular training to ensure any medical emergency can be dealt with in the minimum of time with the maximum beneficial effect for the patient, while lowering the stress to yourself and the other members your dental team.

In addition to your frequent training, your emergency equipment and medication has to be both available and in-date. Therefore, it is important to remind, revise, renew and repeat your training in this core area of your duties.

Some of the medical emergencies are surprisingly common, the Vaso-Vagal Syncope or Faint being one example. Other emergencies are thankfully relatively rare, especially those involving children. Putting this into some context, for a dental team in the UK, there is a medical emergency every 3.5 to 4.5 years, and an emergency necessitating the use of Cardiopulmonary Resuscitation may never occur for many dental team members, the occurrence of that emergency being calculated at one such event in 200 to 250 years per practitioner.[7,8.]

A note of caution should be sounded here as the study from Atherton in 1999 noted a regional difference between Scotland; at one medical emergency every 3.6 practice years, while in England; one medical emergency occurred every 4.5 practice years.[7]

Another study in New Zealand reported one medical emergency for every 10,000 patients who were treated in an outpatient dental care setting.[9]

For the UK, the study of Girdler and Smith is perhaps the most quoted on medical emergencies in dental practice. That study demonstrated a prevalence of 0.7 medical emergencies per dentist per year.[10]

In all of these studies, the most common medical emergency was the vaso-vagal syncope or the common faint. In another European study, this time in Saxony in Germany, published in 2008, the authors also noted that fainting was the most common medical emergency. However, that study of Muller and co-workers revealed some quite striking additional results and these are worthy of comment:

1. There are nearly 3000 dentists in Saxony and all were sent a questionnaire. In a remarkable show of uncharacteristic German inefficiency or something more serious, only around 1/5th responded. It should be emphasised, this study sought information on medical emergencies. This study was of a safety critical nature and not the anodyne market-research questionnaire that dental professionals are inundated with.

2. From those who responded, just over 600 dentists reported almost two faints each (Specifically: 620 dentists and 1238 faints).

3. Perhaps the most noticeable results from this paper were 2 cardiac arrests and 42 severe life-threatening events were noted among those who responded in a 12-month period.

4. While over 90% of dentists reported post qualification training in medical emergencies, just under ¼ did such training once, while just over 2/3rds did so on more than one occasion.

5. This study concluded in some contradiction to Greenwood and Girdler that: Medical emergencies are not rare in dental practice. Although most of them are not life threatening, improvement in competence of emergency management should include repeated participation in life support courses, standardisation of such courses and offering courses designed to meet the needs of dentists[10.]

Another issue worth considering, in addition to the geographical location where you practise, is the area of dentistry you practise. It has been suggested that perhaps specialist referral practices for oral surgery may have a higher risk profile than the hygiene led aesthetic practice.

Certainly for those undertaking oral surgery, the incidence of medical emergencies increases. [12]

With respect to this data, for your continuing professional development, you should be aware if an emergency does occur, it would be:

I.   Unexpected.
II. Stressful for the patient and those accompanying them.
III. Alarming for the dental team.
IV. Possibly life-altering or life-threatening for the patient.
V.   Intense: Documentation will need to be completed afterwards and an enquiry may take place if there was any morbidity or mortality associated with the medical emergency.

As mentioned above, prevention is better than intervention. Your working environment contains many triggers, promoting factors that might lead to a medical emergency eventually occurring. It is important to have as relaxed and as comfortable a work place as possible with friendly supportive colleagues; professional, mature, responsible people on whom you can absolutely rely at all times when working with every one of your patients.

If you do not work in a comfortable relaxed environment with staff displaying a professional attitude to their work, then you should try, in staff meetings; to bring about change towards creating a dental team that not only has self-respect, but shows respect for the work you do and the patients you will be treating.

That is; the culture and climate you create in work should be one that is conducive to safe and stress free work.

In working towards building such a dental team, you will be taking positive steps towards creating an environment that dispels the fears and alleviates the anxieties of nervous patients.

When dealing with patients where an adverse interaction could lead to a stressful situation it is important to remember the following:

> **A principal of preparation is:**
> **Pride, professionalism and partnership.**
> **Practice prudently, predicting and preventing problems.**

As a member of a dental team, you will be well trained, alert and observant to the signs a patient displays and the symptoms about which they will complain. From your training, professional experience and development, together with data from an up to date medical history, you will be able to identify the early warning signs for almost all the medical emergencies.

It follows that you will be able to take appropriate preventive and corrective actions to lessen the impact that a medical emergency will have on the patient, on the practice and on all those in the dental team.

In your dental practice, you will know the location of all emergency equipment and the drugs that you will need and can use. You should be able to request the attendance and assistance of emergency personnel. You need to able to assist in their duties, from their entering your dental practice, through attending to the patient and on to leaving your surgery, if necessary together with the dental patient.

After this, following any medical emergency, you should accurately document the event in the patient's notes and other practice files. If required, you should be prepared to present your data to the medical staff or any other competent authority responsible for the continuing care of the patient.

With every dental patient, it is very important that you update his or her medical history at every visit. Any changes, no matter how insignificant in the medication and medical history are noted down. If you are unsure about something, then clarify your questions and clear your doubts with the patient, their medical practitioner or specialist if they are under specialist care and do so before you begin your dental treatment.

You should be aware that today; more of our patients are taking more medications. Such polypharmacy might prove to be yet another triggering event on the way to a medical emergency. Often a patient will tell you (and they are more often than not; an elderly lady), that she is so full of pills; she will start rattling if you go anywhere near her with a dental drill. That comment may be light-hearted, but it is not flippant and you would be ill advised to ignore it. Such remarks demand further questioning into the patient's medical history and the patient's medication history.

In our experience, almost all patients, not just the above noted elderly ladies attend with a list of the most up to date medications their doctors have given them. Often everyone in the dental team from the receptionist, through the dental nurse and on to the dentist, will be familiar with these lists. We then quite knowingly, yet rather unknowingly begin to type or write the list into the patient's notes. Staring at these ever-lengthening lists of medications, perhaps we do not actively see what is before us or even consider the following:

1. Why is the patient actually taking this medication?
2. What condition or other conditions does the patient have; that they should need this or other medication?
3. Is this a condition that can change? If so how acute or how chronic is the condition and how likely is change to occur?
4. Will change occur during a dental appointment, just how stable is the patient?
5. What is the risk to the patient if their condition does deteriorate?
6. Do we know what to look for, if there is deterioration and what are the clinical signs?
7. If you have to give a drug, any drug; will there be an interaction with the patient's medication?
8. From all of the above, is there a risk of a medical emergency occurring while the patient is in my care?
9. Is this patient at greater or lesser risk of a medical emergency than another patient, who might not be medicated at all or as much...?
10. Do you know how to deal with the particular potential medical emergency this patient will be at risk from?

Obtaining the patient's medication history and their medical history is crucial to determining how you treat them and how a medical emergency involving them will be managed.

Information on the patient's medical history should be gathered at every visit and as noted above: You must be aware of the medication the patient is taking and the effect it will have if an emergency occurs. Please note down any current medical or other health related treatment the patient is undergoing. All of the above information should be entered into the medical history forms. Data must be updated and complete before any dental appointment can begin. Both the patient and the dentist or dental nurse (or hygienist if working alone) should sign such updated forms, before treatment starts; and do so at every visit. The internet is replete with a variety of medical history forms; we will go on to discuss the contents of these and potential deficiencies in these forms in detail in the following pages. If you are not happy with your dental practice's medical history forms for whatever reason, this issue could be a topic of conversation, consultation and collaboration with your colleagues. In your next practice meeting, you might consider creating new ones and convert your stuffy practice principle or stubborn manageress over to your way of thinking with a more appropriate medical history form.

Whatever else you do, do not just sign and then file your completed medical history forms in the patient notes, please actively think about the data you are signing off. The medical forms should be to-hand throughout the course of the treatment. Please do use them and gather as much information from them as you can when treating your patient. Even the smallest signs such as a change in the patient's handwriting or perhaps a change in their medication can give useful clues as to the patient's medical problems and alert you to the higher risk that a medical emergency may occur.

Medical questions

The data gathered in the medical history should include and is not limited to:

1. Asking the patient about the medicines being taken at the time of treatment and the reasons why they are being taken.
2. Questioning the patient about any treatment, operations or illnesses that have been completed or will be needed in the near future and the reasons for such treatment.
3. Does the patient bruise easily or bleed excessively after cutting themselves or having a tooth out?
4. Allergies? What are their causes? How do these affect the patient?
5. Heart condition and blood pressure, are they normal or within normal ranges? Is there a history of heart disease, valve trouble or Rheumatic Fever or Infective Endocarditis?
6. In addition to the heart, what is going on in the chest? With the lungs: Are there any respiratory illnesses; Asthma, Bronchitis, Obstructive Airway disease? Is the patient a smoker and if so, what do they smoke?
7. You can ask about Endocrine problems and functions. Some patients will be familiar with the word: Endocrine, most others might not be. So this question might be reworded to ask about and include Diabetes in all its forms: Type 1, Type 11 or any other variety of Diabetes and the medication your patient will be taking for it. Now is the best time to ask if they have taken it!
8. You might then go on to ask about Epilepsy, any other serious illnesses and perhaps not so serious conditions, such as migraines and so on. An important question to ask: If the patient is nervous and if so, do they faint easily, or have they fainted at the dentist, or do they feel faint right now?
9. With female patients of reproductive age: Are they pregnant? If the answer is yes, then you will now be looking after two (or more) patients in the dental chair!

10. Ask if there are other problems the patient might want to discuss with you. These could be operations, illnesses, or any condition not covered under the preceding nine questions. There may well be specific issues the patient might like to discuss with you in confidence.

Confidence in this case does not mean asking your nurse to step outside, but it could mean the patient's partner or children leaving the room for a few moments, while you and your dental nurse discuss any further issues.

There are so many medical history forms available from the internet as free downloads and you will have your own forms with a layout you are familiar with or as mentioned above, perhaps you might like to introduce a change in the medical history form to improve the way that information is presented.

From the above, you can see the medication and medical history will give you some big pointers towards those medical emergencies to expect when treating the patient. By completing these histories, you will be that little bit more prepared to deal with the patient and any problem they might present with or bring into the dental clinic.

Just before we go on to discuss the drugs and equipment you need to have in your dental practice, my dental nurse, with over 40 years of clinical experience, told me to remind you that trouble in the dental clinic is not like rain; it does not come from the clouds.

Trouble can tumble from a cloudless blue sky.

In our experience, even the fittest of patients with the cleanest of medical history sheets can always be relied upon to provide you with an interesting emergency to deal with. We will return to discuss such a problem in the following sections detailing specific medical emergencies.

Medical Emergency Drugs

In addition to an up to date medical history, in an emergency, you must have immediate access to a minimum level of drugs and equipment in the dental clinic. The section: Prescribing in dental Practice in the 2017 British National Formulary gives a definitive list of drugs that you must be able to access immediately when a medical emergency is declared.[13] This list of drugs is reproduced from that source for your reference:

Drug	Route of Administration	Additional Comments
Adrenaline (Epinephrine) 1 in 1,000 Concentration. 1mg/1ml Acid Tartrate in Automatic dispenser	Intramuscular Injection Outer Quadrant of Buttock or Thigh muscle	For Anaphylaxis
Aspirin 300mg soluble tablet	The tablet is crushed or chewed placed under tongue	For Stroke, Heart attack or Chest Pain where there is a risk that a Heart attack is, or has occurred.
Glucagon. Presented as a hydrochloride salt in a 1ml vial into which the solvent (sterile water) will be injected, and then drawn up immediately before use.	Intramuscular Injection Outer Quadrant of Buttock or Thigh	To be used in the unconscious or semi-conscious Diabetic patient where you cannot administer Glucose orally.
Glucose tablets or Glucose Gel.	Oral route placed in the buccal sulcus or to be chewed.	To be used in the conscious Diabetic patient who is hypoglycaemic.
Glyceryl trinitrate spray. 400 micrograms per dose. Two doses to be used.	Oral or sublingual	To be used in the patient where there is suspected or actual Angina.
Midazolam Liquid for buccal administration Dose is 10mgs/ml Midazolam. Dose is 5mgs/ml Presented as 2ml Ampoules	Oral route or buccal route only	For epileptic seizures. Buccal administration only. DO NOT ATTEMPT IV ROUTE
Oxygen Cylinder (C/D size) Advised to have one in each surgery or a minimum of 2 Cylinders.	Immediate use via a face mask with reservoir bag.	The cylinder must contain 450 litres of Oxygen. This has to be delivered at 15 litres/minute for 30 minutes.
Salbutamol inhaler. Aerosol dose should be 100micrograms every dose and 2 doses are to be given.	Immediate Oral administration	For Asthma and Anaphylaxis. 2 or more doses to be given. A SPACER IS ALMOST ALWAYS NECESSARY.

Medical Emergency Equipment

In addition to the foregoing list of drugs, in 2013, the UK Resuscitation Council recommended that the following equipment should be available for all trained members of the dental team to access immediately if a medical emergency occurs[14]. The list below is reproduced from their website:

http://www.resus.org.uk/pages/QSCPR_PrimaryDentalCare_Equip.htm#equip[14]

The following equipment must be accessible within the first minute of an emergency being declared in the dental practice:

Essential Equipment

Essential Equipment	Availability	Additional Comments
Personal Protective equipment – non latex gloves, aprons, eye protection	Immediate	Note use of non latex gloves and these should be powder free.
Pocket mask with oxygen port	Immediate	Each dental chair should have one of these stuck to the back or side.
Portable suction e.g. Yankauer type.	Immediate	Practise using these!

Equipment to maintain:
Airway and Breathing

Equipment to maintain Airway and Breathing	Availability	Additional Comments
Self-inflating bag with reservoir (Adult)	Immediate	These should be ready to use attached to the face masks
Self-inflating bag with reservoir (Child)	Immediate	As above; ready for use.
Clear face masks for self-inflating bag (sizes: 0,1,2,3 and 4)	Immediate	
Oxygen cylinder (CD size)\n\nAdvised to have one in each surgery or a minimum of 2 Cylinders.	Immediate	This will contain 450 litres of Oxygen that can be delivered at 15 litres/ minute for 30 minutes.
Oxygen masks with reservoir	Immediate	
Oxygen tubing	Immediate	

Equipment to maintain circulation

Equipment to maintain Circulation	Availability	Your Comments
Automated external defibrillator (AED)	Immediate Collapse to Shock time must be less than 3 minutes	The type of AED and its location should be determined by a local risk assessment of your practice. Consider the facilities for paediatric use, especially if your dental practice will treat children.
Adhesive defibrillator pads	Immediate	Spare set of pads also recommended. Also consider paediatric pads and an attenuator to deliver an appropriate level of shock.
Razors or scalpels	Immediate	
Scissors	Immediate	

In a medical emergency, in addition to the drugs and equipment noted above, there are specific protocols you should follow when assessing the dental patient who becomes acutely ill.

You will be expected to use an accepted approach when dealing with a medical emergency.

To remind you the structured approach you will follow are the familiar steps: **A B C D E**, developed from the UK Resuscitation Council guidelines.

These will be considered in detail in the next section.

In a real medical emergency, you should go through these steps several times to assess, and then re-assess your patient. Thus, ensuring no symptoms the patient reports, or the clinical signs you see are overlooked with an incorrect diagnosis being reached.

The following approach is based on the approach detailed in the UK Resuscitation Council's Systematic approach to the acutely ill patient.[15]

In addition to the accepted routine of: **A B C D E**, we need to add: **F** for Follow Up.

Follow up is an important aspect of continuing professional development, where you can reflect and learn from your experience in dealing with a medical emergency and be better prepared to deal with another event in the future.

As with most things in life, medical emergencies are never quite as you expect them to be.

In a dental clinic, it is not a question of: if, but rather, a question of: when a medical emergency arises. You should, from your training; be prepared to deal with every one of them!!

Your approach to medical emergencies in the dental clinic

The correct approach to a medical emergency is to assess and maintain the Airway, Breathing, Circulation, Disability and Exposure (the A B C D E) of the acutely ill patient. Therefore, you must:

1. Undertake a complete initial assessment and periodic re-assessment of the acutely ill patient.
2. Always assess the effects of your treatment on your patient.
3. Life-threatening problems must be dealt with first before any other assessment or procedure is started.
4. You must recognise the circumstances when additional help is required. Attend to the patient first. Then immediately ask for help.
5. Use all members of the dental team to secure the patient's safety and yours if needed.
6. Communicate effectively with the patient, your colleagues and emergency services when required.
7. The aim of your actions in the dental surgery is to be a "holding measure" in the survival chain to keep the patient alive. Your assistance must aim, not only to provide clinical improvement for the patient while in your care; you must aim to be of benefit for their definitive treatment in a secondary care centre too.
8. You must continue with your treatment, even if you see no immediate improvement. It often takes a few minutes for any medical emergency intervention, especially those in Cardio Pulmonary Resuscitation (CPR) to take effect.

The first steps you need to take:

1. Asking the patient the question: How are you? Will provide much needed information with which to begin your emergency treatment.
2. A normal verbal response implies that the patient has a patent airway, is breathing and has brain perfusion. This takes care of the A B C, we will look at this more closely in a moment.
3. If the patient can only speak in short sentences, they may have extreme respiratory distress.
4. If the patient cannot respond to you, this is a clear sign of a serious illness.
5. Monitor as many of the patient's vital signs, doing so as early as possible. Most dental practices will have a pulse oximeter with a basic cardiac monitoring function. Use this to provide additional information to assist with the management of your patient.

Airway (A)

You must treat any obstruction in the airway as a medical emergency and obtain expert help immediately.

Untreated and unchecked, an airway obstruction will lead to a lowering of arterial partial oxygen pressure (Pa 02). Following from this will be a risk of hypoxic damage to the brain, kidneys and heart. If this is uncontrolled, then cardiac arrest and death will follow.

Therefore, you can see the clinical risks to the patient that follow from an airway obstruction may lead to involvement of your medical specialist colleagues.

1. Look for the early signs of airway obstruction:

Airway obstruction leads to paradoxical chest and abdominal movements. You can see these in your patient as the classic "see-saw" inspiration- expiration movements of the chest as the accessory muscles of respiration are being used to force air into and out of the patient's lungs in an attempt to overcome an airway restriction or blockage.

2. **Look for the late signs of airway obstruction:**

Central cyanosis is a late sign of airway obstruction. With a complete airway obstruction, there will be no breath sounds from the patient's mouth or nose. With a partial obstruction, air entry is diminished and often noisy. The most likely cause of airway obstruction in the dental surgery is from a foreign body being inhaled.

In the majority of cases, the straightforward methods of airway clearance are all that are required. You can attempt airway-opening manoeuvres with suction, you will have suction apparatus to hand in a dental surgery. If your simple airway opening measures fail, then emergency medical assistance becomes necessary.

3. **Give oxygen at as high a concentration as possible:**

Provide high concentration oxygen using a mask with an oxygen reservoir. Ensure that the oxygen flow rate is sufficient. Usually, this is in excess of 10 litres per minute, up to a maximum of 15 litres per minute. By providing this level of gas flow, you remove the chances of the reservoir bag collapsing when the patient breathes in.

Breathing (B)

During the immediate assessment of breathing, it is vital to diagnose and treat any immediately life-threatening conditions. In a dental surgery this will be the severe uncontrolled asthmatic attack or (thankfully) rarely the pulmonary oedema caused by a patient whose heart is failing.

Look for the general signs of respiratory distress: sweating, central cyanosis, use of the accessory muscles of respiration and the patient who is breathing using not only the accessory muscles but the abdomen too.

1. Count the respiratory rate. The normal rate is between 12 and 20 breaths per minute. A high rate, and especially an increasing rate, is a warning to you that your patient may suddenly deteriorate.
2. In addition, assess the depth of each breath and the pattern or the rhythm of the patient's breathing.
3. Note any chest abnormality (this may increase the risk of deterioration and the ability to breathe normally.
4. If your patient is having difficulty breathing, look for a raised Jugular Venous Pressure. You will see this sign in your patients with acute severe asthma and again in the patient with cardiac pathologies
5. If you are able to monitor the patient with pulse oximetery, then record their oxygen concentration, this should be within a range of 97-100%. However, remember that the pulse oximeter does not detect increased blood CO_2 (hypercapnia). If you are giving the patient supplemental oxygen or they receive oxygen therapy, their blood saturation O_2 level may be normal in the presence of a very high $PaCO_2$. To determine CO_2 levels, you need to measure: Arterial Blood Gasses (ABGs), such measurements are usually undertaken in hospitals, rarely if ever is capnography (CO_2 measurement) utilised in dental practices.
6. Listen to the sound of the patient breathing at a respectful but short distance from them. In other words, do not cause the patient any more fear, alarm or distress by shoving your finely tuned emergency ear lobe into their panic-stricken face.
7. An airway that is rattling away will indicate excessive secretions within it. The presence of such secretions is usually due to the inability of the patient to cough sufficiently or to take a deep breath.
8. Stridor or wheezing, suggests a partial, but a still significant obstruction of the patient's airway.

9. The specific treatment of respiratory disorders depends upon the cause. Nevertheless, in the dental clinic, all critically ill patients must receive oxygen.

10. There are patients with Chronic Obstructive Pulmonary Disease (COPD), where giving high concentrations of oxygen may have disadvantages. Nevertheless, this group of patients will also sustain end-organ damage or cardiac arrest if their blood oxygen tensions are allowed to decrease. With such patients, when giving oxygen, pulse oximetry is essential and you should aim for and maintain a range of 88% to 92% saturation (SaO_2) levels at the very least.

11. In a medical emergency, if you or a member of your team, decide the depth or rate of breathing of your patient is irregular or inadequate, then you must deliver oxygen using a bag-valve-mask ventilation set up. This will improve the patient's oxygenation and ventilation ability until the medical emergency responders arrive to take over from you.

Circulation (C)

In the dental clinic you can make several useful preliminary and non invasive measurements to assess the state of your patient's circulation. If we step back from the dental clinical environment for a moment and consider circulation in an emergency framework then:

In almost all medical emergencies, consider hypovolaemia to be the primary cause of shock, until proven otherwise.

In any patient with cool peripheries and a fast heart rate, you must maintain their condition until the emergency responders arrive to begin treating the patient intravenously.

Please be aware intravenous treatment is not within your mandated scope of emergency practice.

If shock is of cardiac origin, the clinical signs will become immediately clear to you and we will consider the clinical signs in the subsequent sections on relevant medical emergencies.

In a dental patient who has undergone oral surgery, it is important to exclude haemorrhage; either overt or hidden.

Also, do not forget that respiratory pathology, such as a pneumothorax, can also compromise a patient's circulatory state. Although a tension pneumothorax would be a very rare emergency in an outpatient day care dental setting, there are a few reports in the medical literature identifying dental causes, specifically baro-trauma from the use of a high-speed air turbine in mandibular molar surgical extractions.[16]

Assessing the circulation:

1. Assess the limb temperature by feeling the patient's hands: are they warm or are they cool?
2. Look at the colour of the hands and digits: are they blue, pink, pale or mottled?
3. Measure the capillary refill time (CRT). You can do this by applying pressure on the skin for five seconds on a patient's fingertip held at the level of their heart (or just above) and counting the time it takes for the colour to return (this is capillary refill) after the pressure has been released.

   The normal value for CRT is usually less than two seconds.
4. Assess the state of the veins: they may be under-filled or collapsed when hypovolaemia is present.
5. Count the patient's pulse rate.
6. Feel for the patient's peripheral pulse, assessing for:

> I. **Presence,**
> II. **Rate,**
> III. **Quality,**
> IV. **Regularity**
> V. **Equality.**

Barely palpable pulses suggest a poor cardiac output, whilst a bounding pulse may indicate a spreading infection.

7. In contrast to tension pneumothorax from dental causes being rare, infection and sepsis are almost daily dental events. If a dento-facial infection cannot be appropriately treated (extraction, surgical incision and drainage) or the patient displays a disordered pulse, there must be no hesitation in declaring a medical emergency, with immediate transfer of the dental patient to hospital.

8. While dento-facial infections are common, sepsis, morbidity and associated mortality are in the UK at least; rare events[17,18.] Although there is some evidence to suggest the incidence is increasing in certain deprived areas in the UK.[19]

9. If you are able and you have the means, (the time training and equipment), then measure the patient's blood pressure. Even in shock, the blood pressure may be entirely normal, as compensatory mechanisms increase peripheral resistance in response to reduced cardiac output. Where possible, the diastolic and systolic values must be recorded.

   A low diastolic pressure is suggestive of arterial vasodilatation. This can be due to anaphylaxis or to sepsis.

   A narrowed pulse pressure, (the difference between the systolic and diastolic pressures), (normally in the region of 35-45 mmHg) is indicative of arterial vasoconstriction. If this is the case, you should be alert to the risk of a hypovolaemic patient and the risk of a rapid descent into cardiogenic shock.

   While it is not in your remit to treat these conditions, if you are trained, experienced and able, then all relevant data must be collected to assist in the handover of your patient to the emergency responders. Look for other signs of a poor cardiac output, such as reduced level of consciousness.

10. Another useful sign, which can be gathered from the medical history, is recent or prolonged urinary insufficiency. (Although this measure is perhaps more appropriate to inpatient care, you can still ask your dental patient about frequency of visits to the bathroom.)

11. Examine the patient thoroughly for external haemorrhage from wounds or evidence of concealed haemorrhage from trauma.

Bleeding into the thoracic, intra-peritoneal spaces, cavities or into the gastro-intestinal tract must also be considered.

12. Remember that intra-thoracic, intra-abdominal or pelvic blood loss may be significant and the patient may be unaware of this.

13. The emergency responders will undertake the specific treatment of circulatory or cardiovascular collapse in your patient.

14. After your handover, the emergency treatment is then directed at fluid replacement, controlling haemorrhage and restoration of adequate tissue perfusion levels.

15. In order to facilitate the best care for your patient, you must seek out the clinical signs of those conditions that are immediately life threatening, e.g., cardiac tamponade, massive or continuing haemorrhage or septicaemic shock, then communicate your findings to the attending emergency responders.

Disability (D)

For the avoidance of doubt, in this context: Disability refers to the level of the patient's consciousness.

The possible causes of unconsciousness in a dental patient, aside from fainting, include profound hypoxaemia, hypercapnia and cerebral hypo-perfusion. On the other hand, with specific reference to the practice of sedation services in dentistry; loss of consciousness is related to the administration of sedatives or analgesic medications.

1. Review the ABCs for your patient to exclude hypoxaemia, hypotension or other serious causes of loss of consciousness.

2. Check the patient for both: their medical and their medication history. Where possible if their depressed consciousness can be reversed, then give the appropriate antagonist drug, where available.

3. Examine the patient's pupils, their size, equality and reaction to light and continue to do so throughout your immediate care and when necessary, the recovery phase of the managed medical emergency.

4. Assess the patient's level of consciousness using the AVPU scale. In the outpatient day care setting with an emergency patient, an AVPU grading should be sufficient.

The Glasgow Coma Scale.

Just before we get to the AVPU scale, we should first mention the Glasgow Coma Scale (GCS).[20] After some 40 years use, it is still universally accepted, but in the dental clinic, perhaps it is not as suitable as an AVPU grading of the dental patient or for any paediatric patient less than 3 years old.

However, if you work in a dental practice where conscious sedation is undertaken, together with colleagues who are medically qualified, the GCS is still a valid method to monitor the recovery of your patient, for assessing if complications from the administration of a sedative agent have occurred.

The GCS is mentioned here to illustrate both its simplicity of use, together with the wide range of responses that can be recorded with no specialist training or equipment. Although there has been some recent criticism about both the reproducibility and the recording of clinical signs with the GCS[21], the work of Bryan Jennet and Graham Teasdale some 40 years ago in formulating the GCS, still remains both an acknowledged and an accepted method of patient monitoring for any health care professional.

On balance, the GCS does have validity as a safety monitor for your dental patient if a medical emergency occurs. The Glasgow Coma Scale uses graded scales to measure the patient's response to stimulation.

Response of the patient's: Eyes, their Verbal abilities and their Motor functions are individually graded to determine the patient's level of consciousness.

A clear picture of the patient's conscious state can then be determined from their spontaneous reactions, responses to sensory stimuli and appropriate motor functioning.

In addition to a scale, if the patient's collective responses are summed, giving a total score, this number becomes their Glasgow Coma <u>Score</u>, that is the sum total of all the scaled responses.

This score ranges from 15: being fully alert, down to 3: being moribund, comatose or a patient who is close to death.

Again, such data is useful in your approach to management of the patient who develops an emergency and for the medical emergency responders and secondary care specialists to whom you will hand over care of the patient with as much clinical information as possible, derived from both GCS and AVPU.

Glasgow Coma Scale						
	1	2	3	4	5	6
Eye	Does not open eyes	Opens eyes in response to <u>painful stimuli</u>	Opens eyes in response to voice	Opens eyes spontaneously	N/A	N/A
Verbal	Makes no sounds	Incomprehensible sounds	Utters inappropriate words	Confused, disoriented	Oriented, converses normally	N/A
Motor	Makes no movements	Extension to painful stimuli (<u>decerebrate response</u>)	Abnormal flexion to painful stimuli (<u>decorticate response</u>)	Flexion / Withdrawal to painful stimuli	Localizes painful stimuli	Obeys commands

AVPU

The AVPU scale is a simplified version of the GCS. With AVPU the best score from A to worst score in U is recorded to determine the level of consciousness in the patient. The recordable outcomes are:

Alert . The patient is fully awake, although they may be disoriented. Such a patient will spontaneously open their eyes and respond to your voice. While they may be confused, they will have control of their motor functions.

Voice. The patient is capable of some response when you talk to them. This could be in any of the three components of:

I.   **Eyes:** Opening them when the patient is questioned.
II. **Voice:** Moaning or some limited speech or sounds can be elicited.
III. **Motor:** A movement of an upper limb or hand in response to questioning your patient.

Pain. The patient responds to a centrally or a peripherally applied pain stimulus. With a centrally applied stimulus, a response is more likely to be due to central nervous system activity, rather than a reflex action.

However, centrally applied stimulation needs a constant pressure for up to 30 seconds duration and you might not want to start poking and prodding the patient's head if they have pain, swelling or any cranio-facial injuries, eg: they've fainted and banged their head on a piece of dental furniture on the way down.

In such cases, peripheral stimulation, applying pressure to a finger is a more appropriate measure than pressing on a sore and swollen head. Be sure though, not to press on a finger nail, pressing on or squeezing the side of the patient's finger is sufficient. For some patients (mostly younger women) false finger nails are hideously expensive and pressing on them can be painful for them and expensive for you, even more so if you succeed in breaking one.

With a patient who is only responsive to pain, a broken finger nail would be the least of anyone's worries.

Assuming the patient does not have expensive false nails, you can apply pressure to a finger to elicit a response. Notwithstanding the above, in clinical dentistry, you should be familiar with and be able to elicit a central pain stimulus by:

I. **Mandibular pressure**: The manual stimulation of the <u>mandibular nerve</u>, located within the angle of the jaw.

II. **Supraorbital pressure:** The manual stimulation of the <u>supraorbital nerve</u>. You can achieve this by gently pressing a thumb into the indentation above the eye. Thus is in the line of the patient's eyebrow.

Unresponsive: If your patient cannot respond to any of the above stimuli, an outcome of unresponsive will be recorded. When dealing with any emergency, anything less than an **A,** is an indication that medical assistance will be required.

When the emergency responders arrive, your emergency medical care will finish with your handing over your patient together with an AVPU grading. At this point, the emergency responders will begin with a GCS assessment where necessary.

The AVPU and GC Score (GCS) do correspond as follows:

i. **Alert:** 15 on GCS
ii. **Voice** Responsive: 12 on GCS
iii. **Pain** Responsive: 8 on GCS
iv. **Unresponsive:** 3 on GCS

Disability (D) continued...

5. Where possible, for patients who are Diabetic, especially the Type 1 Insulin Dependent Diabetic, measure their blood glucose levels using a rapid glucose meter or the standard stick method to exclude hypoglycaemia.

If their blood glucose is below 3 mmol l^{-1}, give them 25-50 ml of 50% glucose solution buccally or sublingually. If the patient is unconscious, then draw up and give Intramuscular Glucagon from the emergency drug box.

6. After the nature of the medical emergency is identified, the patient is stabilised, when it is safe to do so; place the unconscious patient in the recovery position.

7. Continue to monitor them until their recovery is fully established.

Exposure / Examination (E)

In order that patients are examined properly, and any details are not missed, your medical colleagues may need to expose the patient to an extent that is greater than that needed for a routine dental examination.

If you or your colleagues have to undertake such an exam, then make sure this is not done alone and any examination on the patient is undertaken in a way that respects their dignity.

Even in hospital wards that are over-heated and under-ventilated, be mindful of the risk of hypothermia as many patients in hospitals through illness and immobility are weak and underweight and have lost muscle mass and fatty tissue.

Re-cover the patient as soon as possible if your exposure and examination reveal nothing of clinical relevance to managing the emergency.

Follow Up /Further Information (F)

1. Take a full clinical history from the patient, their relatives, friends or your colleagues who may have treated the patient before and will be more familiar with them than you are. Often they can shed more light on the possible causes of the emergency, which you are facing.

2. After the medical emergency has been resolved or the hand-over of the patient is complete, now is a good time to:

> I. Review the patient's medical history, their medication history, their dental notes and their charts for any data that might be useful for future treatment and prevention of another emergency.
> II. Study both absolute and trended values of vital signs recorded in the notes.
> III. Check that important and routine medications have been prescribed, have been administered and nothing was missed in the patient's treatment schedules.

3. Review the results of laboratory based tests or other investigations you have asked for.
4. Consider the implications of a medical emergency on the future care of the patient.
5. Decide if the patient might better benefit from being referred to a specialist practice or a hospital environment for their ongoing dental care.
6. Make complete entries in the patient's notes of your findings, assessment and treatment.
7. Record the patient's response to any treatment given to them during the emergency.
8. Consider referral for definitive treatment of the patient's underlying condition.

Medical History Risk Assessment

Before beginning any course of dental treatment...

You will have the patient's medical history signed and updated.

You will have actively considered the information contained in their clinical histories.

These signed forms will undoubtedly contain a wealth of information relevant to clinical dentistry. However, it is unlikely there will be any information contained in those forms that are relevant to how you would handle a medical emergency.

As previously mentioned there are so many medical history forms and formats to choose from.

If you go online and search for: "Dental medical history forms", several hundred images of medical history forms can be seen in your first page of results! Despite a quite bewilderingly broad choice of forms, you will notice three obvious trends among the medical history forms published on the internet:

1. Most, if not all forms set aside a considerable amount of space for enquiries about the means a patient has to pay for their treatment. Many would say this is unacceptable while many more would say perhaps it is acceptable. After all, someone or some-body (either a public or a private body) has to pay for the work you do; sadly such information seems to take priority over more clinically essential data.

2. Enquiries focussing on the desire for the patient to undergo; para-dental activities either; the facial-aesthetic or the dental-cosmetic are also customary, taking up a lot of room in the medical history forms. That is definitely not acceptable. Placing those sorts of enquiries on a medical history form is nothing less than a piece of nonsense.

Lastly but most importantly, the trend of unquestionable importance to this chapter:

3. <u>None</u> of the dental medical history forms seen on the internet had the provision to give a risk assessment of your patient, either at a glance, or in any other acceptable or meaningful way.

From a quick look at the first page of our initial and brief online search into dental medical history forms, this seems to be something of an issue, not only for dental professionals in the UK but also for our dental colleagues worldwide too.

It simply cannot be the case that from reading a dental medical history form we have no capability to risk assesses our patients.

Just before we consider some of the medical emergencies in detail, we might consider the following: Dentistry is a safe activity for both patient and practitioner. This safety is dependent on the patient being in demonstrably good health (the purpose in taking a medical history is to both demonstrate and document this!) and with every one of your dental procedures being controlled and reduced to the least invasive treatment necessary to achieve the best outcome planned for.

You and your dental team must take every care to identify the medically challenged patient. In the dental surgery, your means to do so are somewhat less than those at the disposal of your hospital based colleagues. Nevertheless, an adequate risk assessment is essential in your efforts and energies to predict and prevent an emergency from occurring.

The ASA PS Classification System

One way of assessing and predicting risks is to use an established system such as the American Society of Anaesthesiologists (ASA) Physical State (PS) classification for all of your patients and to implement this in the taking and updating of all your patients medical histories.

The ASA system is like the previously noted AVPU and GCS a graded classification system. However, the ASA is a classification of the Physical Status (PS) of the patient and is not limited to their conscious state.

There are now 6 categories of patient in the ASA system. The 6th category is the patient who has consented or their next of kin have consented for organ donation for the lives of others. This is an important category and one that does not follow from the previous ones. In dentistry we will not have to face this patient, but we will often deal with the others on a daily basis.

The five ASA categories we will work with in dentistry are:

ASA PS Class	Definition
ASA I	**A patient who is healthy with no conditions noted on their Medical History forms.** The ASA Class I patient has no medical history and usually has a family medical history that is also clear.
ASA II	**A patient with mild systemic illness.** Examples you will see in dentistry are: Diabetes that is well controlled. Asthma, Epilepsy, Hypertension. Any Anxiety state.
ASA III	**A patient with severe systemic illness that limits their activity but is not incapacitating.** In contrast to the above Class II, in Class III; the Asthma is severe, the Epilepsy shows frequent seizures, Hypertension is uncontrolled, and there may have been a Heart Attack (MI or Myocardial Infarct) or a Stroke. The above are all ASA Class III patients.
ASA IV	**The patient has an incapacitating illness that presents as a constant threat to their lives.** Cancer that is active, Angina that is unstable, a recent Myocardial Infarct, Cardiac Arrythmia, a Cerebro-Vascular Accident (CVA or Stroke) The above are all ASA Class IV patients.
ASA V	**The patient who is in end of life care, not expected to leave hospital or to live more than another day.** These patients often do not require dental care, but more than anything else they and their next of kin need dignity respect and support. **You don't need to be a dentist to be a human-being**

From the previous table, you can see the simplicity and ease with which you can note the patient's ASA grade or set aside a small amount of space in your medical history forms to copy such a table then grade your patient accordingly.

However, there are some clear limitations in the ASA system:

1. An ASA II patient has a <u>mild</u> illness.
2. An ASA III patient has a <u>severe</u> illness.

3. Conversely, there is no ASA category for patients, with either multiple illnesses, those in various states of disease progression or regression, or for the patient with a <u>moderate</u> illness.

In addition, there are some criticisms of the ASA system as it stands. In assessing patients, there is evidence that the grading system is not entirely reproducible with the different grades being assigned to the same patient by different professionals.[22][23.]

Another issue with the ASA PS system, is that age is not considered in the grading allocation as noted above. Even so, age has a significant impact on the resilience of a patient, the progression of a disease and the risk facing: The patient, yourself and members of your dental team when considering your treatment options.

Most ASA I and II patients are young fit and healthy and can be treated in a general dental practice. Nearly a quarter (23.9%) of all patients aged 65- 74 years are ASA grade III or IV, this figure rising to over one third (34.9%) in the over 75 year olds[24].

If we consider extremes of age in the ASA system, then we might consider the wellness or un-wellness state of the patient too. Further subdivisions of the above noted categories are then possible. Most anaesthetists will classify a fit 80 year old as an ASA PS3.[25]

In addition to age, we must consider other factors. For example, obesity and smoking history are not medical conditions in their own right, yet these can adversely influence how well a patient can tolerate and recover from any clinical procedure, including dental surgery.

If we correctly assess our patients and consider the above, then specialists working in community or hospital clinics, with medical support to reduce the impact of a medical emergency may be better suited to treat certain ASA III and IV dental patients.

Certainly, the ASA PS system can be used to assess a dental patient's pre-procedural physical state. However, on its own, it is not a predictor of operative risk and other factors need to be included in medically risk assessing your patient.

These can include your skill and your dental team's experience, together with the dental patient's physical strength and physiological state on the day of treatment.

While we may not be able to make a risk prediction from the patient's medical history, we can narrow the risk presented, by utilising the ASA PS.

From such risk narrowing, we can reduce the risk even further by focussing our work according to a Prognosis and Assessment of Risk Scale or PARS:

The ASA PARS

ASA Class	Definitions (as previously noted)	PARS Grade	Dental Care
I	**A patient who is healthy with no conditions noted on their Medical History forms.** The ASA Class I patient has no medical history and usually has a family medical history that is also clear.	1	**No changes in dental treatment** and no restriction on choice of anaesthetic drug, pain management or sedation either IV or RA.
II	**A patient with mild systemic illness.** Examples you will see in dentistry are: Diabetes that is well controlled. Asthma, Epilepsy, Hypertension. Any Anxiety state.	2	**Elimination of any dental disease processes that can worsen a medical condition**, ie Oral Hygiene, Periodontal treatment to be completed as routine.
III	**A patient with severe systemic illness that limits their activity, but is not incapacitating.** In contrast to the above Class II, in Class III; the Asthma is severe, the Epilepsy shows frequent seizures, Hypertension is uncontrolled, there may have been a Heart Attack (MI or Myocardial Infarct) or a Stroke. The above are all ASA Class III patients.	3	**As above and consider restricting unnecessary dental treatment.** eg: not doing the non-essential cosmetic or aesthetic procedures before any essential dentistry. Use non-adrenaline containing local anaesthetics. Anxiety reduction is important for cardiac patients.

IV	The patient has an incapacitating illness that presents as a constant threat to their lives. Cancer that is active, Angina that is unstable, a recent Myocardial Infarct, Cardiac Arrythmia, a Cerebro-Vascular Accident (CVA or Stroke) The above are all ASA Class IV patients.	4	Dental treatment must complement the patient's medical care. Surgical or medical procedures make these patients at increased risk of medical emergencies. It is essential to correct poor hygiene and oro-dental health as it influences their medical condition
V	The patient who is in end of life care, not expected to leave hospital or to live more than another day. These patients often do not require dental care, but more than anything else they and their next of kin need dignity respect and support.	5	In addition to items 3 and 4 above, your empathic supportive communication with the patient and their family is essential as is control of acute pain and oral infections. Be a human being

Effectively the combination of ASA and PARS creates our own system; the ASA DS.

The DS represents the patient's Dental State. While not absolutely defining the work we can do, such a system can assist in our focus on the work we should do. The ASA DS may help to reduce the risk of a medical emergency in the dental clinic by modifying any intended dental treatment, not only according to the patient's needs but also in accordance with their physical and psychological ability to tolerate dental treatment. In essence, the ASA DS modifies treatment we might consider undertaking, subordinating almost all dental care in favour of medical care. In doing so, the ASA DS undoubtedly reduces the risk of a medical emergency in the dental clinic for patients who are medically compromised. Ultimately, in patients who are fundamentally medically compromised, we will have to defer care to our specialist medical colleagues. Nevertheless, by following an approach that is both simple and cautious in its nature, we can maintain a high level of care with a low risk profile in such patients.

The Karnofsky Scale

In addition to the ASA and ASA DS, there are two further scales we might consider using for patient assessment. Although in the UK, the first of these is seldom used in dentistry having little application for medical emergency management; it is mentioned for the sake of completeness.

The first is the Karnofsky scale. In a contrast to the previous scales where conscious level or physical state is measured, Karnofsky grades the patient on a linear scale from 100 to 10 in accordance with their <u>functionality and performance.</u> The scale extends from perfect health (100) to moribund (10) in 10 levels. With this numerical system there will be considerable subjectivity and inter operator variability in grading the patient.[26] Despite such criticisms and the fact that Karnofsky does not measure disease progression or prognosis, it is still an incredibly useful method helping to fill out a picture of our patient's abilities, ie: are they flat on their backs, or can they work?[27] Of relevance to you in dentistry, can the patient take their medication eg: use an asthma pump or inject their insulin? If not, will they attend as a dental patient who might also present as a medical emergency?

NEWS: The National Early Warning Score

The second is the National Early Warning Score (NEWS). First introduced in 2012 by the Royal College of Physicians (RCP), it has now been revised and updated from December 2017; for use by all health care staff engaged in the assessment and monitoring of acutely ill patients across the entire NHS.[28.] On balance, while Karnofsky is useful and can be adapted for use in a dental medical history, the second system: NEWS will prove to be more suitable for detecting the deterioration in a patient's condition to a level that urgent medical help is required. NEWS has been developed by the Royal College of Physicians in response to a lack of consistency resulting from the multiplicity of early warning systems presently being used in UK hospitals.[28] This system should prove to be useful in the dental clinic to assess acute illnesses eg: dento-facial infections, abscesses and swellings, to monitor clinical deterioration and to promptly initiate a competent clinical response to any medical emergency arising in the dental clinic. This system is being utilised by first responders. As a dental professional, you should be familiar with NEWS to communicate data during patient handover in the event of a medical emergency. Six simple physiological parameters, which are capable of being measured in your dental clinic are recorded and these are:

1. Respiration rate
2. Oxygen saturation
3. Systolic blood pressure
4. Pulse rate
5. Level of consciousness
6. Temperature

A weighting score is added to each of these measures. This score indicates by how much these results deviate from normal parameters. If your patient requires oxygen, then a weighting score of **2** is added. A final aggregate is complete by adding all the scores together. An illustration of the scoring chart is shown below. The NEWS 2 charts reproduced here are examples only and should not be copied for your clinical use. Please refer to and download the high-quality, full-colour versions on the RCP website before you make any clinical use of the NEWS 2 charts, these can be accessed from:

https://www.rcplondon.ac.uk/projects/outputs/
national-early-warning-score-news-2

National Early Warning Score (NEWS2)

Physiological parameter	Score						
	3	2	1	0	1	2	3
Respiration rate (per minute)	≤8		9–11	12–20		21–24	≥25
SpO$_2$ Scale 1(%)	≤91	92–93	94–95	≥96			
SpO$_2$ Scale 2(%)	≤83	84–85	86–87	88–92 ≥93 on air	93–94 on oxygen	95–96 on oxygen	≥97 on oxygen
Air or oxygen?		Oxygen		Air			
Systolic blood pressure (mmHg)	≤90	91–100	101–110	111–219			≥220
Pulse (per minute)	≤40		41–50	51–90	91–110	111–130	≥131
Consciousness				Alert			CVPU
Temperature (°C)	≤35.0		35.1–36.0	36.1–38.0	38.1–39.0	≥39.1	

Royal College of Physicians. National Early Warning Score (NEWS): Standardising the assessment of acute illness severity in the NHS. Report of a working party. London: RCP, 2017/2108.

From 2017, four trigger levels will determine not only the urgency of response, but which clinician can deliver that required level of response in accordance with the NEWS 2 charting and scoring.

I. **A Low Score:** An aggregate NEW Score of 1-4 should prompt assessment by a trained nurse who will decide if a change in monitoring or an escalation of clinical care is needed. With relevance to dental practise, this could be an unexpected decrease in the post-sedation conscious state of a patient. This will require further monitoring from the dentist or the anaesthetist, *e.g:* possibly requiring oxygen or another drug regimen to be administered to a dental patient.

II. **A Single Red Score:** This can be an extreme variation in an individual physiological parameter; a score of 3 in any one parameter, which is colour coded red in the NEWS 2 chart. This will prompt an urgent review by the clinician to establish the cause of the problem and the need for increased monitoring and an escalation in care.

III. **A Medium Score:** An aggregate NEW Score of 5 or 6. A NEW Score of 5 or more, is a key trigger threshold; being indicative of the risk of an acute deterioration that is serious. In dentistry: Think: SEPSIS!! With this score, an urgent review and the need for critical care must be considered a necessity. In a dental practice this NEWS 2 level almost certainly means the patient will be admitted to a hospital.

IV. **A High Score:** An aggregate NEW Score of 7 or more. This is a key trigger that requires an emergency medical response from the dental practice team. Examples we will deal with in this chapter are: MIs and CVAs (myocardial infarcts and cerebro-vascular accidents). As with the previous level, the dental patient with a High Score NEWS will be hospitalized.

With NEWS 2, a patient observation chart should be used. The chart reproduced here is an example only and should not be copied for clinical use. Please refer to and download the high-quality, full-colour versions of the Patient Observation Chart on the RCP website before you make any clinical use of NEWS 2.

https://tfinews.ocbmedia.com/media/news_obs-2.pdf

I. In the chart, you can see there are 24 columns, enabling a wide range of frequencies to monitor your dental patient.

II. In the out-patient day care setting of the dental surgery there is no specified number of columns that might be used. On one page: a few minutes, an hour, or a day can be recorded.

III. The particular monitoring frequency will be determined by the duration of the procedure, the patient's condition and the 2007 NICE guidance.[29]

IV. In particular, for your patients with hypercapnic respiratory failure due to COPD (of which there are increasing numbers in the out patient population) there is now a dedicated section (SpO_2 Scale 2) where the recommended O_2 saturation of 88% to 92% can be closely recorded during dental treatment.

V. In any medical emergency, or where the NEWS score is 7 or above: Continuous recording in the NEWS 2 rows are now aligned with the ABCDE you will be familiar with, to assist your hand-over to the medical emergency responders.

Observation chart for the National Early Warning Score (NEWS2)

NEWS key	FULL NAME		
0 1 2 3	DATE OF BIRTH	DATE OF ADMISSION	

			Score		DATE	
		DATE				
		TIME				

A+B Respirations Breaths/min

Range	Score
≥25	3
21–24	2
18–20	
15–17	
12–14	
9–11	1
≤8	3

A+B SpO₂ Scale 1 Oxygen saturation (%)

Range	Score
≥96	
94–95	1
92–93	2
≤91	3

SpO₂ Scale 2 Oxygen saturation (%)
Use Scale 2 if target range is 88–92%, eg in hypercapnic respiratory failure

¹ONLY use Scale 2 under the direction of a qualified clinician

Range	Score
≥97 on O₂	3
95–96 on O₂	2
93–94 on O₂	1
≥93 on air	
88–92	
86–87	1
84–85	2
≤83%	3

Air or oxygen?

	Score
A=Air	
O₂ L/min	2
Device	

C Blood pressure mmHg
Score uses systolic BP only

Range	Score
≥220	3
201–219	
181–200	
161–180	
141–160	
121–140	
111–120	
101–110	1
91–100	2
81–90	
71–80	
61–70	3
51–60	
≤50	

C Pulse Beats/min

Range	Score
≥131	3
121–130	2
111–120	
101–110	1
91–100	
81–90	
71–80	
61–70	
51–60	
41–50	1
31–40	
≤30	3

D Consciousness
Score for NEW onset of confusion (no score if chronic)

	Score
Alert	
Confusion	
V	3
P	
U	

E Temperature °C

Range	Score
≥39.1°	2
38.1–39.0°	1
37.1–38.0°	
36.1–37.0°	
35.1–36.0°	1
≤35.0°	3

NEWS TOTAL		TOTAL
Monitoring frequency		Monitoring
Escalation of care Y/N		Escalation
Initials		Initials

National Early Warning Score 2 (NEWS2) © Royal College of Physicians 2017

Royal College of Physicians. National Early Warning Score (NEWS): Standardising the assessment of acute illness severity in the NHS. Report of a working party. London: RCP, 2017. Reproduced with permission.

As noted above, the particular monitoring frequency will be determined by the patient's condition and the findings from the NICE guidance from 2007.[29] In normal circumstances, this might be one set of measurements for the patient being clerked into the dental clinic before a procedure, either with or without sedation, another set of measurements during their recovery and finally, a third set of measurements just before the patient is discharged, when the patient has sufficiently recovered from the effects of sedation and they are fit enough to leave the dental clinic being escorted to their home.

Certainly, with an adverse event, more than two or three columns of patient monitoring would need to be completed. As a dental visit usually lasts only minutes for a simple examination without any treatment and/ or up to an hour or two when procedural or surgical work is undertaken then some modification of the NEWS observational chart may be needed if it is to be routinely applied to dentistry.

With relevance to medicine and to dentistry, the NEWS charting should not be used for pregnant patients or on those less than 16 years of age, due to altered physiological responses in such patients. Whenever there is any clinical concern raised about a patient in a medical emergency, then requesting urgent medical assistance or the attendance of a medical emergency first responder should be sought and this obligation over-rides any patient monitoring.

For patient safety in dental and medical clinics, the NEWS 2 charts are free from copyright restriction being readily available and accessible from:

NEWS@rcplondon.ac.uk

https://tfinews.ocbmedia.com/about/

The permission of the Royal College of Physicians to reproduce their work; bringing it to your attention is gratefully acknowledged. Whatever form or patient monitoring or measuring you undertake, from GCS to AVPU, or Karnofsky to NEWS 2, your results should be recorded both clearly and concisely. By doing so, if any of your colleagues; medical, dental or nursing were to use your data in furthering their care of your patient, there will be no possibility of ambiguity, or confusion with risk to the patient arising from poor communication.

From 2015, NEWS was reviewed and then refined in 2017. It is anticipated that NEWS 2 will be implemented across the entire health care field and not just in the NHS and not just for hospital-based medicine, but for all providers of health care: **including dentistry**. A system such as NEWS 2 is certainly a valuable asset to enhance the safe practice of dentistry. In using such a system, you will bring yourself into line with all health care providers. By doing so, your clinical recording will be standardised, as will your ability to predict and prevent medical emergencies. If a medical emergency does occur, by reverting to standardised data, you and your colleagues in the dental team will be better positioned to deal with it.

To facilitate your understanding and use of NEWS 2 an online training course is available from 2018 from:

https://tfinews.ocbmedia.com/

References: Introduction to Medical Emergencies

1. Kaye W, Mancini ME. Retention of cardiopulmonary resuscitation skills by physicians, registered nurses, and the general public. Critical Care Medicine,14, 620-622. 1986.

2. Hamilton R. Nurses' knowledge and skill retention following cardiopulmonary resuscitation training: a review of the literature. J Adv Nurs. 2005 Aug;51(3):288-97.

3. West H. Basic infant life support retention of knowledge and skill. Paediatric Nursing. 2000; 12 (1) 34-37.

4. Care Quality Commission (CQC) Guidance about compliance: Essential Standards of Quality and Safety. London: CQC; 2010.

5. Greenwood M. Editorial: Medical Emergencies in Dental Practice. Primary Dental Journal. 2014; 3 (1) 4-5.

6. Anders PL, Comeau RL, Hatton M, Neiders ME. Jnl. Dent. Educ. The nature and frequency of medical emergencies among patients in a dental school setting. 2010 Apr;74(4):392-6.

7. Atherton GJ, McCaul JA, Williams SA. Medical emergencies in general dental practice in Great Britain. Part 1: their prevalence over a 10-year period. Br. Dent. Jnl. 1999. 186: 72-79.

8. Thornhill MH, Pemberton MN, Atherton GJ. Equipment and Techniques Introduction pp1-2. Management of Medical Emergencies for the Dental Team 2nd Edition. Stephen Hancocks Ltd London 2010.

9. Broadbent JM, Thomson WM. The readiness of New Zealand general dental practitioners for medical emergencies. N Z Dent. Jnl. 2001; 97: 82-86.

10. Girdler NM, Smith DG, Prevalence of emergency events in British dental practice and emergency management skills of British dentists. Resuscitation. 1999; 41: 159-167.

11. Müller MP, Hänsel M, Stehr SN, Weber S, Koch T A state-wide survey of medical emergency management in dental practices: incidence of emergencies and training experience. Emerg Med J. 2008 May;25(5): 296-300.

12. Atherton GJ, Pemberton MN, Thornhill MH, Medical emergencies: the experience of staff of a UK dental teaching hospital. Br. Dent. Jnl 2000; 188: 320-324.

13. Joint Formulary Committee. British National Formulary. Edition 66. BMJ Group and Pharmaceutical Press; 2013.

14. Resuscitation Council (UK) Quality Standards for Cardiopulmonary Resuscitation Practice and Training. Primary Dental Care. London: Resuscitation Council; 2013. [Online]
Available from: http://www.resus.org.uk/pages/QSCPR Primary DentalCare Equip.htm#equip [Accessed January 2016]

15. Resuscitation Council (UK) A systematic approach to the acutely ill patient. London: Resuscitation Council; 2005. [Online]
Available from: https://www.resus.org.uk/pages/alsABCDE.htm [Accessed January 2016]

16. Barkdull Thad, J. Pneumothorax During Dental Care. J Am Board Fam Med March 1, 2003 vol. 16 no. 2 **165-169 [Online]**
Available from: http://www.jabfm.org/content/16/2/165.full

17. Green AW, Flower EA, New NE. Mortality associated with odontogenic infection! Br Dent J 2001; 190: 529–530.

18. Currie WJR *et al.* An unexpected death associated with an acute dentoalveolar abscess - report of a case. Br J Oral Maxillofac Surg 1993; 31: 296–298.

19. Carter L, Starr D. Alarming increase in dental sepsis. British Dental Journal 200, 243 (2006).

20. Teasdale G, Jennett B. Assessment of coma and impaired consciousness. A practical scale. Lancet 1974 13 (2): 81–4

21. Green, S. M. Cheerio, Laddie! Bidding Farewell to the Glasgow Coma Scale. Annals of emergency medicine, 2011. 58(5), 427-430.

22. Haynes SR, Lawler PG. An assessment of the consistency of ASA physical status classification allocation. Anaesthesia. 1995; 50 (3): 195–9.

23. Harling DW. Consistency of ASA Grading. Anaesthesia. 1995; 50 (7): 659.

24. Scully C. Chapter 2: Medical History and Risk Assessment. in Medical Problems in Dentistry 6th Edition. pp20-22. Edinburgh. Churchill Livingstone. 2010.

25. Fitz-Henry J. The ASA classification and peri-operative risk. Ann R Coll Surg Engl. Apr 2011; 93(3): 185–187.

26. Péus D, Newcomb N, Hofer S. Appraisal of the Karnofsky Performance Status and proposal of a simple algorithmic system for its evaluation BMC Med Inform Decis Mak. 2013; 13: 72.

27. Karnofsky DA, Burchenal JH. In: Evaluation of chemotherapeutic agents. MacLeod CM, editor. New York: Columbia University Press; 1949. The clinical evaluation of chemotherapeutic agents in cancer; pp. 191–205.

28. Royal College of Physicians. National Early Warning Score (NEWS): Standardising the assessment of acute-illness severity in the NHS. Report of a working party. London: RCP,2012.

29. National Institute for Clinical Health and Excellence. Acutely Ill patients in hospital. Recognition of and response to acute illness in adults in hospital. NICE clinical guideline 50. London NICE, 2007.

Following the introduction detailing your assessment of patients, specifically: The acutely ill patient, you might now take a few minutes to revise the dental practice medicines and equipment list. Indeed, at this moment you may be inclined to check the contents of the emergency drug box in your dental practice, just to make sure everything is in date and you are familiar with how the contents are presented, so you know what to use in an emergency, but more importantly; where to find it.

After you have done that, we should really get on with looking at the medical emergencies you will face in dental practice. The best place to begin is with the most common medical emergency. As mentioned in the introduction, the most common and the most easily dealt with is the:

1

The simple faint or Vaso-vagal syncope

Up to 2% of your patients will faint in the dental surgery either before or during treatment[1][2].

This is the most common medical emergency in the dental practice, often it is the young, healthy and physically fit male with no indications of any problems whatsoever in their medical history, who will faint.

These patients will faint at the sight of a needle, during the injection, or immediately after the contents of a local anaesthetic cartridge has been administered to them; usually in response to the dental chair being rapidly sat up, buy an inexperienced nursing colleague as they enthusiastically assist the patient to rinse out....

The symptoms

Your patient will complain of feeling lightheaded or dizzy.
They may tell you they are anxious or are fearful.

The signs

The patient may become pale and you will see a rapid change in colour, as blood quite literally drains from the head, the neck and the face of your patient.

The patient may perspire profusely and feel cold and clammy.

Their pupils will become dilated, like big black saucers in contrast to their skin colour, which appears pale or grey; corpse like.

The clinical colour change, with the forthcoming faint results from a combined but independent; slowing of the heart with a lowering of blood pressure. We will return to discuss this phenomenon in some detail after we have first dealt with the patient who is fainting in front of you.

More signs

As mentioned, the patient will become cold and clammy, as their blood drains away from the head and neck into the thorax and abdomen.

If you have your wits about you and can get a grip of a wrist pulse, you will notice their pulse is slow and weak then suddenly, it becomes noticeably strong and bounding.

Your patient may well feel sick, vomit without warning, or complain of feeling nauseous.

Please note well:

In contrast to the non-fainting child who will unexpectedly vomit in a projectile manner in the dental clinic. The fainting adult will give you plenty of warning before vomiting into the kidney dish you will handily place in their lap, having anticipated they are about to do so from correctly assessing and anticipating the clinical signs noted before.

Placing all of that aside, before you get to this point, somewhat helpfully, your patient will tell you: They feel <u>faint.</u>

It's always beneficial when the patient can correctly diagnose their condition...just before... they

...entirely...

    ... lose...

        ... <u>Consciousness !!</u>

Your Treatment

Just before your patient does lose consciousness, try to catch them and their problem before it becomes a medical emergency with further complications.

In any dental clinic, fainting can easily be dealt with, but only if you act quickly.

However, if you fail to do this and the fainting patient falls, banging their head on something hard or breaking something expensive in your clinic on their way down, you will need to call on your emergency response colleagues and your indemnity provider.

The former are there to help the patient into an ambulance, the latter are here to help you out of a court case.

For these reasons, acting quickly is of the essence.

If the patient is in a dental chair, then you are in some luck; lay the dental chair flat out and get the patient's head lower than their heart to reduce any gravitational resistance to cardiac output. As the chair is going back, maintain the patient's: **Airway**, loosening any clothes around their neck. If the patient is obese and has more than one chin, then tilt their head back to keep their airway open and keep the mass of their neck musculature from constricting their airway.

Your nurse, or if you are a nurse, then your dentist can raise the patient's legs and get some of the blood back from the lower limbs into the heart, around the lungs and up to (or rather down to) the patient's head again.

As you raise the patient's legs two things will happen almost simultaneously:

I.   The patient regains consciousness.
II.   Money falls out of their pockets.

Please note, the patient regains consciousness not from hearing their pockets emptying of change as their coins hit the clinic floor (your Scottish colleagues might disagree) but as a result of their heads filling with blood as cerebral perfusion is regained.

In a post Brexit UK for any patient who faints, Scottish or otherwise, then dust rather than money is more likely to come out of their pockets.

By following these simple measures, the patient should rapidly recover consciousness.

During the immediate recovery phase, you would almost certainly want to make sure the patient's blood is as oxygenated as possible, so get a hold of the Emergency Oxygen cylinder, placing the mask on the patient's nose and mouth and immediately start the delivery of oxygen at 15 litres per minute.

This measure will assist in the patient's: **Breathing**

In some texts, it states that you only need to consider oxygen delivery if the recovery from a faint is delayed.[3] More recently however, an article in 2014, describing four case reports of fainting, does advise that providing oxygen at 15 litres per minute, should be part of the treatment plan for all dental patients who have fainted.[4]

We would agree with the author of that article, principally; as it was stated that there might be some difficulty for an inexperienced dental team member who witnessing a collapse, might not actually correctly determine that a faint had occurred.

It follows if the reason for the collapse was more serious than a simple faint, then having the oxygen already in place can make the continuing treatment of a more serious emergency that little bit more efficient and less stressful for all concerned.

Therefore, for this reason, we consider that giving oxygen, observing the patient and recording their vital signs in a NEWS chart would also be essential.

The patient who has fainted may have been in a state of nervous apprehension prior to their dental appointment and may not have eaten for a considerable time.

Consider on recovery from a faint, that they may be hypoglycaemic and you might provide them with a glucose drink.

On observing vital signs...

Do check the patient's pulse, at their wrist. (That is the radial pulse).

This takes care of the patients: **Circulation**

Please, whatever else you do, do not try grabbing their throat fumbling around for the Carotid pulse. That is neither helpful nor safe. Bear in mind the patient has fainted. A faint is caused by stimulation of the Vagus nerve. Pressing on the Vagus nerve again, no matter how accidental or how well intentioned is not smart.

In your patient's neck, the ever-wandering Cranial Nerve X, the Vagus is located within the Carotid sheath. That sheath is deep to the

Sternocleidomastoid muscles. In feeling for a Carotid pulse, you have to press on or around this muscle, which will exert some pressure on the Internal Jugular Vein and on the Vagus nerve too, before you ever get to feel if there is a pulse in the Carotid artery.

If you do not manage to elicit another inhibitory cardiac event, by physically pressing on the Vagus, with some luck (bad luck this time) you might just massage the Carotid sinus into action, which will slow the patient's heart down once again, or even more. As you need to maintain as much cardiac activity as possible in a patient who has fainted, pressing on the Vagus would simply be the wrong thing and a dangerous thing to do.

So don't do it!

If your luck and that of the patient really runs out, then as you fumble around massaging their neck looking for a Carotid pulse, you might end up dislodging an atheromatous plaque, giving you and your patient more than a medico-legal headache and the need for dental treatment when or if they ever recover.

So when managing a simple medical emergency; keep your management simple.

Although the faint has a simple cause and a simple solution, there is a tremendous risk and capacity to get things badly wrong if the clinical picture isn't recognized and the presentation is misinterpreted then mishandled. For these reasons the faint is and must always be considered as a medical emergency.

To repeat:

Lay the patient flat, raise their legs, give oxygen, and monitor their vital signs until they recover. Make sure you are certain that there are no complications and that the patient had only suffered from a faint.

You will have noticed from the above, with everything else going on; vomiting and money falling on the floor, that you will have followed the **A B C's** taking care of the patient's **Airway, Breathing** and **Circulation.**

As most faints occur in the dental surgery, with the patient in the chair, there was no: Danger to yourself or your colleagues in treating the patient as above.

If there is any doubt, then in addition to the A B C you need to check for any danger to yourself or your colleagues when going to the assistance of a patient.

Fainting Physiology

Fainting is an autonomic reflex. There are two opposed autonomic actions occurring simultaneously leading to the faint that we often see in the dental clinic.

First: there is an increase in Parasympathetic activity: the Vagus Nerve output increases causing heart rate and contraction force to drop.

Second: The Sympathetic activity decreases causing arterial wall dilation with a drop in blood pressure and no compensatory activity from the heart muscle as it is inhibited due to Vagal activity.

The source of these activities has been traced to activity in the Central Nervous System in the Brain Stem Solitary Nucleus where the Vagal Nerve nucleus lies.

The effects of the above are to increase blood flow into the visceral and musculosketal blood vessels and away from the head and neck. Vagal stimulation results in bradycardia, further lowering the flow of blood intra-cranially. While this established physiological process is well understood, what is less than clear, are the reasons why there should be Vagal stimulation in the first place! Precisely at the critical point in a flight or fright response when our dental patient wants to leg it out of the surgery, they end up flat on their backs with their A B and C being attended to.

Further Fainting Factors

As mentioned above, the sitting of a patient upright immediately after you have given them a local anaesthetic is not recommended. If the patient is prone to fainting, a rapid change in posture can result in loss of consciousness. The patient's heart fails to maintain an adequate blood supply to their brain as it tries to pump blood with less vigour into arteries whose walls are relaxed against the force of gravity as the patient is now sitting upright.

In essence, the treatment of fainting means avoiding the actions or triggers that can cause it to happen in the first place.

Some of the triggers and solutions to these are:

I. Inappropriate posture: Standing around for long periods in the waiting room because the dentist is running late. So give the patient a chair and try to see them on time.

II. Loss of appetite: In anticipation of a dental sedation procedure, patients enthusiastically starve themselves. Being deprived of food and water for far too long, resulting in lower blood sugar levels, dehydration and a fainting episode in the dental clinic. So provide clear pre-operative instructions.

III. Lack of sleep: This is caused by anxiety and the patient's nervous anticipation of their dental appointment. You can put the patient at ease by being empathic and supportive in your chair side manner and using simple non-evocative terms to describe what you are going to do.

IV. A poorly ventilated dental clinic, often causes patient to faint. It's easy to open a window.

V. Needle phobia. This is a recognised psycho-pathology with several behaviour modifying strategies. Referral to a clinical psychologist (not a psychiatrist) may be of benefit in such cases.

All of these triggering factors can be avoided with careful preparation, clear instructions for the patient and some foresight in making the dental clinic environment a well ventilated comfortable place to sit and work with a patient whose background is well understood.

As mentioned, fainting is a complex physiological phenomenon. In one study, up to one third of all dental patients have some phobia and may be prone to fainting[5] Fainting in the dental clinic may be part of the blood-injection fear phobia, which is documented in the Diagnostic

Statistical Manual of Mental Disorders (DSM IV TR)[6]. There can be some grave consequences for the patient, if fainting from this cause is not correctly managed in the dental clinic, hence the need to recognise fainting and act quickly. One paper has reported a sinus cardiac arrest resulting from this fear.[7]

From these case reports, we can see that although fainting is common, it should not be life threatening and can be dealt with quite simply. What it lacks in complexity of treatment, it makes up for in the difficulty we still have in trying to understand why it actually happens in the first place.

Preventive Measures

One treatment that is useful in dealing with patients who are prone to faint is: Applied Muscle Tension (AMT).[8] This procedure encourages the patient to tense and relax their leg, arm and torso muscles for periods of 15 to 20 seconds in sets of 5 repetitions. It can take up to one week for a patient to master this technique and to be confident enough to use it in the dental clinic. The purpose of this treatment is to actively use the skeletal muscles to pump blood back into the circulation, encouraging cardiac activity and so increasing the cerebral perfusion, subordinating the Vagal inhibitory activity that causes a faint to occur in the first place.

In overcoming phobias, another useful technique is Applied Relaxation (AR). Your first thought is that it might not seem advisable to use this technique to overcome fainting from needle phobia, due to the reduced peripheral blood flow seen in patients using AR. This technique induces a state of relaxation resulting from lowered heart rate and contraction force, causing skeletal blood flow and pressure to drop, which are initially the causes of fainting in the first place. However, in two studies comparing both AMT and AR, both seem to yield favourable results in preventing fainting in susceptible patients.[9][10]

References: The simple faint or Vaso-vagal syncope

1. Scully C. Chapter 1: Medical Emergencies, Managing Emergencies. in Medical Problems in Dentistry 6th Edition. pp7- 8. Edinburgh. Churchill Livingstone. 2010.

2. Wilson MH, McArdle SS, Fitzpatrick, Stassen LFA. Medical emergencies in dental practice. Jnl Irish Dental Assocn. 2009; 55: 134-143.

3. Greenwood M. Medical Emergencies in Dental Practice: 2 Management of Specific Medical Emergencies. Dental Update; 2009 Jun; 36(5): 262-4, 266-8.

4. Hardwick L. Fainting (Vasovagal Syncope): Case Reports. Primary Dental Journal; 2014 February 3(1): 65-66.

5. Armfield JM, Milgrom P. A clinician guide to patients afraid of dental injections and numbness. SAAD Dig. 2011 Jan;27:33-9.

6. Sokolowski CJ, Giovannitti JA Jr, Boynes SG. Needle phobia: etiology, adverse consequences, and patient management. Dent Clin North Am. 2010 Oct; 54 (4): 731-44.

7. Sadahiro T, Tamura Y, Mitamura H and Fukuda K Blood-injection-injury phobia: Profound sinus arrest. Intnl. Jnl. Cardiol. 2013 Sep 30; 168 (2)

8. Watling A. Chapter 21: Medical Phobias. In Di Tomasso RA Golden BA Morris HJ Handbook of Cognitive Behavioural Approaches in Primary Care pp 472-476. New York Springer Publishing 2010

9. Ducasse D. Capdevielle D. Attal J. Larue A. Macgregor A. Brittner M. Fond G Blood-injection-injury phobia: Physochophysiological and therapeutical specificities. Encephale. 2013 Oct; 39(5):326-31.

10. Ayala ES. Meuret AE. And Ritz T. Treatments for blood-injury-injection phobia: a critical review of current evidence. J Psychiatr Res. 2009 Oct; 43 (15): 1235-42.

2

The Hyperventilating patient

Moving on from the common faint, the next medical emergency we should look at is the hyperventilating patient often appearing either in, or after a state of panic. In many ways, there are similar triggers to the faint, anxiety being the most common of these. Once more, it is a frequent occurrence in the dental practice and can be extremely distressing for the patient. Only very rarely, can hyperventilation lead to complications, but only if this medical emergency is not managed correctly.

The symptoms are:

The patient will feel dizzy and may complain of being anxious or fearful not only of you but from what they think you are about to do to them!

The patient will have tingling or numbness in the face, hands and feet, even before you have laid your healing hands on or near them.

The signs to look for:

I. The patient will be rapidly breathing.
II. There will be a flushed appearance.
III. The patient's pulse will be rapid
IV. There will be tetany and spasticity of the hands and possibly the larynx too.
V. With laryngeal spasm, the patient's airway can become obstructed; this may lead to cerebral vasoconstriction, with collapse of the patient rapidly following from this.

Under no circumstances should a dental patient who is hyperventilating be treated as anything less than a medical emergency.

Treatment of the hyperventilating patient (i)

Your calming, professional and reassuring approach to all patients should reduce to a minimum; if not completely eliminate the presentation of this medical emergency from your dental clinic. If a patient starts to hyperventilate, then stop whatever you are doing, that may have initiated the hyperventilation.

Perhaps you were trying to gain consent for an extraction of a periodontally involved tooth, but to the patient your explanation came across as nothing less than a radical hemi-headectomy. Even trying to explain the need for a hygiene appointment to a nervous patient may seem like a horrible message of doom.

Therefore, a calming empathic approach with a modicum of sympathy as you carefully and actively note the effect your words are having on the patient is essential to avoid a panic attack and ensuing hyperventilation.

If the patient starts to hyperventilate, then after stopping whatever you were doing that was scaring the patient, gently lift the patient's hands to their mouth and while cupping their hands, (not yours), to their mouth; get them to breathe into and out of their cupped hands. Whatever you do, do not put your hands over their mouth. That can be taken as restraint, rather than reducing their radically raised respiratory rate, it will only increase it further.

At present there is a perceived wisdom and a widely accepted opinion that a patient who is hyperventilating should re-breath into a paper bag.[1] [2]. However... there is not a paper bag in your dental practice emergency drug box! Thinking about this critically: Can we accept that attempting to attach a paper bag to a hyperventilating patient's head is perhaps as likely as Scotland winning the world cup? Although we live in hope...it just might not be possible (sorry) Returning to hyperventilation, with sincerity: Convincing your distressed patient to breathe into and then out of a paper bag could be clumsy, it could be difficult and it might be dangerous too.

Certainly, in 2017, the British Thoracic Society Guidelines did not recommend this practice: **Re-breathing from a paper bag can be dangerous and is NOT advised as a treatment for hyperventilation**. (BTS Guideline: 8.13.3; 2017)

Traditionally, re-breathing from a paper bag was thought to allow carbon dioxide levels in the blood to normalize, but doing so can cause hypoxaemia with potentially fatal consequences. (Callaham 1989). Good practice points to considering, then either diagnosing or excluding organic illness in the hyperventilating patient and for monitoring of oxygen saturation to take place.

Despite such evidence, the accepted wisdom of using paper bags remains entrenched in academia, embedded in dental schools and ingrained in textbooks on medical emergencies, where drawings (not photographs) representing such a procedure can be found[2]. Certainly if it works and you can find evidence to support this technique, then a paper bag must be placed in the dental practice emergency drug box. In the absence of a paper bag, then please apply the evidenced and your to support your patients by holding the patient's cupped hands in yours. More than anything else: your empathic manner reduces hyperventilation away from a potential medical emergency towards an occurrence that can be entirely and easily manageable.

Physiology of the Hyperventilating Patient (i)

A patient, who is hyperventilating, is not breathing in either a co-ordinated or an efficient manner. There will be rapid inspiration and expiration of air both into and out of the lungs and the stomach too. Given the different concentrations of oxygen and carbon dioxide in air, more carbon dioxide will be leaving the blood across the alveolar membranes than will be produced by the body. The pH of blood will rise ie: it becomes more alkaline and a state of respiratory alkalosis results, producing the tingling sensations, the dizziness and the other symptoms.

In extreme cases, the involuntary muscle contractions of carpo-pedal spasms will result in uncontrolled movement in the hands and feet. Only in very rare cases, can laryngeal spasm and airway obstruction occur. However, this is an exceedingly rare complication of hyperventilation.

In contrast to fainting, with hyperventilation, the alkalosis results in blood vessel wall constriction. Cerebral blood flow will then rapidly drop. Loss of consciousness does not often follow, as the cerebral hypoxia results in blood vessel dilation and an adequate blood flow returning. Alkalosis reduces the respiratory rate and then breathing slows down as the blood gas ratio of oxygen to carbon dioxide normalises again.[3]

Physiology of the Hyperventilating Patient (ii)

An adult at rest will have a respiratory rate of 8–14 breaths per minute and a mean tidal volume of 500 mL per breath. The arterial carbon dioxide tension, the $Pa\,CO_2$ can be maintained between 4.6 and 6.0 kPa. A useful definition of hyperventilation is that the patient is breathing at a rate in excess of their metabolic requirements[4].

A further description is: An increase in alveolar ventilation that is more than the level required to maintain an ideal balance of blood gasses. This will result in a fall in $Pa\,CO_2$ and the development of respiratory alkalosis. Hyperventilation is not the same as tachypnoea, as patients may have an increased respiratory rate but a low tidal volume, thus maintaining a normal $Pa\,CO_2$.

Despite such physiological explanations, the precise mechanisms behind hyperventilation remain controversial and are often considered to be either; the result of anxiety, hypochondria or both[4]. Alternatively, in those patients displaying chronic idiopathic hyperventilation, there could be a resetting of the patient's sensitivity to their CO_2 levels[5]. Hyperventilation may also be present in patients with chronic respiratory or cardiac disease that is either well controlled or subclinical.

There are three forms of hyperventilation and patients can present with a mixture of these[6]:

1. Acute Hyperventilation, which is episodic and often termed a panic attack.
2. Chronic Hyperventilation during which the Pa CO_2 is always below the normal range but the patient may nevertheless experience a few symptoms.
3. Hyperventilation during or immediately after short intense periods of exercise.

The hyperventilation syndrome

Hyperventilation can be considered as a syndrome of over-breathing when the body does not need more oxygen, yet it receives it. This may be either chronic or recurrent. Your patient associates this syndrome with symptoms which they report as very frightening and unpleasant but if managed correctly are not harmful. The hyperventilation syndrome is very common, being reported more in in females in the age range of 15-55 and in asthmatics. Strong emotions such as anger, fear, excitement or panic can induce hyperventilation[7]. As noted above and for your revision: Hyperventilation causes the concentration of carbon dioxide normally carried in your blood to drop rapidly leading to the sensations and symptoms you will see.

The symptoms of the hyperventilation syndrome are:

I. **Respiratory** symptoms: Breathlessness and chest tightening with fast and frequent breathing.

II. **Tetanic** symptoms: A feeling of tingling in the fingers, arms and mouth, muscle stiffness and trembling in the hands. In addition, the hands and feet can become quite cold with shivering being seen.

III. **Cerebral** symptoms: Dizziness, blurred vision, faintness and headaches. In addition there can be fatigue, lethargy and a feeling of tense anticipation, even a feeling of impending death.

IV. **Cardiac** symptoms: Palpitations, irregular heart beat and Tachycardia.

V. **Gastrointestinal** symptoms: Sickness and abdominal pains.

Should your dental patient present with these symptoms, deal with them as outlined above. In addition, it then becomes incredibly important to exclude any other more serious and life threatening causes. The main cause of the hyperventilation syndrome is anxiety brought on by stress. A dental patient could be a natural worrier and that can be their normal mental state. Or there may be a recent stressful life changing event such as bereavement or any incident that was perceived as being life threatening that can lead towards hyperventilation becoming a chronic feature of their lives.

Different people respond to stress in different ways. People who hyperventilate often tense their upper thoracic musculature in response to stress. As a result, the ability of their diaphragm to function fully and freely will be limited. In turn, this places additional pressure on their already tense thoracic muscles to maintain a normal breathing pattern. After only a few minutes the overuse of these muscles leads to the feelings of breathlessness, tightness in the chest and even a sensation of suffocation.

The innate reaction to these unpleasant symptoms is to hyperventilate; breathing becomes rapid shallow and ineffective and a state of deep anxiety follows. Patients also report being very stressed and frustrated with their symptoms. A cycle of worsening symptoms leads to further hyperventilation and irregular breathing.

Treatment of the hyperventilating patient (ii)

The symptoms of hyperventilation must be recognized then controlled. While the symptoms are very real and are unpleasant; they are not immediately life-threatening.

Controlling the symptoms of hyperventilation is often a matter for the patient's personal management.

Coping and controlling hyperventilation can be achieved with breathing and relaxation exercises.

I.   Firstly, it is necessary to cope with hyperventilation.
II. Secondly, it is necessary for the patient to be in control of potentially stressful situations.

Physiotherapists, clinical psychologists and specialist nurses can all provide the necessary input to help the patient to develop the desired breathing and relaxation skills to prevent hyperventilation.

For our patients and perhaps ourselves; learning to breathe slowly and deeply is especially important for people who are at risk of hyperventilating, this means breathing with the chest muscles and not just the diaphragm.

The following example of an advice sheet contains exercises for the patients to prevent hyperventilation in the dental clinic:

Patient Advice Sheet Before Attending for Treatment
If you begin to feel nervous about your dental visit:

Exercise 1: Practice breathing when sitting
or lying in a comfortable position.

I.   Imagine your lungs are divided into three parts. Breathe in gently through your nose. Imagine the lowest part of your lungs filling with air.

II. If you are using your diaphragm your stomach will come out a little.

III. Imagine the middle part of your lungs now filling with air and your lungs becoming completely full to the top part and your shoulders may rise slightly and move backwards.

IV. Gently and slowly exhale fully and completely.

V.   Repeat the exercise up to five times every day and on the day of the dental appointment too! It is important that you breathe in and out at a steady rate and that you do not have to try too hard while completing this exercise.

Exercise 2: Practice counting while breathing to maintain slow steady breaths.

I.   Take a deep and a full breath.
II.   Exhale slowly fully and completely.
III. Inhale again and count from 1 to 5 or for as long as it feels comfortable and pause for a few seconds.
IV.   Exhale slowly while counting from 1 to 5 or for as long as feels comfortable.
V.   Repeat this exercise up to five times.

As these breathing exercises are practised, try to increase breathing out. To check that you are breathing deeply using your diaphragm, sit or lie with your hands resting across the lowest part of your chest. Your hands should be just slightly above your waistline and your fingertips should just touch.

If you are breathing deeply and expanding the whole of your chest and lungs, then your fingertips will move apart when you breathe in and come together again when you breathe out.

These exercises are the beginning of you helping yourself to deal with the anxiety of your dental visit. You may need further help and support and a clinical psychologist, who can help you.

With perseverance and time, your symptoms will diminish and they may even disappear completely. In this way, you will be able to feel more comfortable about coming for dental treatment.

Lastly if you feel nervous or anxious, then call us and talk to us about your questions, doubts and fears, we are here:

To hear you and to help you

References: The hyperventilating patient

1. Greenwood M. Medical Emergencies in Dental Practice: 2 Management of Specific Medical Emergencies. Dental Update; 2009 Jun; 36(5): 262-4, 266-8.

2. Thornhill MH, Pemberton MN, Atherton GJ. Medical Emergencies in the Conscious Patient. in Management of Medical Emergencies for the Dental Team. 2nd edition pp54-55. London S.Hancocks Ltd 2010.

3. Scully C. Chapter 1: Medical Emergencies, Managing Emergencies. in Medical Problems in Dentistry 6th Edition. pp7- 8. Edinburgh. Churchill Livingstone. 2010.

4. Gardner WN. The pathophysiology of hyperventilation disorders. Chest 1996; 109: 516–534.

5. Jack S, Rossiter HB, Pearson MG. Ventilatory responses to inhaled carbon dioxide, hypoxia and exercise in idiopathic hyperventilation. Am J Respir Crit Care Med 2004; 170: 118–125.

6. Robson A. Dyspnoea, hyperventilation and functional cough: A guide to which tests help sort them out. *Breathe*. 2017; 13(1):45-50. Available from: https://www.ncbi.nlm.nih.gov/pmc/articles/PMC5343732/
Accessed March 2017.

7. Lenfant C. Chest pain of cardiac and non cardiac origin. Metabolism. 2010 Oct; 59

3

Asthma

Moving on from the previous two common medical emergencies that are easily dealt with and are seldom, if ever life threatening, we will now deal with Asthma, one of the most common chronic medical conditions in the UK.[1.]

<u>An asthma attack can be a life-threatening condition.</u>

Therefore, you must always treat an asthma attack with a high degree of urgency, given the serious nature of the problems that will face an asthmatic patient if their condition is not controlled.[2]

As noted above, asthma is a common medical problem with an increasing prevalence affecting some 1 in 50 people in the UK. In some countries, the prevalence of asthma can be as high as 1 in 5 people who are suffering from this condition.[3]

Asthma most frequently develops as a childhood illness. One classic sign is the child who neither plays outside, nor engages with other children in team sports, in other forms of physical activity or in outdoor pursuits. Exposure to cold air, allergens from plants and animals, together with physical exertion are the well known triggers of extrinsic asthma.

You can see from foregoing, that an asthmatic child could suffer the consequences of socially restricting circumstances that arise from their condition; if it is neither recognized early nor managed effectively at a time when it becomes clinically evident.

Notwithstanding this, some 75% of those who suffer from asthma in childhood will improve throughout adolescence and into adulthood.[3]

Pathology of Asthma

Childhood asthma is a common, allergy induced, atopy associated and IgE mediated condition. In this form of asthma, specifically as noted: With Extrinsic Asthma, in response to an allergen; mast cells (tissue resident immune cells): degranulate, releasing: histamines, leukotrines, prostaglandins and a wide range of other immunologically active substances; causing: oedema, bronchospasm and the clinical signs of asthma that will be detailed below.

The other less common form of asthma is intrinsic asthma. This appears in adulthood. Intrinsic asthma is not necessarily always due to an allergic reaction, nor is it associated with atopy, but it is due in part to the development of instability in the patient's immune system. The factors responsible for this volatility can be emotional stress, gastro-oesophageal acid reflux, or as an abnormal physiological reaction to Vagus nerve activity, (with regard to Vagal function please compare asthma with fainting)

With both extrinsic (child) and intrinsic (adult) asthma, the following triggering factors are commonly implicated:

I. Emotional stress or anxiety. This is relevant to many dental patients who are inherently nervous of their dentist, being apprehensive when attending their appointments.

II. Infections of the Upper Respiratory Tract. These can be from viral, bacterial or fungal sources.

III. Irritating vapours. These can be seen in the dental surgery in the spray from high-speed water-cooled hand pieces, or the ultra-sonic scalers the hygienists use. In addition, uncured methyl methacrylate monomer, is a known cause of asthma.

IV. Exercise. Especially out-doors in the winter with exposure to cold air and in spring and summer with exposure to pollen. Exercise induced asthma is common in those patients not used to physical exercise, especially those patients who are literally if not actually "running late" to their dental appointments.

V. <u>Food products.</u> This is a well-known and well-documented category of asthma inducing and exacerbating factors. Among the most common are nuts, food additives and food colourants.

VI. <u>Medication.</u> Again this is a well known category, with the NSAID (Non Steroidal Anti-Inflammatory Drug) Ibuprofen, being a well proven causative initiator of asthma in the susceptible patient. Other NSAIDs are implicated too, as are Beta-Blockers and Angiotensin Converting Enzyme (ACE) Inhibitors.

Between attacks of asthma, patients are often completely asymptomatic. However, there may be other allergic conditions such as; hay fever, eczema and drug sensitivities that can develop in the absence of an asthma attack.

The signs of Asthma

In patients who regularly take their medication, there may well be no signs of asthma. However, the following list of signs will identify a patient of being at risk of an asthma attack:

I.   With an updated and accurate medical history, you will note the patient takes medication for asthma.

II. This will be either a Beta 2 Agonist such as salbutamol or a Corticosteroid such as beclomethasone. These are often referred to respectively by the patient as: their **Blue Inhaler** or: their **Brown Inhaler**. These drugs respectively; relieve and prevent asthma.

III. Data in an updated medication history is the first indication the patient is at risk from asthma. So please do take care when taking and updating the patient's medical and medication histories. In a patient whose asthma is well controlled, the clinical signs may well be absent. In a patient who does not take medication (often a child where their condition has not yet been diagnosed) you may see the following signs in the clinic:

IV. A noticeable conciseness of speech that cannot be ascribed to shyness or that the patient is genuinely uncommunicative: The asthmatic's speech pattern will be abrupt with short sentences punctuated by frequent long pauses for breath.

V. This is Paroxysmal breathing, the asthmatic patient struggles to exhale but in comparison; inhalation will be markedly easier for them.

VI. Wheezing and coughing: In the asthmatic patient, this is noticeable and is not the result of a cold. The asthmatic patient will be susceptible to frequent colds that easily develop into Upper Respiratory Tract Infections (URTIs).

VII. The asthmatic patient will frequently use their accessory muscles to assist in breathing while at rest. You will see this in the clinic as you sit facing the patient observing them breathing.

VIII. With a prolonged asthma attack, the patient will become quite anxious and distressed.

IX. Their heart rate will increase (tachycardia).

X. There will be tiredness, listlessness and the chronic asthmatic can become quite exhausted due to the expenditure of energy from the accessory muscles and other skeletal muscles being recruited into their efforts just to keep breathing.

Treatment of the Asthma Attack

Your treatment is based on correctly diagnosing that the patient has asthma and is suffering from an asthma attack. You must be able to identify this and that the patient is neither hyperventilating nor choking (we will deal with choking in the next section).

As noted previously, if you refer to the patient's medical history, this will assist in your diagnosis. In asthma and many medical conditions, the medication the patient takes is indicative of their illness. Therefore, once you are certain of your diagnosis, your treatment should be straightforward:

> I. Go to the dental practice drug box and take out the Blue Inhaler.
> II. As you shake this, you will feel the contents being mixed up to give the most effective aerosol.
> III. You can then apply this to the patient's mouth. As you press down on the button to dispense the salbutamol, try to co-ordinate this as the patient breathes in.
> IV. Invariably the first one or two attempts will not be in time with the patient's breathing and they will exhale just as you really need them to inhale.
> V. After a minute or two, with some perseverance, the patient's rate of breathing will slow down as the salbutamol dilates their bronchioles, allowing an increased airflow both out of and into the patient's lungs.

In contrast to the well-worn fable of the hyperventilating paper bag, paper cups can be found in dental practices, patients do use them and they are useful in managing asthma attacks.

In addition to shaking the asthma inhaler, a cup used as a spacer can further improve the aerosol flow and the effectiveness of salbutamol. A hole is made in the base of a cup and the inhaler is placed in this opening. The top of the cup is placed against the patient's mouth and two to three doses of salbutamol are given. An improvement in clinical signs should be seen in two to three minutes.

But honestly, as a professional health care worker, do yourself a favour: Stop the nonsense, go to any chemist (dispensing pharmacist) and buy yourself a spacer and put it in your dental practice drug box.

Managing the Severe Asthma Attack

Most asthma attacks do respond to the patient's or the practice's inhaler, however if there is no improvement in a few minutes, then oxygen must be given and an ambulance should be called.

The signs to be aware of are that the patient becomes increasingly distressed, their breathing rate increases as will their heart rate and the salbutamol has no immediate effect.

At this point: You will be giving 15 litres of oxygen per minute via a bag valve mask set up and getting ready to transfer your patient to the paramedics in the ambulance.

You will continue to use the salbutamol. By this stage the salbutamol can be administered into the bag simultaneously with the oxygen.

You will refer to the NEWS observation chart, monitor the patient's vital signs and add 2 to the weighting aggregate (as you are now giving oxygen). You will need to keep an eye on the AVPU level and their rate of breathing. In addition, you should have access to a pulse oximeter and so you can monitor the patient's oxygen saturation and heart rate too. The four physiological parameters:

1. **AVPU**
2. **Breathing**
3. **Oxygenation saturation**
4. **Pulse**

should provide adequate information for the ambulance crew on handover to the emergency responders.

It must be noted that although deaths from asthma are rare, they do occur, often from a failure to recognize the deterioration in the condition and from a prior reluctance to use corticosteroids.[3.] For those reasons updating medical histories and NEWS monitoring are essential tasks for all asthmatic dental patients.

Asthma Deaths and Dentistry

The National Review on Asthma Deaths (NRAD) published in 2014 reveals some significant facts about asthma.[4] While the condition remains both diverse and common and this in itself may have created a degree of complacency in how we deal with it, it is of note that not only severe asthmatics died from asthma, those for whom the disease was not well controlled with prescribed medications not being taken, or for whom preventive drug regimens were not being followed also died.

This may be more indicative of a failure in the health care system to actively involve patients in their care and effectively communicate the need for their compliance, rather than the fault of the patient who doesn't take their medicines for no good reason.

The following are of relevance to safety in dentistry when treating a patient with asthma and are based on the evidence from the NRAD report:

I. Nearly half of all those who die from asthma do not seek medical care at the time of an attack, with the majority of those having had no specialist care in the preceding year.

   ie: The patient's knowledge of their medical history was insufficient.

II. Of those dying from asthma 1/5 were in a hospital with the patient having had a history of attendance at an A and E unit in the previous year.

   ie: If your dental patient has attended hospital with asthma this must be noted in your medical history as there could be repetition.

III. Triggering factors (of which as previously stated, there are many in the dental surgery) contributed to nearly half of all deaths.

   ie: There are risks present in the dental surgery for the asthmatic patient.

IV. A lack of knowledge in the health care professional's ability to deal with the asthmatic patient were contributory to nearly half of all deaths.

    ie: Your ability to recognize and treat this condition is critical to your patient's survival.

V. Less than ¼ of those dying from asthma were in receipt of a Personal Asthma Action Plan (PAAP) something that is acknowledged to improve asthma care.

    ie: In all of your asthmatic dental patients, ensure they have a PAAP, if not then you must contact their doctors to make sure they implement a PAAP ASAP.

VI. There was an over-emphasis on asthma relief medication rather than asthma preventive medication. Even to the point that Long Acting Beta Agonists (LABA) were being used without simultaneous corticosteroid prescription.

    ie: Your giving Salbutamol in an emergency may not succeed in saving a patient in status asthmaticus. Prevention is key and early appropriate management is critical.

Further information on Asthma

If a patient is a severe asthmatic, then the timing and nature of dental treatment you propose should be co-ordinated with the patient's medical practitioner. The risk of an asthma attack in the surgery while undergoing dental treatment can be reduced by deferring dental treatment to a time when the patient is in a more stable phase of their condition.

Only the simplest dental treatments should be attempted and completed using local anaesthesia where necessary.

In asthmatic patients taking salbutamol, the beta agonistic action of this drug, when combined with the adrenaline contained in a dental local anaesthetic cartridge may cause cardiac arrhythmias.[3.] In patients taking methyl-xanthines, such as theophylline, a slow acting drug for prolonged prevention of nocturnal asthma, the risk is even more pronounced.[5] This published evidence suggests that adrenaline containing local anaesthetics are contra-indicated in dental patients taking these medications.[3.]

Due to the adverse risk: benefit ratio, referral for a general anaesthetic is always best avoided for any dental procedure. In the patient with asthma, any uncontrolled increase in blood CO_2 with a decrease in O_2 during a general anaesthetic might result in pulmonary oedema precipitating further inflammation in the patient who is already predisposed to such problems.

Other strategies to reduce anxiety such as using Nitrous Oxide and Oxygen for conscious sedation are preferable and not contra-indicated in the asthmatic patient. However, intravenous sedation using benzodiazepines or other IV drugs are best avoided as they may precipitate an asthma attack.[3 6.] In addition to the above noted drug interactions, patients with extrinsic asthma are often allergic to Penicillin. These drugs will be considered in greater detail in the next chapter on drug actions and interactions.

Anxiety is a common problem affecting many dental patients and in those patients with asthma, this problem carries an added significance[7,8]. It has been reported in the anxious asthmatic patient that attending for a routine dental appointment can result in a 15% reduction in their lung function[7,8,9]. Taking this into consideration, your safe and appropriate management of the asthmatic dental patient can be achieved not only by an understanding of their condition, but also by communicating your understanding of the problems they face to the patient with an empathic supportive manner that demonstrates your care, compassion and clinical skills.

Such an approach must be adopted before any of the problems associated with asthma begin to emerge in this avoidable, serious, but entirely manageable medical emergency.

References to Asthma

1. Mukherjee M, Gupta R, Farr A et al Estimating the incidence, prevalence and true cost of asthma in the UK: secondary analysis of national stand-alone and linked databases in England, Northern Ireland, Scotland and Wales-a study protocol. Brit. Med. Jnl BMJ open.-2014-006647.
   Online available from: http://www.ncbi.nlm.nih.gov/pmc/articles/PMC4225242/
   [Accessed: January 2015].

2. Shafer DM Respiratory emergencies in the dental office. Dent Clin North Am. 1995 Jul;39(3):541- 54.

3. Scully C. Chapter 15: Respiratory Medicine; Asthma. in Medical Problems in Dentistry 6th Edition. pp 365-366. Edinburgh. Churchill Livingstone. 2010.

4. The Royal College of Physicians. Why Asthma Still Kills. The National Review of Asthma Deaths 2014.
   Online available from:
   https://www.rcplondon.ac.uk/sites/default/files/why_asthma_still_kills_executive_summary.pdf
   [Accessed: January 2015]

5. Radenne F. Verkindre C. Tonnel AB. Asthma in the elderly. Rev Mal Respir. 2003 Feb; 20 (1 Pt 1):95-103.

6. Coke JM. Karaki DT. The asthma patient and dental management. Gen Dent. 2002 Nov-Dec; 50(6): 504-7.

7. M.S. Thomas, A. Parolia, M. Kundabala, M. Vikram Asthma and oral health: a review Aust. Dent. J., 55 (2010), pp. 128–133

8. T. Mathew, P.S. Casamassimo, S. Wilson, J. Preisch, E. Allen, J.R. Hayes. Effect of dental treatment on the lung function of children with asthma J. Am. Dent. Assoc., 129 (8) (1998), pp. 1120–1128

9. D.M. Steinbacher and M. Glick The dental patient with asthma. An update and oral health considerations J. Am. Dent. Assoc., 132 (2001), pp. 1229–1239

4

Choking and Foreign Body Inhalation or Ingestion

In contrast to the previous three medical emergencies; all having essentials of psychology, physiology and pharmacology in their cause and cure, the accidental ingestion or inhalation of a foreign body does not.

This medical emergency is not such a complicated event to understand, to deal with, or to prevent from occurring in the first place.

This medical emergency is rare, but the horribly ignominious involvement of your medical colleagues fishing your patient and yourself out of trouble as they trawl around the patient's right main bronchus to retrieve the evidence of your negligence, could pale into a dento-legal irrelevance for you if further medical complications arise from this emergency and the GDC decide to wade in...

> **This medical emergency is entirely preventable.**

If you are a dentist, you work in a dental surgery, repeatedly putting things into your patient's mouths and taking things out again, all day and every day of your working life.

Alternatively, if you are a nurse, you will be assisting your dentist with their insertions and extractions, all day and every day of your working life. The best thing all dental professionals can do is to make sure that accidental ingestion or inhalation does not happen. However, the very nature of dental treatment places patients at an increased risk of swallowing, ingesting or aspirating and then choking on foreign bodies that are constantly being put into and taken out of their mouths.

Although ingestion is more common than aspiration, the mortality associated with the latter far outweighs the morbidity associated with the former.

Foreign body airway obstruction is a well-known and documented phenomenon, with its own abbreviation: FBAO.

It must be emphasized: With adequate safety measures: FBAO is entirely preventable.

Despite the simplicity of the above statement, FBAO still occurs and so we will now look at this emergency and ways of dealing with it. By the end of this section, you will know what to do if this medical emergency should happen to a dental patient while they are in your care.

The following results of clinical research should not come as a series of astounding revelations to you:

I. Food is the most common accidentally inhaled foreign object, with children being the most susceptible.

II. After food, dental appliances are the second most common accidentally aspirated objects in adults.[1,2]

III. Aspiration and ingestion are both recognized complications of dentistry.[3]

IV. Accidental ingestion is more common than accidental aspiration.[4]

V. In the former, complications are rare and hardly ever serious whereas in the latter, if an object is inhaled, a complication will be more common and more serious.[5]

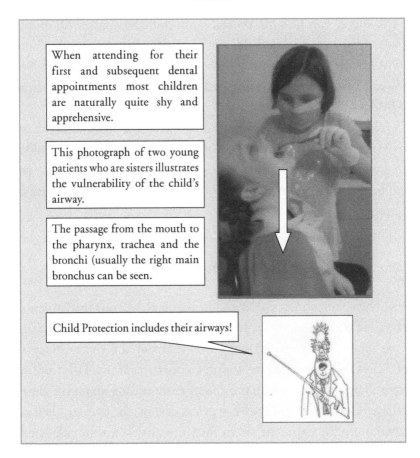

When attending for their first and subsequent dental appointments most children are naturally quite shy and apprehensive.

This photograph of two young patients who are sisters illustrates the vulnerability of the child's airway.

The passage from the mouth to the pharynx, trachea and the bronchi (usually the right main bronchus can be seen.

Child Protection includes their airways!

While the focus of this section will be with FBAO, the complications of ingestion do occur but as stated, they are rare. Most foreign bodies do pass quite harmlessly through the patient's gastro-intestinal tract. If an impaction were to occur, this would be most frequently at the level of the oesophagus. If this were to occur, your specialist medical colleagues can undertake endoscopy and retrieval.

In CUSPID Volume 2, Chapter 5, in the section: End of Life Care, some of the problems of patients with COPD; of: dysphagia and the risks of oro-pharyngeal impaction and aspiration will also be considered.

In dentistry, the most commonly inhaled foreign bodies are teeth or fragments of teeth, crowns, fillings and chemicals, root canal instruments and other materials used to restore teeth.

Looking deeper into this problem, you could be forgiven for thinking patients were being treated like wishing-wells for the prosthodontists who were most likely to drop things into a patient's oro-pharynx. Some 3.6% to 27.7% of all objects dropped or lost were precious metal crowns and bridges.[6.]

Following from the prosthodontists were the orthodontists who, with a frequency that was qite alarming did lose appliances in children; with some rather dire consequences for all concerned. At best, there could be litigation against the practitioner, while at worst children were hospitalised.

Prevention of FBAO

Rubber-dam, throat packs and tying up all of your instruments all of the time with dental floss, seem to work. However, orthodontists do not use rubber-dam ever and seldom, if ever secured their bracketry with dental floss. Rubber-dams are useful; an instrument that falls from your grasp will bounce around on the dam, before ending up on the floor. If you have remembered to place eye protection on the patient, then after bouncing off the dam, the sharp instrument will not impale itself in one of your patient's eyeballs.

However, dentists do not always use rubber-dam (or eye protection) all of the time. A recent study was enlightening: 63% of dentists did not use rubber-dam at all.[7.] The results of that study being in agreement with later work where overall; more than 70% of dentists surveyed stated they did not use rubber-dam[7,8].

Every dental practice has rubber-dam and the dentists working there do have the ability to use them, but for some reason; they do not.

This is a good example of risk normalisation and we as a profession seem content to accept that. We engage in a risk on behalf of our patients who will suffer the consequences when <u>our risk</u> becomes <u>their reality</u> and only then do we seem to wake up to the hazards of undertaking dentistry without any due regard to the safety critical nature of what we are doing to our patients.

In addition to having protective equipment in the dental practice, we need to engage in preventive behaviours; so we actually use the equipment.

I cannot think of any other preventive measure, where the cost: benefit ratio is as favourable as it is for rubber dam. That is, if we compare the cost of using rubber-dam against the impact of an emergency medical intervention up to and including; chest radiography, bronchoscopy and thoracotomy to recover the patient, your dental equipment and your career from the patient's lungs and lawyers... It really doesn't bear thinking about does it?

Despite all of that, the protection afforded by rubber is not universally embraced either by dentistry or other professions whose activities I am not qualified to comment on, neither being an expert on rubber or experienced in the activities of those professions using these products.

The signs of FBAO:

I.	This is most likely to occur while eating or in the middle of a dental procedure.
II.	Your patient will almost certainly clutch at their throat; this is the most common sign.
III.	There will be a nod or an indication, communicated to you, when asked if they are choking: That they are in difficulty and they are choking.
IV.	Your patient will be coughing repeatedly and have difficulty breathing.
V.	In severe airway obstruction your patient cannot speak and cannot breathe effectively.
VI.	There will be wheezing, coughing will be silent and is not at all effective.
VII.	The patient may lose consciousness.

The treatment of FBAO

In the first instance, your patient should be encouraged to cough repeatedly and to do so forcefully if they still can. Effective coughing may yet dislodge the foreign body. Clearing the airway in this way is the simplest method using the patient's normal responses and air in their lungs to remove the problem.

If this does not work, then your patient should lean forward and with you standing to one side, supporting their chest, you must deliver up to five firm back blows between the patient's shoulder blades, forcing air out of the lungs to clear the obstruction.

Failing to dislodge the blockage with the above procedure, you must now use abdominal thrusts. Stand behind the patient, lean them forward and clench one hand, hold your fist with the other and rapidly draw your locked hands and arms upwards, towards you and into the patient's diaphragm. This process should be completed five times. This procedure uses the mass of the patient's visceral organs to force residual air out of the lungs with a force sufficient to dislodge the blockage.

If these procedures do not work, an ambulance should be called immediately. AVPU and NEWS monitoring of the patient should begin as you administer **Oxygen at 15 litres per minute** from the bag valve mask set up. The patient should be placed in the supine position and supported as you lower them.

Remember the order **of A B C** and **A V P U**, to record the essential clinical data in NEWS and to hand over the patient to the emergency responders with as much relevant clinical data in a concise orderly manner.

The following algorithm is used for a choking adult. The 2015 UK Resuscitation Council Algorithm is reproduced below with their permission. This algorithm is available online from:

file:///C:/Users/Owner/Downloads/G2015_Adult_Choking_
Treatment%20(1).pdf

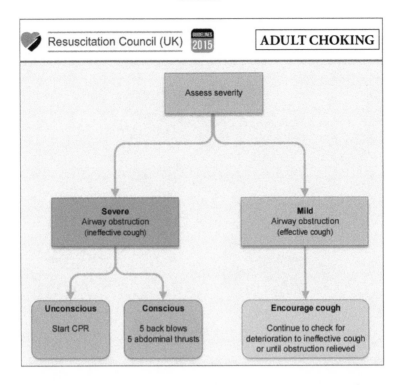

The previous algorithm is for use when an adult is choking. As noted above, children are more at risk than adults from FBAO with some 80% of all accident and emergency admissions for this problem being children.[1,5]. In a study of 500 cases of inhalation of foreign bodies, the most common age was 1 to 3 years old with nearly a 2% mortality rate and foreign objects that were inhaled and "forgotten about" resulting in considerable morbidity in 1.4% of cases. Another study of children up to 12 months noted a 6% mortality rate.[9.] Such morbidity and mortality resulted from laryngeal oedema and post bronchoscopic tracheostomy, with granulation and scar tissue formation.[10]. To re-enforce the point on prevention and protection, these studies looked at: <u>children.</u>

The following algorithm detailing your approach to paediatric care is reproduced with permission from the UK 2015 Resuscitation Council Guidelines. This algorithm is available online from:

<u>https://www.resus.org.uk/resuscitation-guidelines/</u>
<u>paediatric-basic-life-support/#process</u>

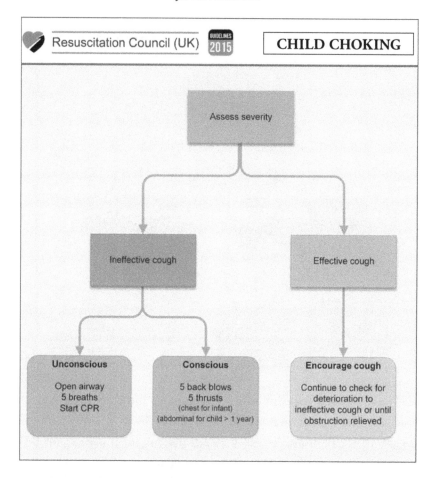

I. For adults and children if the 5X back blows and 5X abdominal thrusts do not work then the cycle of 5 X back blows and 5X abdominal thrusts must be repeated.

II. The patient with FBAO will need Oxygenation and Emergency transport to hospital

III. The total number of back blows addominal thrusts must be noted on patient handover.

IV. There is a risk of trauma to the liver and viscera from back blows and abdominal thrusts.

V. The patient may need to have a full examination including MRI in hospital to exclude visceral trauma.

FBAO: the full Picture

When you consider the outcomes below including inspecting stools, using rubber dam seems far more appealing. The complexity of this diagram shows in one picture why you need to be safety critical with respect to FBAO.[5]

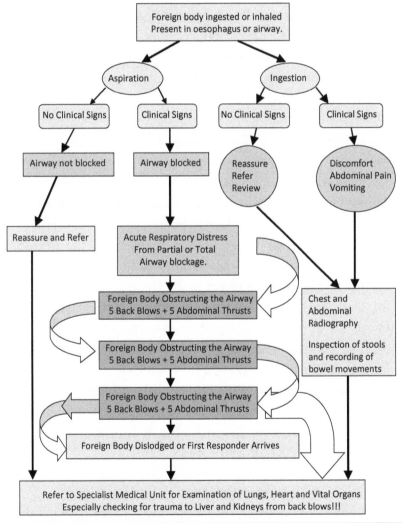

References: Choking and Foreign Body Inhalation or Ingestion

1. Aytaç A, Yurdakul Y, Ikizler C, Olga R, Saylam A. Inhalation of foreign bodies in children. Report of 500 cases. J Thorac Cardiovasc Surg. 1977;74(1):145–151.

2. Tiwana KK, Morton T, Tiwana PS. Aspiration and ingestion in dental practice: a 10-year institutional review. J Am Dent Assoc. 2004;135(9):1287–1291.

3. Milton TM, Hearing SD, Ireland AJ. Ingested foreign bodies associated with orthodontic treatment: report of three cases and review of ingestion/aspiration incident management. Br Dent J. 2001;190(11):592–596.

4. Kürkciyan I, Frossard M, Kettenbach J, Meron G, Sterz F, Röggla M, et al. Conservative management of foreign bodies in the gastrointestinal tract. Z Gastroenterol. 1996; 34 (3):173–177

5. Kumar Umesan U, Chua, KL and Balakrishnan P Prevention and management of accidental foreign body ingestion and aspiration in orthodontic practice. Ther Clin Risk Manag. 2012; 8: 245–252.

6. Tamura N, Nakajima T, Matsumoto S, Ohyama T, Ohashi Y. Foreign bodies of dental origin in the air and food passages. Intnl. Jnl. Oral Maxillofac Surg. 1986; 15 (6):739–751.

7. Lynch CD, McConnell RJ. Attitudes and use of rubber dam by Irish general dental practitioners. International Endodontic Journal. 2007; 40 (6):427–432

8. G S, Jena A, Maity AB, Panda PK. Prevalence of Rubber Dam Usage during Endodontic Procedure: A Questionnaire Survey. Journal of Clinical and Diagnostic Research : JCDR 2014;8(6):ZC01-ZC03. doi:10.7860/JCDR/2014/9011.4425.

9. Blazer S, Naveh Y, Friedman A Foreign body in the airway. A review of 200 cases. Am J Dis Child. 1980 Jan; 134(1): 68-71.

10. Dibiase AT, Samuels RH, Ozdiler E, Akcam MO, Turkkahraman H. Hazards of orthodontics appliances and the oropharynx. J Orthod. 2000; 27(4): 295–302

5

Angioedema and Anaphylaxis

Just before going on to deal with angioedema and anaphylaxis, in quickly reviewing the first four medical emergencies, fundamentally; they arise from problems in <u>Circulation</u>, <u>Breathing</u> and the <u>Airways</u>:

1. **Fainting** was the first of the emergencies, it is a common condition and the clinical effects are seen after a rapid collapse in cerebral circulation and that can be easily reversed.
2. **Hyperventilation** was the second emergency. Empathy, support and understanding go a long way to alleviating this condition by returning the patient's breathing to a normal rate again.
3. **Asthma** is more complicated, but with effective medical management, prevention and co-ordinated timing of medical and dental care, we can successfully limit or avoid the life threatening complications associated with that problem too.
4. **FBAO** the fourth medical emergency is entirely preventable. If it occurs and develops into a medical emergency, it is more complex than the previous three to deal with. In asthma, FBAO and for all these and the following medical emergencies: Management of the patient's airway is crucial.

We need to build on the basics of dealing with these first four medical emergencies to now deal with two more medical emergencies that could compromise the patient's airway. Given the causes and complications of angioedema and anaphylaxis; before any intervention is attempted, these emergencies must be accurately diagnosed.

Fortunately, medical emergencies arising from angioedema and anaphylaxis are rare, nevertheless, we should be prepared to both face and deal with them in the same way we have approached and dealt with the first four medical emergencies we have looked at.

Angioedema and Anaphylaxis

Angioedema is common, with one in five people experiencing localised urticaria (nettle rash) and oro-facial angioedema (an abrupt non-pitting swelling of the skin of the face, especially around the eyes and lips) at some point in their lives.[1,2]

The risk from these common conditions arises when a localised allergic reaction triggers the uncontrolled degranulation of mast cells. The effects of histamine being released and inflammatory mediators spreading into local tissue spaces and around the blood stream can rapidly overwhelm the susceptible patient. This results in the medical emergency of anaphylaxis, where a Type 1 Hypersensitivity reaction to common precipitants such as:

Latex, food products; often nuts, medicines and insect bites has been reported to affect up to 15% of the general population.[1]

Angioedema can be caused either by an IgE antibody mediated response, or following the activation of the inflammatory products of the kinin-kallikrein cascade. With the latter mechanism, a similar clinical picture is seen, either with or without urticaria. Whereas the former mechanism is an allergic reaction most commonly to food or drugs, the latter mechanism is often caused by the reaction to drugs alone, most commonly to the Non Steroidal Anti-inflammatory Drug (NSAID) family.

Once such an immune reaction has begun, tissue swelling will quickly follow from the increased permeability of dilated capillaries.

If the swelling involves tissues surrounding, or in any part of the patient's airway, a life threatening medical emergency will rapidly develop after a few seconds, or at the very most: within minutes after your patient has been exposed to the causative agent.

The risk of a medical emergency developing is far greater if there is a family history of urticaria, angioedema or any other allergy.

Of safety critical importance:

> **You must be aware of allergy or a history of allergy in your patient's medical history. This information must be documented for you to act upon in an emergency.**

The most common allergy you will see in your patients is to Penicillin. A recent study revealed some 11.5% of patients with an allergy to Penicillin. Over one third (37%) of these patients showing a rash, and some 11.8% showing angioedema. 6.8% of those patients allergic to Penicillin had a medical history demonstrating anaphylaxis.[4]. What was remarkable about that study was that only 6% of those patients allergic to Penicillin had previously referred themselves for specialist care.

So please, once again: Check your patient's medical history for any statement of a declared allergy. If the results of the above reported study are anything to go by, and we extrapolate the data, then 94% of all patients who are at risk of angioedema or anaphylaxis will have no documented medical evidence of their risk.

So you must be prepared to deal with this emergency in anyone of your patients and not just those for whom a risk factor has been documented.

1. The Clinical Signs of Angioedema:

I.   Most strikingly, the clinical signs will develop rapidly from seconds, certainly within minutes, so you must keep a regular and close observation of your patient at all times.

II. There will be swelling around the eyes, the lips and the patient's tongue may swell too.

III. The floor of mouth and throat can become involved.

IV. The larynx and pharynx can become compromised.

V.   If the angioedema involves the head and neck, then a rapidly fatal respiratory obstruction will occur.

In addition to the signs of angioedema as noted above there will be:

2. The Clinical Signs of Anaphylaxis:

I. Flushing or Pallor of the patient's face, possibly with presentation of a rash too.

II. Hoarseness, wheezing and your patient will have difficulty in breathing.

III. Bronchial involvement and bronchospasm are present.

IV. Vasodilation and acute hypotension follows.

V. The patient will become grey or white as a rapid collapse in their peripheral circulation now occurs.

VI. The patient will rapidly become unconscious and cardiac arrest may follow in minutes.

The treatment of Angioedema and Anaphylaxis

In order to treat angioedema and anaphylaxis successfully, (in common with all medical emergencies); the emergency must be correctly identified the moment clinical signs start to develop in your patient.

If you observe any of the signs listed above, then you can be certain these medical emergencies are happening. In the dental clinic, angioedema will most likely occur in response to a precipitant in your dental practice to which your patient is allergic.

These are noted to be: latex, chemicals used for cleaning or disinfecting and medications such as:

Penicillin, Aspirin, Ibuprofen, or Angiotensin Converting Enzyme (ACE) Inhibitors.

In addition to the above, in patients who are dentally phobic or generally nervous, the stress of a dental appointment is sufficient to precipitate urticaria and angioedema. Although these are likely to be self-limiting, their appearance may herald another medical emergency such as a faint that you should be prepared to deal with having revised this in the first of the medical emergencies we have considered.

As you are working in a dental team, either yourself or one of your colleagues will alert the medical emergency responders: informing them of the specific emergency you have identified: so upon arrival they will be well briefed to deal with the patient's hand-over.

Before you follow the **A B C D E** pattern in dealing with angioedema and anaphylaxis, the causative allergen or precipitant if identified must be removed, by washing with a stream of running water.

After this, your approach should focus on the first three of these five steps, the **A, B** and **C** to secure and maintain the patient's Airway, their Breathing and their Circulation.

Oxygen should be given to the patient at 15 litres per minute via the bag-valve-mask.

Laying the patient flat and raising their legs slightly will restore the blood pressure to their heart and brain thus counteracting the physiological effects of hypotension in the advent of the anaphylaxis developing.

Two items must now be taken from the Dental Practice Drug Box:

First, from the medical emergency drug box, the automatic dispenser with the Epinephrine (Adrenaline) is taken and this is firmly inserted into the patient's thigh muscle in the outer aspect of their leg: The entire contents will be administered to the patient.

In order to given an optimum response to epinephrine, there are variations in dose with age from children, through adolescents and to adults. However, as you are dealing with a medical emergency, invariably, the entire contents of the Epinephrine dispenser will be given to your patient.

The Epipen will dispense a median dose of 0.3ml or 300 micrograms of adrenaline intramuscularly.

However, the ideal age dependent doses of Adrenaline are:

Your Patient is:	Age Range of Patient	Ideal Adrenaline Dose is:
A Child	Less than 6 Years old	0.15ml (150 ugms)
An Adolescent	6 to 12 Years old	0.3ml (300 ugms)
An Adult	Over 12 Years old	0.5ml (500ugms)

Second, if the patient is wheezing and in respiratory distress then the Salbutamol is administered either directly to the patient or via the bag-mask set up together with oxygen. As stated in the previous medical emergency, this will cause broncho-dilation, improving the patient's airflow and oxygenation.

It must be noted that adrenaline will cause bronchodilation by non-specific binding to the beta 2 adrenergic receptors (in contrast to the beta 2 adrenergic specific binding of salbutamol). However, this is a non-specific but beneficial side effect.

The principle reason for the use of adrenaline in anaphylaxis is to increase peripheral resistance via α_1 receptor-dependent vasoconstriction and to increase cardiac output via its binding to β_1 receptors. The aim of reducing peripheral circulation is to increase both coronary and cerebral perfusion pressures and by doing so, increase the availability of oxygen for the patient.

The Initial Treatment for Anaphylaxis and Angioedema

The following algorithm is available online from the UK Resuscitation Council. From:

file:///C:/Users/Owner/Downloads/G2010Poster_Anaphylaxis-Initil.pdf

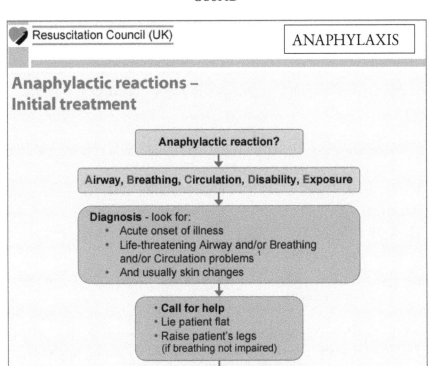

Resuscitation Council (UK)

ANAPHYLAXIS

Anaphylactic reactions – Initial treatment

Anaphylactic reaction?

↓

Airway, Breathing, Circulation, Disability, Exposure

↓

Diagnosis - look for:
- Acute onset of illness
- Life-threatening Airway and/or Breathing and/or Circulation problems [1]
- And usually skin changes

↓

- **Call for help**
- Lie patient flat
- Raise patient's legs (if breathing not impaired)

↓

Intramuscular Adrenaline [2]

---

[1] **Life-threatening problems:**

Airway: swelling, hoarseness, stridor
Breathing: rapid breathing, wheeze, fatigue, cyanosis, SpO_2 < 92%, confusion
Circulation: pale, clammy, low blood pressure, faintness, drowsy/coma

[2] **Intramuscular Adrenaline**

IM doses of 1:1000 adrenaline (repeat after 5 min if no better)

- Adult   500 micrograms IM (0.5 mL)
- Child more than 12 years: 500 micrograms IM (0.5 mL)
- Child 6 -12 years: 300 micrograms IM (0.3 mL)
- Child less than 6 years: 150 micrograms IM (0.15 mL)

Further treatment of Angioedema and Anaphylaxis

From this stage in your treatment, until the arrival of the medical emergency first responders, you should follow the **M O V E** protocol, this is:

I.   **Monitor** the patient, to observe the patient and run through the **A B C D E** as above.

II. **Oxygen.** Continue with 15 litres per minute via bag-valve-mask set up.

III. **Verify** the medical emergency responders are coming and know what they will find on arrival.

IV. **Epinephrine**, repeat the Epipen administration every 5 minutes if no improvement.

You will need to monitor the patient with regard to their **AVPU** status and **NEWS** scores, remember adjust the aggregate **NEW S**core by a factor of 2 as Oxygen is being given. On patient handover, the full medical history and event data will be given to the emergency responders to enable the most effective continuing care of your dental patient.

Further notes on Angioedema and Anaphylaxis

As mentioned previously, these conditions are thought to affect up to 15% of the population[1,2]. However, given the exposure of your patients to an assortment of chemicals that can act as precipitants, the numbers of patients we see with the clinical signs of an incipient angioedema, seem to be higher than the quoted figures.

There are a broad range of precipitants implicated in angioedema and anaphylaxis, however there is a significant group of patients for whom no cause can be identified.[5,6,7]. These are the non-allergic or non IgE mediated anaphylactoid cases.

It should be remembered that only 6% of those who were Penicillin allergic (the most common form of allergy) had previous specialist care[4].

Some 1 in 1,333 of the UK population will have experienced anaphylaxis at some point in their lives.[7]. In view of this, we must maintain a high index of awareness and suspicion when faced with the clinical signs as listed above.

Treatment of anaphylaxis demonstrates a good rate of recovery, the ratio of fatalities to cases being less than 1%.[8]. The mortality increases in those with asthma, especially poorly controlled asthma or in those who fail to use preventive measures or delay interventional treatment (as noted in the previous section on asthma). Putting all of this into some context, in the UK there are some 20 deaths from anaphylaxis annually.[7]

It has been suggested that patients with anaphylaxis are regularly not given the correct treatment, due to a failure to identify the condition either promptly or correctly.[9]. In several cases in a state of converse clinical confusion: Patients who have fainted or were hyperventilating, have been injected with adrenaline![10].

Diagnostic problems have arisen particularly in children. There must be an emphasis on the need for safety, when diagnosing anaphylaxis. There are a range of signs and symptoms, none of which are specific for any one anaphylactic reaction; a single set of clinical signs will not identify all anaphylactic reactions. However, the combination of multiple related clinical signs will make your diagnosis of an anaphylactic reaction more probable.[11].

Lastly, even after a successful patient hand-over, there is a risk of relapse especially in the patient who has a drug induced anaphylaxis or angioedema, notably from exposure to ACE inhibitors.

In such cases, the anaphylaxis is a class based reaction and not a reaction due to one specific drug or drug interaction.

Ongoing medical care in an ITU is necessary for 24 hours after anaphylaxis. Follow up care is essential with the need for the patient to carry a Medic Alert bracelet and an Epipen and for you to update your dental patient's medical notes.[12,13].

References to Angioedema and Anaphylaxis

1. Scully C. Chapter 17: Urticaria and Acute Allergic Angioedema. in Medical Problems in Dentistry 6th Edition. pp 414-416. Edinburgh. Churchill Livingstone. 2010.
2. NHS Choices. Angioedema Overview Online Available from: http://www.nhs.uk/conditions/Angioedema/Pages/Introduction. aspx
   [Accessed January 2015]
3. Kaplan AP. Angioedema. The World Allergy Organization Journal 2008; 1(6):103-113.
4. Albin S, Agarwal S Prevalence and characteristics of reported penicillin allergy in an urban outpatient adult population. Allergy Asthma Proc. 2014 Nov; 35 6): 489-94.
5. Pumphrey RS. Fatal anaphylaxis in the UK, 1992-2001. Novartis Found Symp 2004;257:116-28; discussion 128-32, 157-60, 276-85
6. Ewan PW. Anaphylaxis. BMJ 1998;316(7142):1442-5
7. Working group of the Resuscitation Council UK. Emergency treatment of anaphylactic reactions. Guidelines for healthcare providers. 2008. London Resuscitation Council UK
   Online Available from: http://www.resus.org.uk/pages/reaction.pdf
   [Accessed January 2015]
8. Bohlke K, Davis RL, DeStefano F, Marcy SM, Braun MM, Thompson RS. Epidemiology of anaphylaxis among children and adolescents enrolled in a health maintenance organization. J Allergy Clin Immunol 2004; 113(3):536- 42.
9. Haymore BR, Carr WW, Frank WT. Anaphylaxis and epinephrine prescribing patterns in a military hospital: underutilization of the intramuscular route. Allergy Asthma Proc 2005; 26(5):361-5
10. Johnston SL, Unsworth J, Gompels MM. Adrenaline given outside the context of life threatening allergic reactions. BMJ 2003;326(7389):589-90.
11. Brown SG. Clinical features and severity grading of anaphylaxis. J Allergy Clin Immunol 2004;114(2):371-6.

12. Oike Y, Ogata Y, Higashi D, Matsumura T, Numata Y. Fatal angioedema associated with enalapril. Int Med. 1993;1:308–310.
13. Thompson T, Frable M. Drug-induced, life-threatening angioedema revisited. Laryngoscope.1993;1:10–12.

6

Adrenal insufficiency and crisis

The effective treatment for the previous medical emergency was by injecting adrenaline. Once administered with other measures, that medical emergency can be effectively dealt with. Adrenaline is a naturally occurring catecholamine and neurotransmitter produced in the inner area or medulla of the adrenal glands, of which there are two, sited on the upper aspect of your kidneys. They are small glands and shaped like little pyramids.

We will now turn our attention to the outer area of these glands or the adrenal cortex, which under a series of feedback loops from the Hypothalamus to the Pituitary and into the adrenal cortex, are responsible for the production of a variety of steroids.

These steroids are essential factors in the human body's response to physiological, physical and psychological stresses such as hypoglycaemia, trauma, infection and most forms of pain sensations, from the physical to the emotional, together with responses to social stresses too. The level of these corticosteroids produced, will be directly proportional to the stress level your patient encounters and can deal with.

The corticosteroids

I. **Cortisol.** A glucocorticoid released in response to stress and low blood sugar levels. It can also suppress the immune system, decrease bone formation and aid the metabolism of fat and protein.
II. **Corticosterone.** A primary intermediate metabolite important in the steroid pathway from glucocorticoid to mineralocorticoid production.

III. **Aldosterone**. A mineralocorticoid produced in the adrenal cortex, it works in the kidneys, increasing sodium retention and excreting potassium. This physiological squeezing of capillaries increases urine flow and then you will feel thirsty (quite simple really!)

IV. **ANP**. Atrial Natriuretic Peptide it is produced in the right sided heart muscle cells, increases sodium loss and works against Aldosterone action.

It is of some importance that we remind ourselves of this clinical knowledge, the actions of the adrenal cortex and the effects of these corticosteroids on your patient, before moving on to the less common but slightly more complex medical emergency of Adrenal Insufficiency and Crisis.

This medical emergency is not so common but we should be prepared to deal with it, principally because more of our patients are taking more medications and corticosteroid medication is perhaps the main cause of adrenal insufficiency in our patients. With relevance to this, two further issues must be considered:

First, more of our patients will be living for longer. Older patients have higher ASA profiles and the risks presented when we treat them will be greater.

Second, with more medications being taken by more patients, the risk of an adverse interaction either from dental prescriptions or from a medical practitioner's prescriptions will similarly increase. Many of these drug actions and interactions will be considered in the next chapter.

The causes of adrenal insufficiency and crisis

Medication with systemic corticosteroids is the most common cause of adrenal insufficiency and crisis. This effect suppresses the activity in the adrenal cortex. This is <u>Secondary Hypoadrenocorticism.</u>

A rarer cause is that the patient's adrenal cortex is fundamentally diseased. This could arise from an infection such as Tuberculosis, HIV and/or AIDS, or that a secondary tumour has arisen, especially from Breast Cancer, or rarely from oral cancer metastates, these will be considered in greater detail in Chapter 5.

Physiological causes might follow from failed hormone secretion, or an endocrine deficiency can follow from auto-immune disease. With these causes, the patient develops antibodies against their own adrenal cortex cells. This is Primary Hypoadrenocorticism.

The clinical features leading to a potential medical problem will be uncovered in your medical history. That is, by asking sensitive yet inquiring questions that are both appropriate and unique, you will be able to build a comprehensive safety focussed medical and medication history from and for each of your patients. Regardless of the causes being either primary or secondary hypoadrenocorticism, the clinical signs we need to be aware of in a medical emergency will always be the same:

The clinical observations of adrenal insufficiency

I. Often, the patient is underweight, with a history of anorexia, nausea and vomiting.

II. Their blood pressure is low and hypotension is a constant feature.

III. A pulse that is thready, weak and rapid will be detected and hopefully documented too.

IV. There is both mucosal and cutaneous pigmentation.

V. There could be signs of mucocutaneous candidosis.

VI. Muscle tremor, weakness and loss of muscle bulk are also commonly seen.

The clinical signs of an adrenal crisis

I. The patient's inability to concentrate with already low and rapidly diminishing levels of consciousness.
II. Their pulse might be very slow or might not be discernible at all.
III. Hypoglycaemia, with dangerously low blood sugar levels may be noted. **Less than 3 mmol/L**
IV. Dehydration is seen.
V. Collapse and total loss of consciousness will soon follow.

Although an adrenal crisis presenting in the dental clinic is a rare event, adrenocortical hypofunction can lead to shock and can rapidly prove to be fatal if your patient has already suffered stress from an operation, an illness, infection or the combined stress and trauma from extensive oral or dental surgery.

Prevention of adrenal insufficiency and crisis

From your updated medical history, you will know if your patient has used or is currently using corticosteroids and for the specific condition these are being taken.

Some patients will carry a **Blue** Steroid Warning Card.

With experience you may come across the relatively rare condition of Addison's Disease. This is Primary Hypo-adrenocorticism caused in 70% to 80% of cases by auto-antibodies directed against cells in the adrenal cortex. If your patient has Addison's disease, then they will be taking: Hydrocortisone to replace Cortisol and Fludrocortosone to replace Aldosterone.[2] Such patient's may require an increased dose of their medication prior to their dental visit. Another more common example is the dental patient who is on long-term immunosuppressive steroids after organ transplantation. In these cases, high doses of steroids are used and these will cause a Secondary Hypo-adrenocorticism.

There are recent studies suggesting that supplemental steroid cover is not needed for routine dentistry with these patients.[3,4] However, where a dental procedure is more involved, the patient's condition is not well stabilised, or they are of a nervous or anxious disposition, then you must defer to the patient's endocrinologist for an expert specialist opinion on how best to proceed.

Patients who are systemically unwell, presenting with dental abscesses including raised temperature and facial swelling, in addition to following the best evidence based practice for antibiotic stewardship, there is an established recommendation to provide a pre-operative increase in the dose of corticosteroids the patient is already taking.[5] Although this guideline has now been updated by the UK Resuscitation Council, the most up to date information is from the December 2015 ACAP (the Addison's Clinical Advisory Panel) recommendations, which broadly agrees with those guidelines. These are reproduced below and are available online from:

www.addisons.org.uk/surgery

Major Dental Surgery	100mgs Hydrocortisone Intramuscular injection before anaesthesia	Double dose of oral medication 24 hours before procedure, then return to normal.
Dental Surgery	Double oral dose up to 20mgs Hydrocortisone one hour before surgery.	Double dose of oral medication 24 hours before procedure, then return to normal.
Minor Dental Surgery	Take an extra oral dose 60 minutes before the procedure.	If there are hypo-adrenal symptoms then take an extra oral dose and then return to normal.

I. Intramuscular hydrocortisone is preferable to intravenous injection due to a more sustained duration of action.

II. The hydrocortisone should be administered in a bolus over a minimum of 10 minutes to prevent vascular damage.

III. Hydrocortisone acetate cannot be used due to its slow-release, microcrystalline formulation. Ensure the parenteral drug administered is hydrocortisone sodium phosphate or hydrocortisone sodium Succinate at 100mg.

IV. Monitor electrolytes and blood pressure post-operatively for all procedures requiring parenteral steroid cover. If your patient becomes hypotensive, drowsy or peripherally shut down, administer 100mg hydrocortisone IV or IM bolus immediately.

V. Ensure back-up supplies of oral and injectable hydrocortisone are available for resuscitation before commencing surgery. Even at full steroid cover, postoperative resuscitation may occasionally be required.

These guidelines are not only for primary adrenal insufficiency, they also apply to potentially life threatening steroid dependency too. Certainly prevention is better than intervention, should a steroid crisis develop while a patient is in your care the following procedures must be followed:

The treatment of an adrenal crisis

I. **Monitor** the patient's AVPU and NEWS. Check the A B C D repeating every 2 to 3 minutes.

II. **Oxygen** at 15 litres per minute is given to a clear Airway.

III. **Verify** that an ambulance has been called and help is coming.

IV. **Elevate** the legs as the patient is laid flat to assist in maintaining cerebral blood flow.

Maintain the MOVE Protocol as above until the medical emergency first responders arrive and you can arrange handover of the patient with relevant clinical data with AVPU and NEWS. The event should then be recorded and documented.

Further notes on adrenal insufficiency and crisis

In the medical histories you obtain from dental patients, a particular emphasis must be placed on documenting and noting their long-term use of systemic corticosteroids. Adrenal suppression is likely to occur if a dose exceeding 10mgs/day of Prednisolone has been taken for longer than 3 months.[1] The function of the adrenal cortex may be suppressed if a patient has been taking daily systemic corticosteroids in excess of 5mgs/day for more than 1 month in the past year.

Although it is unlikely that routine outpatient day care dentistry is sufficiently stressful to cause an adrenal crisis, it is recommended that you consider steroid cover and monitoring of the patient's blood pressure for any signs of incipient or developing adrenal insufficiency and to intervene promptly if a crisis begins to develop.

Intravenous sedation and general anaesthesia are particularly risky and you must avoid unnecessary haemorrhage and hypotension as well as being vigilant to prevent hypoxia. One further risk is that of pathological fracturing of the dento-facial skeletal structures as corticosteroid treatment does result in osteoporosis.

Any dental patient who has Addison's disease should have an emergency injection kit containing 100mgs Hydrocortisone to be injected intramuscularly in the event of a crisis. In an emergency, a dental patient who has Addison's disease may experience the following symptoms:

Muscle weakness, tremor, a rapid drop in blood pressure, mental confusion and loss of consciousness.

If your patient vomits more than once during a crisis, then extra steroid medication is urgently needed. As a member of the dental team, even though the Hydrocortisone 100mgs IM, is not part of your medical emergency drug box, you must be prepared to assist your patient if they need help in administering their medication as their life may now depend on it.

In any event, the **A B C D E** and **MOVE** protocols must be followed for this emergency as they are for others.

References for adrenal insufficiency and crisis

1. Scully C. Chapter 6: Endocrinology. Adrenal Cortex. in Medical Problems in Dentistry 6th Edition. pp 148-149. Edinburgh. Churchill Livingstone. 2010.

2. National Health Service. NHS Choices Website. Addison's Disease Treatment. Online Available from: http://www.nhs.uk/Conditions/Addisons-disease/Pages/Treatment.aspx
[Accessed January 2015].

3. Thomason JM, Girdler NM, Kendall-Taylor P, Wastell H, Weddel A, Seymour RA An investigation into the need for supplementary steroids in organ transplant patients undergoing gingival surgery. A double-blind, split-mouth, cross-over study. J Clin Periodontol. 1999 Sep; 26(9):577-82.

4. Greenwood M. Medical Emergencies in Dental Practice. Management of specific medical emergencies. 2009. Dental Update. Jun. 36 (5) 262-264. 266-268.

5. UK Resuscitation Council. Medical Emergencies and Resuscitation Standards for Clinical Practice and Training for Dental Practitioners and Dental Care Practitioners in General Dental Practice. – A statement from the Resuscitation Council (UK) July 2006. Revision 2008.

7

Hypoglycaemia and diabetic collapse

As we progress through the medical conditions, you will have noticed their increasing complexity; not only in their origins, but also in their treatments too. Despite this, the measures and management strategies we must follow to prevent a medical emergency from developing do need to be kept as simple as possible and such an approach applies to the next medical emergency we will look at.

With Hypoglycaemia and Diabetic Collapse, it is critically important that we know and recognize the clinical signs identifying these medical emergencies and the symptoms distinguishing them from the preceding conditions of Adrenal Insufficiency and Crisis. In those conditions, hypoglycaemia is only one of many clinical signs following from an adrenal endocrine imbalance, whereas in diabetes, hypoglycaemia is the direct result of the pancreatic endocrine imbalance itself.

In the previous section on Adrenal Insufficiency and Crisis, suppression in the function of the adrenal cortex most commonly resulted from systemic corticosteroid use, occasionally from acquired adrenal disease or very rarely from a congenital defect in the biochemical pathways that produce the hormones of the adrenal cortex.

Despite some quite different causes, the clinical features of Adrenal insufficiency and Diabetes can be similar with hypotension and hypoglycaemia being seen[1]. In contrast, if there is adrenocortical hyperfunction, either Cushing's disease or Cushing's syndrome can be seen:

i. The former (Cushing's disease) is caused by an increase in Adrenocorticotrophic hormone (ACTH) released from the anterior pituitary gland or from a tumour.
ii. Whereas the latter (Cushing's syndrome) often does not have an ACTH derived stimulus and hyperglycaemia is also seen[2,3].

Just to clarify one important point, in those patients taking long-term corticosteroids, hyperglycaemia may also arise: This may be due to insulin resistance precipitating diabetes.

In such cases this is: Non Insulin Dependent Steroid Induced Diabetes: **NOSID** rather than an opportunistic unmasking effect of an underlying diabetic susceptibility[4,5].

The diabetic collapse caused by hypoglycaemia

In this medical emergency as with the previous five emergencies, an up to date medical history is vital.

This will reveal if the patient is diabetic, the type of diabetes the patient has and the degree of control both they and their medical practitioner (or endocrinologist) have over their condition.

There are several forms of diabetes, it is important to know the specific form of diabetes our patient has. Broadly, when dealing with a diabetic patient we can classify their condition as follows:

Form of Diabetes	Type of Diabetes	Clinical Features in the Diabetes	Abbreviation
Primary Diabetes	Type 1 Diabetes	Child Onset. Insulin Dependent Diabetes Mellitus	IDDM
	Type 1 ½ Diabetes	Latent Autoimmune Diabetes in Adults	LADA
	Type 2 Diabetes	Adult Onset Non Insulin Dependent Diabetes Mellitus	NIDDM
	Type 2 ½ Diabetes	Maturity Onset Diabetes in the Young	MODY
Secondary Diabetes	Pregnancy Diabetes	2nd or 3rd Trimester Insulin resistant	
	Endocrine Diabetes	Associated with Cushings Syndrome.	
	Iatrogenic Diabetes	Non Insulin Dependent Steroid Induced Diabetes	NOSID.

We think it is helpful to classify diabetes in this way, broadly into two forms with four primary and three secondary types. Please note, although the types 1 and 2 and 1 ½ diabetes are recognized clinical entities, the type 2 ½ diabetes is labelled as such in this context for convenience only. Until there is a consensus on the classification of the range of conditions spanning the diabetic spectrum, please refer to this form as **MODY**.

Prevention of the hypoglycaemic collapse

It is important to gain an accurate and up to date medical history from your patient. Specifically, if there is a history of hypoglycaemic episodes or evidence of wide variations in their blood glucose levels. Almost all **IDDM** patients have access to accurate glucose measuring equipment. If there is proof of hypoglycaemia or poor diabetic control, then the risk of diabetic collapse is increased. Diabetic patients with these problems should be the first to be treated in any clinical session and not kept waiting. You must ensure and verify their medication has been taken and they have eaten adequately before you begin any treatment.

It should be borne in mind that even if your patient's diabetes is well controlled, trauma, stress and dento-facial infections can impact on how they balance their health against disease. In the spectrum of diabetic problems, in dental practice, you are more likely to come across complications from hypoglycaemia, rather than from hyperglycaemia.

i. The former has an acute and striking presentation.
ii. Whereas the latter displays a slower course over many hours with reduced levels of consciousness eventually being seen.

Unconsciousness is rarely observed with a hyperglycaemic coma. If a diabetic patient is unconscious, you must assume it is from hypoglycaemia. Before this state of affairs is reached, the following clinical signs are seen:

The clinical signs of hypoglycaemia

I. The patient may not have eaten, being hungry, irritable with tremors, and trembling.
II. Their speech may be garbled, slurred or incoherent.
III. Sweating, pallor or a loss of colour is seen.
IV. The pulse will be rapid and bounding in response to adrenaline release.
V. A lowered level of consciousness is seen with seizures and convulsions.

Collapse and loss of consciousness will result if you do not intervene.

Clinical Symptoms of Hypoglycaemia:

I. Hypoglycaemic patients complain of:
II. Headache
III. Hunger
IV. Heat
V. Hands with pins and needles.

Treatment of hypoglycaemia in the conscious patient:

1. An **AVPU** and **NEWS** assessment must be undertaken and the patient is laid flat. If they are still conscious, then help must be summoned and the patient is given glucose orally, either in gel form, or sugar or a drink.
2. The **A B C, D** and **E** approach that you apply to any of the previous medical emergencies is also applied to a conscious diabetic patient in your care who presents with any difficulties.

That is you must secure the patient's:

> **I. Airway**: Loosen any clothes or surgical aprons from around their neck.
>
> **II. Breathing**: Make sure the patient can breathe and is comfortable.
>
> **III. Circulation**: Check their wrist pulse.

3. The diabetic patient who is conscious and has been given glucose must be monitored every two to three minutes with a note being made of their **AVPU,** and their **NEWS**. If the patient has a blood glucose monitor, this could be useful to determine their blood glucose levels.

4. However, do not rely wholly on the patient's blood glucose monitor, better still if you have a certified recently calibrated one in the dental clinic: **Then use it NOW.**

5. Note and document the patient's blood glucose level.

6. If the patient's blood glucose level drops below 3.0 mmol/L and they are not responding, despite you giving oral glucose, then you must consider repeating the oral dose of glucose every few minutes and do so <u>again and again,</u> until assistance arrives.

7. Before doing anything else, even if the patient is still conscious you must be prepared to summon help from an emergency medical first responder *ie* dial 999 or 911.

8. Be prepared to use Oxygen at 15 litres per minute and collect the Glucagon from the emergency medical drug box

Treatment of hypoglycaemia in the unconscious patient:

1. Before your patient loses consciousness, you and/or your colleague will already have drawn up the sterile water injecting 1ml of this into the vial containing 1mg of powdered Glucagon.

2. If the patient becomes completely unresponsive losing consciousness, summon help and administer the Glucagon NOW.

3. Unless you are particularly gifted; being skilled at dealing with simultaneous emergencies in one patient:

> **DO NOT ATTEMPT TO GIVE ANY**
> **MORE GLUCOSE BY MOUTH.**

(Please refer to the FBAO Medical Emergency for the reasons not to give a semi-conscious patient anything by mouth!!)

4. Attach a Green Needle (21 Gauge 0.8mm dia.) to a fresh 1ml syringe then inject the Glucagon solution intramuscularly into the outer thigh muscle of the unconscious patient.

5. It will take some 5 to 10 minutes for the patient to regain consciousness, continue to monitor their AVPU and NEWS.

6. At this stage be prepared to hand over the patient to the medical emergency responders with any relevant clinical data from the patient's medical history and the incident itself which will assist with the hospital care of the patient.

Throughout your management of the hypoglycaemic diabetic collapse continue to **MOVE** your patient, that is:

> I. **Monitor** the patient's AVPU and NEWS. Check their **A B C** repeating every 2 to 3 minutes.
>
> II. **Oxygen** at 15 litres per minute is given to a clear Airway. Secure and clear the Airway.
>
> III. **Verify** that an ambulance has been called and help is coming. Be prepared for handover.
>
> IV. **Emergency Actions** Lay the patient flat maintain A B C and ensure their safety and security.

If you can act promptly and properly then hypoglycaemia and diabetic collapse can be avoided in the dental surgery. If it should happen and you don't have to resort to use of Glucagon, then the patient must be accompanied home, the incident documented and the patient's general medical practitioner must be informed of the event.

The diabetic collapse caused by hyperglycaemia

The hyperglycaemic collapse is a much rarer event with a slower onset than hypoglycaemia, perhaps taking place over many days. Most, if not all medical emergency training for dental practice deals with hypoglycaemia, however we must be aware of the possibility that hyperglycaemia is occurring, especially in a paediatric patient where there may be MODY or IDDM.

In addition to the clinical signs being different, there will be dry skin, a weak pulse and classically and worryingly in children: an osmotic diuresis with polyuria resulting in dehydration.

The hyperglycaemic collapse is a medical emergency demanding an urgent hospital admission. The main differences between hypoglycaemia and hyperglycaemia are detailed below:

A comparison of hypoglycaemia and hyperglycaemia

Hypoglycaemic collapse	Hyperglycaemic collapse
The patient often has a medical history with diabetes being noted.	There is often no previous medical history, especially in children or diabetes of the new born.
Alcohol, Insulin, Exercise, Stress, Infection and Starvation are causative.	Limited Insulin, Infection or Heart Attack are causative.
Clinical signs of rapid pulse, sweating dilated pupils muscle tremors, fitting and facial muscle twitching are indicative	Ketones in the breath, sweat and urine, dry skin, dry mouth and hypotension are indicative.
Rapid descent into unconsciousness. Treat with Glucagon in Dental Practice, then refer to hospital for follow up care and observation.	Slow descent into unconsciousness and Ketoacidotic coma. Urgent Emergency Referral needed. Hospital treatment by IV rehydration with Insulin.

The patient who presents with hyperglycaemia must be urgently referred to an accident and emergency unit where rapid IV rehydration, correction of electrolyte imbalance and potassium loss, together with insulin is given.

Further notes to hypoglycaemia and diabetic collapse

Diabetes is an extremely common condition. It affects some 3% to 4% of the UK population, with Type 2 diabetes accounting for some 80% to 90% of all known cases, however only 75% of those with diabetes have been diagnosed[2]. The prevalence of people with diabetes is currently rising, possibly in response to two factors[8]:

I.   Life style: More children and more adolescents are becoming overweight.
II. Family History: More incidental diagnoses of diabetes are being made on hospital attendance, when presenting with conditions related to diabetes.

Although we have focussed on the acute complications of diabetes, specifically: hypoglycaemia, with regard to chronic conditions related to diabetes, it is a major cause of disability and death.

Complications of Chronic Hyperglycaemia

I.   Microvascular complications such as retinopathy and nephropathy.
II. Macrovascular complications such as atherosclerosis resulting in poor distal circulation causing ischaemia and gangrene in the toes. Poor proximal circulation resulting in Ischaemic Heart Disease.

Another rare but notable example is swelling of the major salivary glands from diabetic autoimmune neuropathy, perhaps involving the Cranial Nerves. If and when a healthy patient of yours presents with symptoms of a burning mouth, if no other cause can be found, then referral to an endocrinologist may reveal diabetes.

If not causative, then diabetes would certainly be an incidental but important finding for you to make on behalf of your patient. From your patient's medical histories, you will be able to document almost all of the risk factors for diabetes. These are:

I.   Family history: the risk rises if a close relative has diabetes.
II. Lack of exercise: obesity is often present with an increase risk of diabetes developing.
III. Age: the risk increases if your patient is over 45 years old.
IV. Race: Type I diabetes is more common in Caucasians. Type 2 diabetes is more common in Africans and Asians.

Although there are no conditions specifically associated with diabetes, there are some clinical signs which, if present, should alert you to your patient being at risk of diabetes or, if already diagnosed with this condition, then being at risk from further complications from it. These are:

I.   Periodontal disease, the diabetic patient is susceptible to more severe periodontal disease that might cause an imbalance in their diabetic control.
II. Oral presentations of candidosis and angular stomatitis are seen.
III. Uncontrollable dento-facial infections with spread through the fascial spaces.

From the above, you can see many quite serious complications are associated with diabetes. In an emergency the acute complications from hypoglycaemia can be prevented by properly planning your procedure. Your patient's food intake pattern must not interrupted; with adequate carbohydrates being consumed beforehand.

i. A well-controlled diabetic should tolerate routine out-patient day care treatment.
ii. A poorly controlled diabetic will not and may require in-patient specialist supervision.

In diabetes as with all medical emergencies, as noted in the introduction to this emergency:

Simple prevention is preferable to complex intervention.

Point of care glucose monitoring is possible, but only with a device that is both approved and calibrated and you have been trained to use. Most if not all Type 1 diabetics have such devices. Should you refer to data from such a device when treating your patient the key points are:

I. Avoid hypoglycaemia keeping blood glucose levels at the correct level but avoid hyperglycaemia that can delay wound healing.
II. For surgical procedures blood glucose should be between 3 and 5 mmol/L.
III. If blood glucose is lower than 5mmol/L then consider giving the patient carbohydrates before you begin a procedure.

Drug interactions may precipitate a diabetic collapse or enhance diabetic complications and you must be aware of the following interactions:

I. Corticosteroids may increase blood glucose by increasing insulin resistance.
II. Conversely some dental antibiotics: Tetracycline and Doxycycline can cause hypoglycaemia.

III. Use Amoxycillin or Metronidazole as your first choice, but only where necessary and not as a substitute for: (where indicated) extraction, incision or drainage.

IV. NSAIDS can interact with aspirin that many diabetics take, causing GI tract bleeding. Caution is urged in their use.

V. Local Anaesthetic (LA) either with or without adrenaline is safe, the risk of hyperglycaemia being at the least: theoretical from using LA containing adrenaline.

VI. With dental sedation, Relative Analgesia (RA) should be promoted in preference to Intravenous (IV) sedation (due to no food being taken pre-operatively with IV sedation). However, a well-controlled diabetic should be able to tolerate IV sedation.

With the above firmly in mind you should be able to safely treat your diabetic patients and avoid the potential for hypoglycaemia and diabetic collapse and the medical complications from occurring.

References to hypoglycaemia and diabetic collapse

1. Guignat L, Bertherat J. Cushing syndrome: When to suspect and how to confirm? Presse Med. 2014 Apr; 43 (4 Pt 1):366-75.

2. Scully C. Chapter 6: Endocrinology. Pancreas. in Medical Problems in Dentistry 6th Edition. pp 138-139. Edinburgh. Churchill Livingstone. 2010

3. Ericson-Neilsen W, Kaye AD. Steroids: Pharmacology, Complications, and Practice Delivery Issues. The Ochsner Journal 2014;14(2):203-207.

4. Stewart PM, Krone NP. The adrenal cortex. In: Melmed S, Polonsky K, Larsen PR, Kronenberg H, editors. Williams Textbook of Endocrinology. 12th ed. Philadelphia, PA: Saunders. 2011.

5. Simmons LR, Molyneaux L, Yue DK, Chua EL. Steroid-Induced Diabetes: Is It Just Unmasking of Type 2 Diabetes? ISRN Endocrinology 2012; 2012:910905. doi:10.5402/2012/910905
   Available online from: http://www.ncbi.nlm.nih.gov/pmc/articles/PMC3398625/
   [Accessed February 2016]

6. Chandu A, Macisaac RJ, Smith AC, Bach LA. Diabetic ketoacidosis secondary to dento-alveolar infection Int J Oral Maxillofac Surg. 2002 Feb; 31(1): 57-9.

7. Newton CA, Raskin P. Diabetic ketoacidosis in type 1 and type 2 diabetes mellitus: clinical and biochemical differences. Arch Intern Med. 2004 Sep 27; 164(17): 1925-31.

8. National Health Service. NHS Choices web site Diabetes.
   Online Available from: http://www.nhs.uk/conditions/diabetes/pages/diabetes.aspx
   [Accessed February 2016]

8

Epilepsy

Moving on from the previous two endocrine-based medical emergencies to one with a neurological basis, some of the clinical signs of epilepsy may resemble those signs we have noted in hypoglycaemic collapse, adrenal crises or vaso-vagal syncope.

However, as similar as the initial signs may appear and as familiar as the symptoms the patient complains of may seem to you, it is important that you are able to make an immediate and accurate assessment of the problem facing your patient.

In addition to correctly diagnosing an epileptic fit or seizure, your ability to do so will permit your prompt and proper management of their medical emergency, removing or reducing the risk of further complications arising from this condition.

An up to date medical history from your patient must be available. This will confirm whether they have epilepsy. Not only should this be to hand, but further data on; the type of epilepsy and the effectiveness of any medication must also be present in this medical history.

Several potential causes of seizure may resemble an epileptic fit. These can be:

I. Stroke or Transient Ischaemic Attack. (TIA)
II. Panic Attack and hyperventilation leading to respiratory alkalosis.
III. Diabetic Collapse, either hypoglycaemic or hyperglycaemic.
IV. Cerebral Hypoxia.
V. Recreational drug use, especially cocaine, opioids, or any one of the hallucinogenic drugs, either naturally occurring or artificially produced.

In taking a medical history, it is important to gain as much information as possible from your patient and not limit your data down to merely clinical criteria, the possibility of your patient taking recreational drugs <u>must be sensitively explored</u>, as these can provide a triggering action leading to the initiation of epileptic seizures. Other triggers of a seizure that your dental patient may encounter in addition to drugs from prescription or recreation are: Anxiety and deprivation of sleep and food.

The Signs and Symptoms of an Epileptic Seizure

The signals your patient is about to have an epileptic seizure are:

I. Lowered level of consciousness with lowered responsiveness.
II. The patient may have an aura or premonition that a seizure is forthcoming.
III. There will be loss of consciousness.
IV. The tonic phase is seen the patient becomes rigid and if not seated may fall down.
V. The clonic phase follows with the patient having jerking movements of the limbs.
VI. The tongue may be bitten; teeth, dentures or other dental work may be damaged.
VII. There will be excess salivation, noticeable drooling, frothing or foaming of saliva.
VIII. Urinary incontinence is also seen.

The initial treatment of a patient with an epileptic seizure

It is important that you **do not** attempt to physically restrain a patient in the grip of a seizure. In addition to being extremely unsafe, with a risk of trauma to the patient and yourself, such an approach would be a waste of your time and a further needless waste of the patient's energies. Nevertheless, you must support and if possible, protect the patient to ensure they do not incur serious injuries by striking anything with their head or limbs.

It would be quite pointless to attempt to monitor the patient with either an **AVPU** grading or **NEWS** during a seizure.

It should be clear that an epileptic seizure is in progress. After a few minutes, of progression, the seizure will abate and then you will be able to monitor the patient's **NEWS** and **AVPU** as they regain their full faculties.

Post Ictal Confusion

In a simple solitary seizure, the patient will slowly regain consciousness; they may be in a state of post ictal confusion that can last for several minutes. In addition to this confusion, they may be quite alarmed or in our clinical experience; often somewhat embarrassed as it dawns on them what has just happened.

At this point, you must be prepared deal with another seizure, should one occur. If not, then your warm, empathic and supportive clinical manner is crucial and you must display such professional attributes to support your patient as they recover.

Be prepared to deal with the socially stigmatizing consequences if the patient has suffered either urinary or other incontinence in your clinic.

<u>As a health care professional, both you and other members of the dental team must be able to sensitively and skilfully deal with this.</u>

The patient who has just suffered an epileptic seizure should be monitored and accompanied home. Once there, they must be placed in the care of a responsible person, with the episode being documented and the patient's medical practitioner being notified.

Status Epilepticus

If after a solitary seizure, if the patient enters into another one, there are a series of seizures, or an extended seizure lasting more than 5 minutes occurs, then a medical emergency is taking place. This is status epilepticus. This condition has been noted to be particularly dangerous, with a mortality rate of one in five patients in this state.[1]

With this medical emergency as before, the **A B C** approach must be adopted to safeguard the patient. During the tonic phase of the seizure, with extreme extension of the neck and head, the patient's airway may become narrowed. Although you should not attempt restraint, measures to support the patient's head and secure the airway should be made.

After the tonic phase, the clonic phase will follow. There will be uncontrollable repetitive muscular spasticity. During this period, the patient may show excessive saliva flow, together with vomiting and these may present a choking hazard.

The continued treatment of the patient suffering an epileptic seizure

You must be prepared to deal with this risk, keeping the patient's airway clear by using high volume suction.

Oxygen should be delivered at 15 litres per minute via a bag-valve-mask and administration of Midazolam via the buccal sulcus must be attempted, when the clonic phase has abated somewhat.

The Midazolam contained in the dental practice emergency drug box should be used. The following age dependent doses must be administered onto the patient's buccal sulcus mucosa:

Age of patient in status epilepticus	Dose of Midazolam to be placed in Buccal Sulcus
Adult over 10 years old	10mgs ie 1ml
Child 5 to 10 years old	7.5mgs ie 0.75ml
Child under 5 years old	5mgs ie 0.5ml

If you have to use Midazolam for a patient in status epilepticus, your dental team colleagues will already have summoned the medical emergency first responders advising them of the nature of the medical emergency. You should be prepared for the handover of the patient upon their arrival to give any necessary supporting data to them.

With prolonged or recurrent seizures, the emergency medical responders may administer Diazepam intravenously. This is rapidly effective in stopping any seizure. It has been noted that the buccal route of administering midazolam is not as effective as IV Diazepam in stopping a seizure.[2].

Essential further actions

Until the medical emergency first responders arrive, you must monitor if possible, the patient's **AVPU** and **NEWS**, documenting these for hand-over.

The MOVE protocol for fitting and convulsions should be used:

I.   **Monitor** the patient safeguarding their Airway Breathing and Circulation

II. **Oxygen** at 15 litres/minute must be given through the bag-valve-mask

III. **Verify** that the medical emergency responders are aware and will arrive.

IV. **Essential** actions are to prevent further injury to the patient by placing them in the recovery position and continue to protect their airway.

In addition to the management of the status epilepticus, you should be prepared to deal with associated traumatic injuries, the patient may have bitten their tongue or lip, or as mentioned previously, there may be damage to their dentition, dentures, crown or bridge work.

The episode should be fully documented including any injuries and possible triggers or causative factors that should be noted and avoided in future.

Further notes to epilepsy

Epilepsy is one of the most common and widespread of all the neurological disorders with current publications stating an estimated 1% of the adult population have this condition.[1,3.] Of specific interest and importance, there is an increased prevalence of epilepsy in countries where resources to treat and control the condition are limited. In those countries, some 90% of people with epilepsy have not received treatment for their condition. This fact is of relevance for the dental professional working in any resource-limited environment, irrespective of the country or community where dentistry is practiced. In such circumstances, it is important to be able to co-ordinate care with medical specialists, so the dental patient at risk from an epileptic seizure can be treated promptly and properly, should a medical emergency occur.

In countries where resources are less limited, some accurate figures on the prevalence of epilepsy are available. In the European Union, epilepsy shows a prevalence of 4.3 to 7.8 /1,000 population, with the condition now costing in excess of 15.5 Billion Euros in terms of its overall impact.[4]. Perhaps the most interesting point being the cost to treat epilepsy actually plays a small part in the total budget for epilepsy care, a budget that costs every European citizen some 33 Euros per year. Most of the cost arises from the non-clinical complications that epilepsy brings to the patient, practitioner and the public, in terms of disability and adjustments to their living and working conditions.

Mortality rates in epileptic patients are 2x to 3x higher than the general population.[5] Patients with physical and mental disabilities are also more likely to have epilepsy and even more likely to succumb to the Sudden Unexpected Death in Epilepsy syndrome (SUDEP) which is the most likely cause of death in epileptic patients[6]. These patients are more likely to die prematurely than your other dental patients in the general population.

By taking an accurate and up to date medical history, we can safely treat patients with epilepsy in dental practice and reduce the risk of seizure, with the associated morbidity and mortality. This approach if coordinated as part of a multidisciplinary framework would be beneficial in reducing the mortality associated with SUDEP in our dental patients who are intellectually disabled.

There are some common age related causes of epilepsy and these are summarised in the table below. The condition is most prevalent in the young patient between the ages of 5 and 20 who may present with additional mental and physical disabilities as previously mentioned. There may be triggering factors initiating the epilepsy, but in many cases, there are no identifiable causes. With reference to dental practice, an epileptic patient who is anxious, who has neither slept nor eaten in nervous anticipation of their dental visit, is more likely to succumb to a seizure, than your dental patient who is relaxed and confident in your abilities to treat them.

Your abilities to both effectively and empathically communicate your concerns, while at the same time demonstrating your professionalism, are perhaps just as important as the anti-epileptic drugs the patient takes to prevent a seizure from occurring in the first place.

The age of onset and triggers for epilepsy

Age of patient	Commonly noted initiators of epilepsy
Paediatric	Genetic syndrome, Congenital condition, Intra-uterine or Post partum trauma; hypoxia, childhood illness such as Febrile convulsions or Diabetes (IDDM) or infection such as Meningitis.
Adolescent	Acquired infection, Metabolic or Physiological disorder, Brain injury following physical trauma
Young adult	Injury following physical trauma, drug or alcohol abuse, HIV associated infection
Adult	Brain tumour HIV or AIDS associated lesions, drug or alcohol abuse
Geriatric	Disturbances of cerebro-vascular function following from brain tumour or strokes. Pathological advances of the dementing processes, or age related changed in brain form and function

There are other patients who may display the clinical signs of seizure but do not have epilepsy. In those cases, it is important to identify the causes of the seizure, to treat these conditions accordingly, and not to assume, by default, that every seizure in every patient is caused by the abnormal cortical cerebral electrical activity of epilepsy.

Noted causes of non-epileptic seizure may be panic attacks, the transient ischaemic attack and hypoglycaemia. In these cases, if you or a colleague witness such a seizure in your patient who has no history of epilepsy, it is important not only to go through the emergency medical management procedures as above, but to refer the patient for the necessary specialist investigations to determine the precise cause of their seizure.

In these cases, investigations are undertaken to identify specific disease markers arising from infection of the brain, diabetes, liver or kidney disease, alcohol or drug use as being the reason for a non-epileptic seizure being reported.[1,7,8].

Classification of epilepsy

While managing a medical emergency caused by an epileptic seizure, it is of limited value or no practical use, to suddenly stop assisting the patient while attempting to learn of the precise form of epilepsy your patient is now (involuntarily) demonstrating to you.

However, if a patient indicates in their medical history they are epileptic, you must make inquiries into the nature of the epilepsy they have, how well controlled it is, what medication is being used for control and for how long (if at all) they have been fit-free.

In having such knowledge to hand, you will be better prepared to prevent a seizure by removing the potential triggering factors, to recognize the signs indicating an epileptic seizure is about to occur and not risk confusing such important signs with those belonging to another medical emergency.

There are several classifications of epilepsy, the 2013 Commission Report from the International League Against Epilepsy (ILAE) made no significant departures from the already established 1989 classification of epilepsy.[9]

That classification of epilepsy being:

I. Localized, originating from one part of the brain.

II. Generalized, originating from multiple parts of the brain.

III. Undetermined origin being either localized or generalized.

IV. Associated with syndromic involvement.

V. Epilepsy may be associated with clinical signs of memory loss, confusion or headache.

VI. Rarely: Generalised seizures are seen with rapid loss of consciousness.

VII. Commonly: Partial seizures are seen with a lowered but not a total loss of consciousness.

With respect to the patient's control of epilepsy, it has been documented that non-adherence to their Anti Epileptic Drugs (also known as AED!) regimen is an ongoing area of concern. This non-compliance is a major risk factor with epilepsy associated mortality.[10] In addition to such non-compliance, in the patient with epilepsy, the dental practitioner may have a role to play too. There are a number of potential drug interactions from routinely prescribed dental medications. While these may not result in a greater risk of seizure from lowered anticonvulsant efficacy, the converse is often seen. Sodium -Valproate, Phenytoin and Carbamazepine may all induce an excessive bleeding tendency if the patient is prescribed aspirins, antifungals or antimicrobials.

IV sedation using midazolam is quite safe, RA sedation with nitrous oxide is also routinely used but there may be an additional cerebral CNS depression if the patient is taking anticonvulsant medication.

Lastly, patients with epilepsy may sometimes have antisocial or psychopathic behaviour patterns making them quite challenging to treat, even in the absence of a seizure. In children with febrile convulsions, which are not in themselves caused by or related to epilepsy, some 3% subsequently go on to develop epilepsy in later life.

This is very sadly due to brain damage from the childhood illness, in many cases this being viral meningitis.

References to Epilepsy

1. Scully C. Chapter 13: Neurology. Epilepsy. in Medical Problems in Dentistry 6th Edition. pp 344-346. Edinburgh. Churchill Livingstone. 2010

2. UK Resuscitation Council. Medical emergencies and resuscitation. Standards for clinical practice and training for dental practitioners and dental care professionals in general dental practice. December 2012. Online available from: http://www.resus.org.uk/pages/MEdental.pdf [Accessed February 2015]

3. Caraballo R, Fejerman N Management of epilepsy in resource-limited settings Epileptic Disord. 2015 Jan 30. (In press.)

4. Pugliatti M, Beghi E, Forsgren L, Ekman M, Sobocki P Estimating the cost of epilepsy in Europe: a review with economic modeling. Epilepsia. 2007 Dec; 48 (12):2224-33.

5. Johnston A, Smith P Sudden unexpected death in epilepsy. Expert. Rev. Neurother. 2007 Dec; 7(12):1751-61.

6. Kiani R, Tyrer F, Jesu A, Bhaumik S, Gangavati S, Walker G, Kazmi S, Barrett M Mortality from sudden unexpected death in epilepsy (SUDEP) in a cohort of adults with intellectual disability. J Intellect Disabil Res. 2014 Jun;58 (6):508-20

7. D'Ambrosio R, Miller JW. What Is an Epileptic Seizure? Unifying Definitions in Clinical Practice and Animal Research to Develop Novel Treatments. Epilepsy Currents 2010;10(3):61-66.

8. Martiniskova Z, Kollar B, Vachalova I, Klobucnikova K, Waczulikova I, Goldenberg Z Solitary epileptic seizures in the clinical practice. Part I: etiological factors responsible for their occurrence. Neuro Endocrinol Lett. 2009; 30(4):482-6.

9   International League Against Epilepsy. Commission on Classification and Terminology. Commission Annual Report 2013. Online Available from: http://www.ilae.org/Commission/Class/reports.cfm [Accessed February 2015]

10. Lathers CM, Koehler SA, Wecht CH, Schraeder PL Forensic antiepileptic drug levels in autopsy cases of epilepsy. Epilepsy Behav. 2011 Dec;22(4):778-85.

9

Chest Pains

In your patient's medical notes, if there is history of heart disease or their family have a history of heart disease, when they complain of chest pain, there is a fair chance that such pain is of cardiac origin.

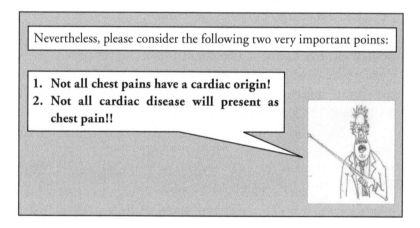

Nevertheless, please consider the following two very important points:

1. Not all chest pains have a cardiac origin!
2. Not all cardiac disease will present as chest pain!!

In addition to the symptoms of chest pain, we have to recognize all of the patient's clinical signs, so we can arrive at a firm conclusion about the nature of the problem or the potential medical emergency we are now facing.

In addition to the medical history, the patient's medication history is extremely important in your ability to come to a definitive diagnosis. If the patient is taking medication to control a cardiac condition and they complain of chest pains, then you might be inclined to draw the obvious conclusion, declare a medical emergency and manage the patient accordingly.

In particular, if the patient is taking medication such as glyceryl trinitrate (GTN) to control angina, this is usually carried with them and can be used to treat their problem. Failing this, the dental practice emergency drug box has GTN spray that should be used, together with oxygen as you monitor their **NEWS**, their **AVPU**, then summon help as necessary.

In this section, we will look at the medical emergencies arising from cardiac problems, beginning with simple and stable angina and working through unstable angina, building our revision of this subject. We will finish the section with the management of the myocardial infarct and the resuscitation protocols to be followed, both with and without the use of an Automatic External Defibrillator: the AED.

Angina Pectoris

Angina pectoris (usually referred to simply as: angina) is the name given to chest pains caused when the oxygen demands of the heart muscle (the myocardium) exceed their blood supply from the coronary arteries.

This condition develops due to the arteries supplying the myocardium narrowing or being blocked, either commonly through atheroma because of Coronary Artery Disease (CAD) or rarely through spasm in the smooth muscle cells of the arterial walls.

As a result of this, some 1% of adults will have myocardial ischaemia. In addition to the risk factors listed below, the prevalence of this condition rises with increasing age of the patient.[1]

Preventable Risk Factors for Coronary Artery Disease.
I.   Smoking
II.   Poor Diet
III. Excess Alcohol intake
IV. Lack of exercise
V.   A stressful environment: both at work and at home.

Inevitable Risk Factors for Coronary Artery Disease
I.   Congenital defects of the heart. eg: Stenosis, Shunts and Septal Defects.
II.   Family history
III. Physiology favouring increased Low Density Lipoprotein metabolism
IV. Type A Personality
V.   Ethnicity in conjunction with socioeconomic background and geographical location

In the industrialised countries of UK, Europe and North America some 45% of young adult males have atheromatous plaques with 20% showing signs of ischaemic heart disease. This condition accounts for 35% of the total mortality in the UK and the USA[1.] These atheromatous plaques are often seen post-mortem as lipid accumulations, together with deposits of inflammatory residues and cholesterol crystallised onto the inner surface of arterial walls. Thromboses or clots frequently break away from well developed atheromatous plaques. Such emboli result in strokes, the cerebrovascular accidents with associated degenerative conditions. Angina, coronary insufficiency and myocardical infarctions being other common sequalae.

The reduction in blood flow to the heart muscle will lessen both its functional efficiency together with its ability to withstand any physiological or pathological stresses placed upon it. A reduction in blood supply to the heart will result in lower levels of oxygen perfusion to the myocardium and so the heart becomes susceptible to the onset of degenerative disease processes. Coronary ischaemia often eventually results in myocardial infarction.

Ischaemia of the heart muscles is most commonly seen following coronary artery disease. The severity and outlook for the patient with this condition depends on the degree of arterial narrowing or extent of blockage of the coronary arteries. The mortality rate from angina is in the region of 4% per year.[1] Complete blockage of a coronary artery or arteries causes the myocardial infarct: the heart attack.

Many patients go through life and then suffer a heart attack with no previous family or personal history. In other patients, in those for whom cardiac disease has been diagnosed, their symptoms and signs are so well controlled, that only your vigilance and adherence to both updating, then actively looking into their medical and medication histories reveals the true extent of the cardiac illness your patient both lives with and brings with them into your dental clinic.

In other patients with coronary artery disease, the most common symptom is the chest pain of angina.

The two common forms of angina:

I.   **Stable angina.** This form is seen only if the patient experiences physical stress from exertion or is placed under emotional or psychological stress arising from fear or anxiety. The dentally phobic patient with CAD is especially susceptible while in your care. Reassurance, monitoring and treatment with the patient's GTN being sprayed sublingually will all be necessary to alleviate their symptoms. This form of angina is not an immediate medical emergency and the symptoms will abate on rest. Stable angina is a sign of insufficient blood supply to the heart and a warning of possible future problems.

II. **Unstable angina.** This is also known as the Acute Coronary Syndrome, the onset is indeed acute, with the symptoms rapidly increasing in severity. In contrast to stable angina, this is a medical emergency, due to the coronary blood supply being reduced to a critical level even when the patient is resting. Although the blockage might be only momentary, it could immediately lead to further complications including myocardial infarction.

The three uncommon forms of angina:

I.   **Decubitus angina**. This form presents only when the patient is lying down, eg; prone in the dental chair.

II. **Vaso-spastic angina**. This form results from the release of catecholamines (adrenaline and nor adrenaline) causing:
   i.   An increase in heart rate and force of contraction,
   ii. With narrowing of arterial walls,
   iii. Both resulting in a rapid increase in blood pressure.
        The symptoms of angina, usually follow this triad of physiological responses.

III. **Cardiac syndrome X angina.** In this rare syndrome, the gross anatomy of the heart and its blood supply are normal, however the microanatomy and capillary circulation are not. Ultimately blood flow to the heart muscles is inadequate and angina will be both seen and felt.

Although all five forms of angina should be considered, in a medical emergency involving chest pains, we should perhaps restrict our initial considerations to whether the angina is either:

I.   **Stable angina** and we can manage the patient, with sublingual GTN, reassurance and empathic support
     or:

II. **Unstable angina** and we then declare a medical emergency, stabilise the patient, use GTN and Oxygen, support the patient as above and summon the medical emergency responders.

The clinical symptoms and signs of angina:

I.   The patient will complain of a tight band of pain across their chest.

II. This pain is described as crushing and tight and will be <u>longer than 30 seconds</u> in duration, *i.e:* it is neither a fleeting nor a momentary pain.

III. There will be the classic radiation of pain to the arm and jaw.

IV. Usually the left arm and mandible are involved but the right side can be involved too.

V.   Nausea, sweating and pallor are seen. The patient appears fearful and alarmed about what is happening to them (often stated to be: A sense of impending doom)

The treatment of stable angina:

If you are treating the patient and they complain of chest pains, immediately stop what you are doing. Return the patient in the dental chair to the seated position. Assess and observe both their symptoms and their clinical signs:

I.   Monitor the patient's AVPU and NEWS. Note: The pulse may be very slow: <u>Less than 40 bpm.</u> or rapid: <u>More than 120 bpm</u> or: <u>Irregular.</u>

II. Assess from the clinical signs whether the chest pain is of cardiac origin and if you suspect Angina, then your approach will follow the **A B C** protocol.

III. **Airway.** <u>Protect</u> the patient's airway at all times, only remove dentures if they are loose.

IV. **Breathing.** Observe and monitor the patient's breathing.

V.   **Circulation.** If you have a pulse oximeter; then use this now.

Continue to observe and document the **AVPU** and **NEWS**. If the angina is <u>stable </u>and resolves, then refer the patient to their General Medical Practitioner. Whatever else you do, if the angina passes, DO NOT conveniently return to treating the patient as if nothing has happened.

Your dentistry really can wait for another day. If you carry on regardless; then the patient may not have another day. As a matter of professional courtesy and perhaps a clinical necessity: Ensure the patient is taken home in a taxi. Never allow them to get on a bus, drive home or waltz out the door unattended (ok, more like a shuffle than a waltz, whatever...but please ensure your patient is placed in the care of a responsible adult).

Patients who have stable angina, present with quite mild symptoms and they will be quite relieved to have survived another dental appointment. Their misplaced emphasis on the chance avoidance of your healing talents being directed at them seems, at least, in their minds, to make their angina fade into an insignificant inconvenience. However, cardiovascular health is slightly more significant than dental health and you must act on the patient's symptoms and signs.

You must document in your notes what has happened and alert the patient's medical practitioner about what you have just witnessed.

If nothing else, your follow-up actions confirm for both the patient and their medical practitioner that you are a safety conscious dentist, the health of your patients being at the forefront of how you practise; as it should be.

Unstable Angina

If the symptoms do not pass, potentially you are facing a patient with <u>unstable angina.</u> Consequently, your patient is now in a more uncertain and perilous state of survival. As noted previously, studies generally specify a mortality rate for stable angina of 4%[1]. However, a documented annual mortality rate of 0.9% to 6.5% has been reported for angina, both stable and unstable. This range reflecting the age and other risk factors for those with all forms of this condition[2.] Should your patient specifically have unstable angina, the mortality rate is significantly higher. Two reviews of angina resulted in the data noted below. These should, at the very least, make you sit up, take notice and undertake the learning necessary to become more aware of the clinical signs of angina that might present in your dental patient[3,4]:

I.   Stable angina is <u>not</u> a benign condition.
II. 10% of those with stable angina will suffer a myocardial infarct either fatal or non-fatal within one year of being diagnosed with angina.
III. The annual mortality rate is between 2.8% to 6.6%, cardiovascular death rate is 1.4% to 6.5% and non-fatal myocardial infarct rate is 0.3% to 5.5%.

The treatment of angina that does not abate

If the symptoms of angina do not abate by stopping what you are doing, sitting the patient upright and reassuring them, then continue your management of your patient, who is still in some distress as follows:

I. Collect the GTN spray and Aspirin from the dental practice medical emergency drug box and administer:

II. **GTN 2 Sprays at 400 µgms/** actuation given sublingually to the patient.

III. Now use **Oxygen at 15 litres/minute** delivered from the bag-valve-mask.

IV. Give **Aspirin 300mgs** and order the patient to chew this placing under the tongue.

V. After 5 minutes, if the pain does not abate, repeat the GTN spray and do so at 5 minute intervals. Do so two more times only.

VI. If after a third attempt to alleviate the symptoms and there is still no easing of symptoms Then you must:

VII. CALL FOR EMERGENCY MEDICAL ASSISTANCE

<u>**MOVE**</u> the patient.

I. **Monitor.** Observe them and reassess their **AVPU,** their **NEWS** and their **A B C.**

II. **Oxygen.** Ensure this is delivered at 15 litres per minute.

III. **Verify.** That the medical emergency first responders are coming.

IV. **Ensure.** In this emergency, the patient is both comfortable, safe and is not left alone.

The event should be documented and you must prepare the patient for handover to the medical emergency first responders as they arrive in a matter of minutes. When calling for the medical emergency responders the following protocol should be used. Please note it is crucial to clearly inform the attending ambulance personnel that you have given aspirin as the hospital based medical team will need to consider this when planning any further anticoagulant or thrombolytic treatment for your patient.

Communicating Angina to the Medical Emergency First Responders:

Dial:	999, 911 or 112 from any mobile
Ask:	For the Ambulance Service
Give:	Your name and location.
State the following:	
1. I have a patient with Cardiac Chest Pain	
2. I have given: **GTN, Aspirin** and **Oxygen**; with no improvement	
3. Send an ambulance now.	
4. Our location is:	
5. Please read back this data to me.	

Angina: The Differential Diagnoses

As stated previously, not all chest pains have a cardiac origin and not all cardiac disease will present as chest pain. The following is a list of possible alternative causes of chest pain other than angina, stable or unstable:

I.   **Prinzmetal's angina:** occurs only at rest exhibiting a circadian pattern, with most episodes occurring in the early hours of the morning. Seen in 2% of all angina patients, the narrowing is caused by vaso-spasticity in the smooth muscles of coronary artery walls and not by atheroma.

II. **Acute pericarditis:** tends to be a more constant pain than angina. Pericarditis is aggravated by inspiration, lying flat, swallowing and movement.

III. **Musculoskeletal pain:** is made worse when moving. Sudden movement rather than general exercise cause the worst pain. There may be an injury to the chest wall or pain from the thoracic spine. Deep inspiration and rotation are likely to aggravate the pain and there may be local tenderness.

IV. **Gastro-oesophageal reflux:** this is often a burning pain, most commonly seen on lying down or after meals. Exercise may aggravate the pain, which is relieved by use of alginates or reducing stomach acid production with proton pump inhibitors.

V. **Pleuritic chest pain:** the pain is sharp on breathing in. It may occur with infection, especially pneumonia, or with an infarction following a pulmonary embolism. If there is a pulmonary embolism then Oxygen must be given but GTN is absolutely contraindicated. In addition, there may be a productive cough and the patient will be coughing blood.

VI. **Aortic dissection**: This is a life threatening condition, the pain is constant.

VII. **Gallstones** These cause acute cholecystitis, the pain is not related to exercise.

Lastly:

VIII. **Myocardial infarction:** The pain lasts longer than 5 minutes, is neither relieved by rest, nor by use of GTN. After three attempts to alleviate the pain with GTN and the use of high flow Oxygen, you can be certain the patient is suffering from a heart attack. Give aspirin, call the emergency medical first responders and advise of the condition of your patient and that you have given aspirin.

If there is any doubt any chest pain should be treated as being of cardiac origin until proven otherwise.

Myocardial Infarction

This medical emergency may follow from angina as described above. In such instances, you will be fortunate to have the time to be able to gather your wits and your dental team about you as you consider how to manage this medical emergency. In other circumstances, a myocardial infarct may arise quite unexpectedly with no symptoms and no signs whatsoever.

In some 10% to 20% of cases of myocardial infarct, the first and only sign is loss of consciousness following the overwhelming obstruction of blood supply to the left ventricle[1]. In these cases, the swift cardiogenic hypotensive shock leading to death is the inescapable grim conclusion. As shocking as this may be, it is a mercifully quick ending for your patient.

In other instances of myocardial infarct, only partial obstruction of blood supply to the myocardium occurs. In such cases, the coronary arteries are able to maintain at least something of the blood supply to keep the heart and the patient alive for some time and the myocardial infarct may result in distress for many hours. Other clinical signs of myocardial infarct are pulmonary oedema from left ventricular dysfunction, in such cases, the symptoms of pulmonary oedema will present as:

I.   The patient will cough up blood or bloody froth
II. There will be shortness of breath and difficulty breathing when lying down.
III. The patient will be grunting, gurgling, or show wheezing sounds when breathing

These clinical signs must not be confused with those of Asthma, where there is an expiratory wheeze.

Due to the high pressure of blood flow in the coronary arteries, atherosclerotic plaques are unstable. The presence of plaques causes platelet adherence and activation, or the plaques can rupture, with fragments detaching from the artery wall. Once activated, platelets and platelet derived inflammatory mediators result in further growth of the existing thrombus and formation of new thrombi. This cycle continues with inflammatory processes and fatty deposits causing further platelet adhesion and activation. These may eventually completely obstruct the blood flow in a coronary artery. Perhaps worse than the blockage of a coronary vessel, is the breakaway of an occlusive thrombus to embolise in the systemic circulation, resulting in the Cerebro-Vascular Accident (CVA) or stroke.

The Symptoms and Signs of a Myocardial Infarct:

I.   Your patient will complain of a pain that is deep; that is pressing into the middle of their chest.

II. This pain spreads to the shoulder arm and jaw to the left (mostly) or the right too.

III. This pain spreads to the shoulder, to the arm and to their jaw; commonly to the left side or occasionally, to the right side too.

IV. Stomach cramps, nausea, vomiting and extreme discomfort are also seen.

V.   Your patient will become pale or appear grey and will be sweating.

VI. If you have access to Nitrous Oxide and the patient is in-extremis, giving N2O would be a kindness. (Although this is not in the 2013 UK Resuscitation Council Guidelines). You should be qualified and experienced in administering N20 at an appropriate concentration of up to 50% Oxygen and 50% Nitrous Oxide for analgesia. Use a pulse oximeter and: **Monitor their response**

VII. If 3 attempts to stop pain with GTN do not work: <u>Your patient has a Myocardial Infarct</u>.

The Treatment of Myocardial Infarct

Even if you are not certain but you strongly suspect your patient is suffering from a myocardial infarct then:

<u>**IMMEDIATELY** CALL FOR EMERGENCY</u>
<u>MEDICAL ASSISTANCE "MOVE" the patient.</u>

I. **Monitor**. Observe them and reassess their **AVPU,** their **NEWS** and their **A B C.**

II. **Oxygen.** Ensure this is delivered at 15 litres per minute.

III. **Verify.** That the medical emergency first responders are coming.

IV. **Ensure.** In this emergency, the patient is both comfortable, safe and is not left alone.

Communicating Myocardial Infarct to the Medical Emergency Services:

Dial:	999, 911 or 112 from any mobile
Ask:	For the Ambulance Service
Give:	Your name and location.

State the following:
1. I have a patient with a suspected Heart Attack
2. I have given: **GTN, Aspirin** and **Oxygen. I am monitoring the patient** The patient has an AVPU level of: ... ...
3. Send an ambulance now. This is an EMERGENCY.
4. Our location is: ... ...
5. Please read back this data to me.

While your patient remains conscious, continue your treatment of the Myocardial Infarct:

I.	Sit your patient up, to reduce their distress from orthopnoea (if there is a left ventricular infarct and failure).
II.	Reassure your patient the ambulance will be here shortly and they will be OK.
III.	Give **Oxygen at 15 litres/minute** from the bag-valve-mask. Monitor their response.
IV.	Give **GTN spray sublingually**, continuing at 5 minute intervals. Monitor their response.
V.	Give **Aspirin 300mgs**, order the patient to chew this, placing it under their tongue. Monitor their response.
VI.	If you have access to Nitrous Oxide and the patient is in-extremis, giving N2O would be a kindness. (Although this is not in the 2013 UK Resuscitation Council Guidelines). You will be qualified and experienced in administering N20 at a concentration of 30% Oxygen and 70% Nitrous Oxide. Monitor their response.
VII.	Be prepared to expedite the handover of your patient to the medical emergency first responders.
VIII.	Advise them on your use of aspirin so further thrombolytic treatment can be co-ordinated in the hospital.
IX.	Until the medical emergency first responders arrive, continue to **MOVE**
X.	**NEWS** and **AVPU** should be undertaken every two minutes and the data noted down.

After you have dialled 999, the medical emergency first responders might not be able to arrive before a myocardial infarct develops into a cardiac arrest.

In the UK: 75% of requests for assistance in **immediately life threatening** emergencies will be responded to within eight minutes.

Where onward transportation is required: 95% of calls for assistance in life-threatening cases will receive an ambulance capable of transporting the patient safely within 19 minutes of the request for transport being made.[5]

Therefore, for a period of 20 minutes from your diagnosing a myocardial infarct, that may lead to cardiac arrest you must be capable and be able as a dental team to give basic life support to every one of your patients.

Cardiac Arrest Basic Life Support

If the myocardial infarct continues unabated, the patient will lose consciousness and stop breathing. The UK Resuscitation Council Algorithm should be used. The flow chart details the steps you must take to ensure your patient has the best possible chance of survival.

This is available online from: file:///C:/Users/Owner/Downloads/ G2015_Adult_BLS.pdf and is reproduced with the permission of the UK Resuscitation Council.

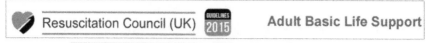

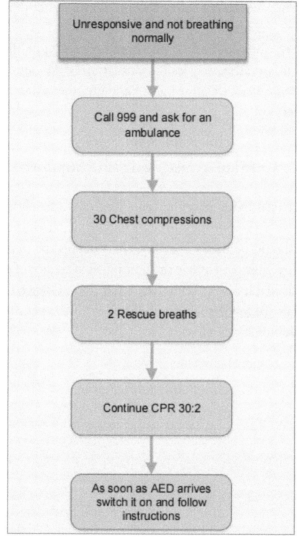

While this algorithm somewhat inconveniently, or inconsiderately begins with the patient who has already collapsed, it is more likely in the dental surgery that either you or your colleagues will already be attending to the conscious patient and will witness their descent and collapse into unconsciousness.

Despite the slight inconvenient start to this algorithm, begin your management by first checking the responsiveness of the patient, *i.e:* don't wait for them to collapse!

Check the patient is responsive by taking hold of their shoulders and asking if they are: OK? If there is a response, then you can continue with your emergency clinical monitoring as follows:

The patient's **A V P U** and **NEWS** should be assessed and this is repeated and help summoned as necessary.

If the patient appears to be unconscious, lay the patient on their back, either in the dental chair or on the ground. If there is no response from your gently shaking the patient, begin the steps as listed in the algorithm, going through the routine of **A B C:**

Airway. Check your patient' airway for any sign of obstruction, this can be achieved by placing one hand on the forehead, tilting the head back and lifting the chin to open the airway.

Breathing. Keep the airway open and look for any sign of normal breathing. Look for movement in the chest. Listen for sounds of breathing. Feel for exhaled air on your cheek. Do not take longer than 10 seconds to determine if the patient is breathing and if this is normal. If your patient is breathing, then turn them into the recovery position and continue to monitor **AVPU NEWS** and **MOVE** the patient.

If the breathing is agonal, abnormal or absent, then assume the patient is in cardiac arrest. Some 55% of those in cardiac arrest will show signs of agonal gasping, this is not normal and must not be confused with normal breathing, this is a sign of cardiac arrest and CPR must begin now[6].

Circulation. In cardiac arrest your patient will not have the ability to circulate or oxygenate blood themselves (now due to cardiac dysfunction or complete non-function). You must be prepared to support their circulation and do so for up to 20 minutes while you await the medical emergency first aid responders (see above).

I.   Begin chest compressions NOW: Kneeling to one side of your patient, place the heel of one hand in the centre of the patient's chest, your other hand is placed on top of the first hand. Interlock your fingers ensuring your hands are in the centre of the chest.

II.   Do not apply any pressure over the upper abdomen or the lower sternum. Position yourself above the patient's chest, now press down on the sternum to a depth of 5 to 6 cms only and no more. Do so with straight arms and push from your shoulders. Following each compression, release all the pressure, allowing the patient's chest to re-inflate. Repeat this 30 X at rate of 100 - 120 per minute.

III. The compression and relaxation strokes should be equal in timing, force and depth.

VERIFY that your call for the medical emergency first responders has been acted on, If not then dial 999 and repeat the procedure as outlined in the previous pages on communicating with the medical emergency services. To repeat: this should be done before commencing CPR

Chest compressions must be combined with rescue breaths:

I.   After the first 30 X compressions open the airway by using the head tilt and chin lift. Pinch the patient's nose closed. Maintain a chin lift to open the mouth. Place your lips around the patient's mouth and making sure that you have a good seal, blow steadily into the patient's mouth, check for chest inflation.

II.   In one second the chest will rise. This shows an effective rescue breath. Maintain the head tilt and chin lift, take your mouth away from the patient, their chest will fall as exhalation occurs. Take another breath and blow into the victim's mouth to give 2X effective rescue breaths. Do not take more than 5 seconds to complete these 2 breaths.

III. Now return to giving a further 30 X chest compressions. Continue with chest compressions and rescue breaths in a

> ratio of: <u>30 X Compressions to 2 X Breaths.</u> Monitor your patient continually.
>
> IV. Only if there are signs of regaining consciousness: Coughing, opening eyes, speaking, or moving purposefully. Or your patient begins to breathe normally, can you stop this procedure. Otherwise, be prepared to continue chest compressions and rescue breaths for up to 20 minutes. Do not interrupt resuscitation and do not break from what you are doing until the medical emergency responders arrive.
>
> V. Be prepared for the handover of your patient to the medical emergency first aid responders.

Anticipate working together with your colleagues for up to, or possibly more than <u>20 minutes</u>, delegating responsibility for a team member to summon help and to co-ordinate the medical emergency first responders as they arrive in your dental practice. If there are two dental team members, then chest compressions and breathing is a shared responsibility.

In your dental practice you will also have access to Oxygen and an Automatic External Defibrillator (AED).

Cardiac Arrest and the use of an Automatic External Defibrillator

An AED can be used safely and effectively without previous training. With advances in technology and ease of use, it is now expected that every UK dental practice will have an AED on their premises. Their use is not restricted to GDC registrants or trained rescuers. Despite advances in technology, training in the use of AEDs must be undertaken on a regular basis. This will improve the efficiency with which they will be used, reducing the time from correctly assessing that a cardiac arrest has happened, through correctly placing the AED pads to delivering a shock to your patient.

If an AED is to be used, there has to be minimal interruption in the chest compressions and rescue breaths while the AED is collected and the pads are attached to the patient. Do not stop to check your patient or discontinue cardiopulmonary resuscitation (CPR) unless as stated before, your patient shows signs of regaining consciousness. These signs could be coughing, opening of the eyes, speaking, intentional movement and normal breathing.

AEDs will administer an appropriate shock, but only when a patient in cardiac arrest will respond. AED pads have sensors that detect residual electrical activity in your patient, if such activity is indicative that a shock can defibrillate the heart, then a shock will be delivered.

As stated: Ease of use is essential and AEDs can be safely and reliably used by all members of the dental team. The following flowchart should be followed.

This flow-chart is available from the UK Resuscitation Council, or online from: file:///C:/Users/Owner/Downloads/AEDflowchart%20(3).pdf

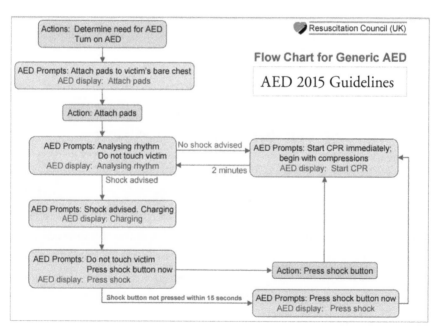

Event Sequence for AED
Cardiopulmonary Resuscitation

Collect the AED and continue CPR while a member of the dental team switches the AED on. Follow the audio and visual prompts from the AED. Attach the electrode pads to the patient's bare chest as illustrated here:

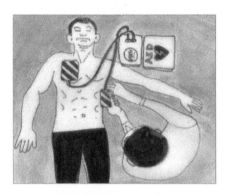

Placement of AED pads

I.   One AED pad is placed to the right of the sternum (breastbone), below the clavicle (collarbone).
II. The other pad is placed in the left mid-axillary line.
III. It is important that this pad is located sufficiently laterally and that it is clear of any breast tissue. AED pads are labelled left and right with a picture of their correct placement.
IV. It does not matter if their positions are reversed. If the pads are incorrectly placed, they should not be removed or repositioned, this wastes time and the pads will not stick once peeled off and re-attached.
V.   Your patient's chest must be exposed to enable correct pad placement. Chest hair will prevent the pads adhering to the skin and will interfere with electrical conduction, excessive hair needs to be shaved off.

Defibrillation

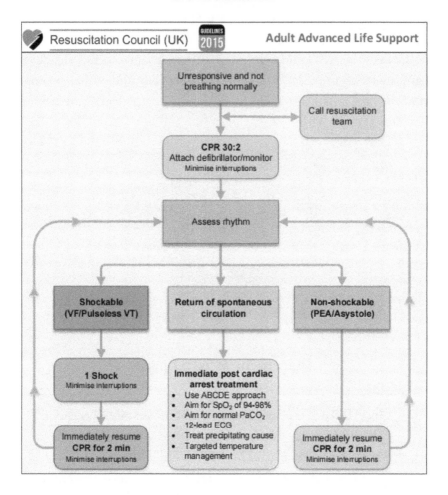

This flow-chart is reproduced with the permission of the UK Resuscitation Council and is available from: file:///C:/Users/Owner/Downloads/G2015_Adult_ALS%20(1).pdf

Make sure nobody is in contact with the patient after the AED pads have been placed. The AED will now assess the patient's residual cardiac electrical activity. If a shock is indicated, again, make sure nobody is in contact with the patient. Now push the shock button as directed, or with the fully automatic AED, a shock will be given, but only when necessary. Continue in accordance with the audio and visual prompts as given.

When safe to do so, continue the chest compressions and rescue breaths.

If no shock is indicated, then resume CPR immediately using the ratio of 30 X Compressions to 2 X Rescue breaths. Continue to follow the AED prompts until the medical emergency responders arrive. If the patient shows signs of regaining consciousness, such as coughing, opening the eyes, or breathing normally, then CPR can stop. There are no other reasons to cease CPR. Becoming exhausted is not a reason as you will be working in a team and your colleagues will carry on if you cannot. As stated above, you must be prepared to carry out CPR for up to 20 minutes, possibly more, until the medical emergency first responders arrive.

Further notes to Chest Pains and Cardiac Arrest

Every year in the UK, outside of hospitals, emergency responders treat more than 30,000 cardiac arrests. The latest figures for 2013 set this figure at 28,000 for Out of Hospital Cardiac Arrests (OHCA) in England alone.[6,7] Although the total number of cardiac arrests in England is not precisely known, the 1/1,000 incidence of cardiac arrests in the European population might be taken as an indication of the extent of the problem we face.[8] The figure quoted by the Ambulance Services Association from 2006 of 57,345 OHCA's, would therefore be accurate in demonstrating the true extent of cardiac arrests among the UK population[9].

Electrical defibrillation is well established as the only effective means of treating cardiac arrest caused by ventricular fibrillation (VF) or pulseless ventricular tachycardia (VT). The earlier that you can start defibrillation, the greater the chance of your patient surviving a myocardial infarct will be. If there is delay from collapse to the delivery of the first shock, the chances of survival will be lower.

One fifth and one fifth

One fifth of all OHCAs occur in a public place, the remainder in the patient's home[10.] However, only a fifth of these patients will present with residual electrical activity that an AED would detect and respond to, delivering a defibrillatory shock. This is principally due to delay in commencing CPR. This is either due to a failure to recognize the signs and symptoms of cardiac arrest, on the part of trained responders, or reluctance on the part of bystanders to become involved. This comes from fear of causing harm to the patient or harm to themselves, eg: apprehension of being sued or fear from contracting a blood borne illness. Hence, the opportunity to commence effective and what might be successful CPR has been missed.

For any registered health care professional, there is a duty to respond to a medical emergency and to do so in a competent manner. It is known that skills in basic life support deteriorate after some three to six months following training.[11] So refresher courses must be attended to maintain then improve both your skills and your abilities to recognize and react not only to cardiac arrests, but to all the medical emergencies.

The safety of both patient and practitioner are paramount in medical emergencies. While there have been cases of adverse events during CPR, with acute respiratory syndromes being reported, the transmission of HIV during CPR has never been reported[12]. While there have been no human studies investigating barrier devices during CPR, laboratory studies do show that barrier devices with one-way valves can prevent transmission of oral bacteria from the patient during mouth-to-mouth CPR. Rescuers must take appropriate safety precautions, especially if the patient is noted to have a transmissible illness such as TB[13].

With regard to the proportion of patients who will respond to CPR and an AED, both you and emergency medical responders can successfully treat this proportion of patients. Not only can you increase their chance of survival by immediate and effective CPR either with or without an AED, you may also be able to increase the numbers of patients in that proportion (the one fifth of the fifth) by immediately calling 999, immediately beginning CPR and immediately recognizing the signs and symptoms of cardiac arrest.[14] If defibrillation is delivered promptly, survival rates as high as 75% have been reported.[13] The chances of successful defibrillation decline at a rate of about 10% with each minute of delay. Basic life support will help to maintain a shockable rhythm but is not a definitive treatment.[15.]

With a cardiac arrest the outlook for the patient can be broadly determined by the clinical signs in relation to the patient's symptoms and their medical history.

In cases of sudden cardiac arrest with no premonitory symptoms where there is only a loss of pulse following from arrhythmia the prognosis is very good, with increasing symptoms and a history of cardiovascular and heart disease the outlook worsens. In those who survive, re-infarction valvular incompetence and myocardial rupture are common complications. The Killip classification of myocardial infarct gives some context by placing the survival rates into the following categories.[16]

The Killip Classification

Killip Class	Clinical Signs	Mortality Rate
I	No previous history and no current clinical signs	**5%** (6%)
II	Increased jugulo-venous pressure and lung and heart (S3) sounds (from Left Ventricular Failure)	**15%** (17%)
III	Acute Severe Pulmonary Oedema (from Left Ventricular Failure)	**45%** (38%)
IV	Cardiogenic Shock Hypotension Cyanosis Peripheral Vasoconstriction and Sweating are all seen.	**90%** (81%)

The figures in brackets are those from the original 1967 study, the figures in bold are those within the survival rate-range, adjusted to the nearest 5% percentiles for your ease of recall and notation. For prognosis the bracketed figures need to be quoted.

Although the Killip–Kimball classification is now 50 years old and was based on an immediate physical (bedside) examination of patients who had suffered a Myocardial Infarct (MI) to determine those patients who would best benefit from further care and onwards referral to a coronary care unit, a very recent re-evaluation with a five year follow up has emphatically proven the concept and classification to be sound and thus it performs a highly useful prognostic role in mean mortality for patients who have had an MI[17].

What is striking if we think about these figures for a moment, is that after 50 years of medical advances in reperfusion, together with antithrombotic therapies and the availability of AEDs, the prognosis for those suffering an MI with prior clinical symptoms remains the same.

The relevance to dentistry is twofold:

i.   Firstly the Killip-Kimball classification might be usefully included in the medical histories of our patients who have had an MI to heighten our safety critical approach to their care. These can be coupled to an ASA grading to narrow the patient's risk status.

ii. Secondly, the table gives both perspective and comfort to those of you who have had to administer CPR to a patient in cardiac arrest and the result wasn't the best you or the patient's family could have hoped for either at the time or in the days or weeks after the event.

It has been noted from the 28,000 OHCAs in England treated by emergency medical responders the survival rate was 8.6%.[7,10,18.] This figure is lower than in North Holland 21%, Seattle 20% and Norway 25%.[18] In the UK, there is an absolute need to improve the OHCA survival rates in the UK and doing so is a priority for the Resuscitation Council (UK), the British Heart Foundation and NHS England. This priority was also identified by the Department of Health in the Cardiovascular Disease Outcomes Strategy of 2013. In order to achieve better outcomes one proposal was to focus on the chain of survival:

The Chain of Survival

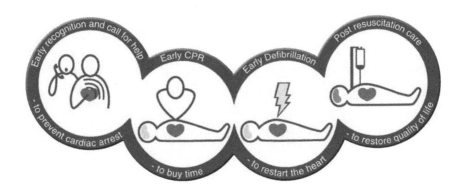

This chain of survival philosophy has resulted in countries with some strikingly high CPR survival rates. In Norway, there was a 74% participation in bystander CPR, compared to only 43% in the UK.[18]

This figure dropped to 1.74% of bystanders prepared to use an AED in OHCA cases in a South of England study.[19]

The reasons for this poor level were given above and are again listed below, with some suggestions to improve your ability to gain the best result for your patient who requires CPR either with or without an AED.

Reasons for poor CPR outcomes	Measures you can take to mitigate deficiencies
Failure to recognise cardiac arrest.	Regularly revise and update clinical knowledge.
Lack of knowledge on managing emergencies.	Repeatedly practice emergency procedures.
Fear of causing harm.	Administer CPR correctly.
Fear of being harmed or acquiring an illness	Document incidents and use barriers.
Fear of being sued.	Unlikely due to Good Samaritan Act
No access to an AED in public area.	All UK dental practices will now have an AED.

With further training and revision of your established knowledge, the impact from poor CPR outcomes can be reduced while the chain of survival for your patient can be strengthened.

As you are not a bystander, but rather a trained professional working within a team of health care providers, it is your duty to ensure you can maintain the chain of survival to give the best chance of success for your patient in a medical emergency, whether they are inside or they are outside of the hospital environment.

It is better to do something than to do nothing.

References to Chest Pains

1. Scully C. Chapter 5: Cardiovascular Medicine. Acquired Heart Disease. in Medical Problems in Dentistry 6th Edition. pp 106-108. Edinburgh. Churchill Livingstone. 2010.

2. Arden C. The management of stable angina October 2011 Br J Cardiol. 2011;18 (Suppl 3).
Available online from: http://bjcardio.co.uk/2011/10/ the-management-of-stable-angina/
[Accessed February 2016]

3. Gandhi MM, Lampe FC, Wood DA; Incidence, clinical characteristics, and short-term prognosis of angina pectoris; Br Heart J. 1995 Feb;73(2):193-8

4. Jones M, Rait G, Falconer J, et al; Systematic review: prognosis of angina in primary care. Fam Pract. 2006 Oct;23(5):520-8.

5. NHS Choices. Emergency and Urgent Care Services. NHS Ambulance Services.
Available online from:
http://www.nhs.uk/NHSEngland/AboutNHSservices/ Emergencyandurgentcareservices/Pages/Ambulanceservices.aspx
[Accessed February 2016].

6. Eisenberg MS. Incidence and significance of gasping or agonal respirations in cardiac arrest patients. Curr Opin Crit Care. 2006 Jun;12(3):204-6.

7. NHS England Ambulance Quality Indicators.
Data Available online from:
www.england.nhs.uk/statistics/stasistical-work-areas/ ambulance-quality-indicators/
[Accessed February 2016]

8. Ambulance Service Association. National Out-of-Hospital Cardiac Arrest Project 2006.

9. de Vreede-Swagemakers JJ, Gorgels AP, Dubois-Arbouw WI et al. Out-of-hospital cardiac arrest in the 1990s: a population-based study in the Maastricht area on incidence, characteristics and survival. J Am Coll Cardiol 1997; 30:1500-1505.

10. London Ambulance Service Cardiac Arrest Annual Report 2012/2013.

    Available online from www.londonambulance.nhs.uk

    Accessed February 2015.

11. Soar J, Monsieurs KG, Ballance JH European Resuscitation Council Guidelines for Resuscitation 2010 Section 9. Principles of education in resuscitation. Resuscitation. 2010 Oct;81(10):1434-44.

12. Koster RW, Baubin MA, Caballero A, et al. European Resuscitation Council Guidelines for Resuscitation 2010. Section 2. Adult basic life support and use of automated external defibrillators. Resuscitation 2010; 81

13. The Resuscitation Council UK. Adult Basic Life Support Guidelines 2010.

    Online Available from:

    https://www.resus.org.uk/pages/bls.pdf

    [Accessed February 2017]

14. Waalewijn RA, Tijssen JGP, Koster RW. Bystander initiated actions in out-of-hospital cardiopulmonary resuscitation: results from the Amsterdam Resuscitation Study (ARREST). Resuscitation 2001; 50:273–279.

15. Valenzuela TD, Roe DJ, Cretin S, Spaite DW, Larsen MP. Estimating effectiveness of cardiac arrest interventions: a logistic regression survival model. Circulation 1997;96:3308-13

16. Killip T, Kimball JT. Treatment of myocardial infarction in a coronary care unit. A two year experience with 250 patients. Am J Cardiol. 1967. 20 (4): 457–64.

17. De Mello BHG, Oliveira GBF, Ramos RF, et al. Validation of the Killip-Kimball Classification and Late Mortality after Acute Myocardial Infarction. Arquivos Brasileiros de Cardiologia. 2014; 103(2):107-117.

    Available online from: https://www.ncbi.nlm.nih.gov/pmc/articles/PMC4150661/

    Accessed March 2017.

18. British Heart Foundation, NHS England, UK Resuscitation Council. Consensus Paper on Out of Hospital Cardiac Arrest in England. 2014. Resuscitation Council UK 2015.
Available online from: https://www.resus.org.uk/pages/OHCA_consensus_paper.pdf
Accessed February 2017

19. Deakin CD, Shewry E, Gray H, Public access defibrillation remains out of reach for most victims of out-of-hospital sudden cardiac arrest. Heart 2014; 100:619-623

10

Paediatric CPR and Defibrillation

In dental practise, paediatric medical emergencies are rare events, nevertheless they do occur and the team approach to managing any medical emergency, whether paediatric or adult, is essential to ensure the best possible outcome for your patient.[1] The incidence of cardiac arrest in children is thankfully very much lower than in the adult population. However, in common with adult cardiac arrest, most paediatric emergencies occur outside the hospital environment, where bystanders attending to the child patient may have little or no knowledge of paediatric medical matters.

There is a preconception that a child suffering cardiac difficulties may suffer more harm from the effects of CPR, than if nothing was done[2]. Consequently, bystanders, both lay and professional, might be inclined under such a notion, to stand around doing nothing until the medical emergency responders arrive. Such an approach from a member of the public would be reprehensible, but from a registered health care professional it is unthinkable, indefensible and inconceivable that you would do nothing while a child struggles for their life in an emergency. Or for that matter that any health care professional would stand and do nothing while anyone struggles in any situation, emergency or otherwise.

Therefore, any medical emergency involving a child must be managed both promptly and properly. From your history taking, whenever you discover that a paediatric patient has any condition with the potential to develop into a medical emergency, your dental notes and your medical history must clearly attest to your findings. Accurate and where necessary; in depth history taking, is an important measure alerting you to the clinical risks involved in treating a paediatric patient with demonstrable medical risk factors. Whenever you treat an at-risk paediatric patient, you must be observant to the clinical signs and symptoms alerting you to a medical emergency that could be developing.

Recognizing the signs and symptoms enabling the interception of a medical emergency, is preferable to stabilizing your patient, then attempting to correct their problems once an emergency has developed, after you failed to heed the warning signs. Early identification of paediatric emergencies, forestalling them, is perhaps the most important measure you can take.

The three reasons to be vigilant when treating children

I.   In a paediatric cardiac emergency, in the face of extreme stress to the respiratory and circulatory systems: physiological decompensation is more rapid than in adults.

II. In children, asphyxial arrest occurs more commonly before cardiac arrest does.

III. With asphyxial arrest, lowered oxygen perfusion and the risk of irreversible brain damage to a child is extremely high.

Even if the child can be resuscitated successfully, the catastrophic effects of brain damage from cerebral hypoxia will condemn a previously healthy child, their parents and their family to a lifetime of managed care. In short, the earlier you can identify a problem, the faster medical emergency responders can be called upon to transport the child to hospital for specialist care.

Initial examination and treatment of a child in cardiac arrest

The paediatric patient should have **NEWS** monitoring if possible and **AVPU** assessment as a necessity. If the child does not respond to stimulation or demonstrates absences of the signs of life:

I. No response to clear verbal or physical stimulation.
II. Shows abnormal breathing such as agonal gasps
III. Has no spontaneous movement or demonstrates movements that are abnormal.
IV. Has no detectable pulse.

Then CPR must commence <u>within 10 seconds of your examination</u>.

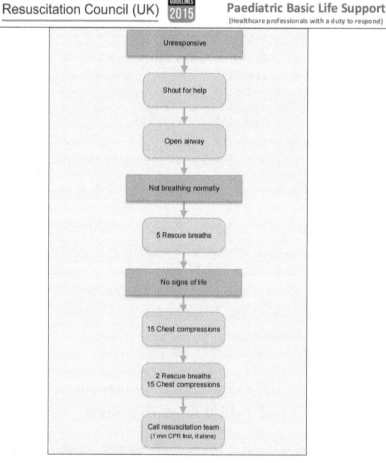

Reproduced with permission of Resuscitation Council UK ©2017. Available online from: file:///C:/Users/Owner/Downloads/G2015_Paediatric_BLS.pdf

With paediatric patients, if there are any doubts, start CPR, as less harm will be caused by your use of CPR that is redundant, than withholding CPR that is essential.

The presence of a pulse cannot be the sole determinant for not initiating CPR. You need to verify the presence or absence of signs of life as listed above, before making a decision not to initiate CPR.

If any member of your dental team considers that there are no signs of life, then commence CPR.

The Sequence for Paediatric CPR

I.   First: Ensure it is safe for you to assist with the medical emergency ie you are not at risk.
II. Make an AVPU assessment of the child. Move gently while asking: *"Are you all right?"*
III. Do not shake children with suspected cervical or spinal cord injuries.

With an AVPU response of A:Stabilise the child, monitoring them until they recover.

You must reassess regularly and summon help if the **AVPU** becomes **V, P** or **U** or their **NEWS** falls. Just because the child is alert and responds to verbal prompts, this does not mean that deterioration might not occur; you must continue to monitor your patient until hand-over to the medical emergency responders can be achieved.

With an AVPU of U: Shout for help, then follow the A B C D E protocol

---

I.   Opening the airway and keeping it open is more important than any other consideration.
II. Turn the child onto their back, open their airway by lifting the chin and tilting the head.

III. Place one hand on the forehead to tilt the head back. Lift the chin by using your fingers, but do not push on the soft tissues under the chin as this may block the airway.

IV. Use a jaw thrust if there is difficulty in opening the airway. Do this by placing the first two fingers of each hand behind each side of the child's lower jaw pushing forward.

V. Listen at the child's nose and mouth for breathing sounds and feel for air on your cheek. Do not confuse agonal gasping with normal breathing.

VI. If after 10 seconds you have doubts and the breathing is not normal, then start CPR.

If the child is breathing normally, then turn the child into the recovery position.

The Recovery Position

An unconscious child with a clear airway, who is breathing normally, should be turned into the recovery position.

The child should be placed in as near a true lateral position as possible with their mouth open to allow drainage of fluid.

The child should be supervised, supported and stable.

The risk of cervical spinal injury must be considered at all times when moving the unconscious child.

In an infant, this may mean using a small pillow or a rolled-up blanket to maintain this position. There should be no pressure on the chest that might impede breathing.

The airway should be accessible and easily observed at all times, the adult recovery position is entirely suitable for use in children:

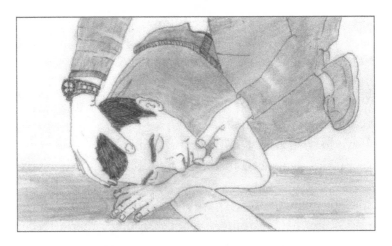

**If the breathing is not normal: Shout for
help and do not leave the child!**

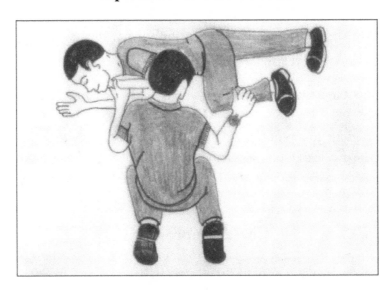

Your colleagues in the dental team can summon the medical emergency responders while you attend to the child. Check for continued normal breathing. If the breathing is not normal or is absent, you must remove any obstruction in the child's airway but do so carefully, taking care not to lodge any debris in the child's mouth or throat that can be aspirated or ingested.

Give FIVE Rescue breaths as follows:

I.   Note any gag or cough responses and check again for any *"signs of life."*

II.   With the head tilt and chin lift, open the child's mouth and blow steadily for 1 to 2 seconds.

III. Watch for the chest to fall on exhalation.

IV.   Repeat this sequence a further FOUR TIMES.

Continue to look for signs of life. These include: movement, coughing, or normal breathing. Do not take longer than 10 seconds to check for a pulse, a brachial pulse on the inner aspect of the upper arm can be used. If you detect signs of circulation within 10 seconds, then continue rescue breaths, until the child starts breathing effectively on their own.

Turn the child into the recovery position if they start breathing effectively but remain unconscious.

Now Give Oxygen via a bag-valve -mask at 10 to 15 litres per minute.

Continue to monitor the **AVPU** and **NEWS** supervising the child until the medical responders arrive. Be prepared to repeat the sequence of Rescue breaths if there is any relapse in the child's condition.

Chest compressions

If there are no signs of life, then start chest compressions: Now. The compressions should be combined with rescue breaths. For all children, compress the lower half of the sternum and avoid compressing the upper abdomen.

Locate the xiphisternum by finding the angle where the lowest ribs join in the middle.

Compress the child's sternum, one finger's breadth above this point.

Compress the child's chest as follows:

I. Compression should depress the sternum by at least one third of the depth of the chest.
II. Push **HARD and FAST**
III. Release the pressure completely, then repeat at a rate of **100 – 120 pushes per minute**
IV. After **15 compressions**, tilt the head, lift the chin, and give two effective breaths.
V. Continue compressions and breaths in a ratio of **15 X Compressions: 2 X Breaths**

Compression methods vary between infants and children.

Chest Compression in an Infant (less than 1 year old)

I. Place both thumbs flat, side by side, on the lower half of the sternum.
II. Your thumb tips should point towards the infant's head.
III. Spread both hands, with fingers together, encircling the lower part of the infant's rib cage.
IV. Your fingertips should support the infant's back.
V. Press down on the lower sternum with your thumbs.
VI. Compress the chest to one-third of the antero-posterior depth.

Chest compression in Child (over 1 year old)

I. Place the heel of one hand over the lower half of the sternum.
II. Lift your fingers to ensure that pressure is not applied on the ribs.
III. Interlock your fingers as necessary.
IV. Position yourself vertically above the child's chest.
V. With your arms straight, compress the sternum by one-third of its antero-posterior depth.

These procedures should be carried out for one minute, cycling the **15 X Compressions: 2 X Rescue** breaths. You or your colleagues must reassess the patient's **AVPU** and **NEWS** after one minute.

Verify that the medical emergency responders have been summoned. Either you or one of your colleagues will need to co-ordinate their arrival. Be prepared to carry out CPR for up to 20 minutes until the medical emergency responders arrive.

The only exception to performing 1 minute of CPR before going for help is in the case of a child with a witnessed, sudden collapse. In this situation, a shockable rhythm is likely to be present and you should go straight to defibrillation.

The differences between adult and paediatric CPR are largely based on their different causes, with primary cardiac arrest being more common in adults, whereas children usually suffer a cardiac arrest secondary to asphyxia.

Hence the need for the initial and immediate 5X Rescue Breaths in children.[3]

Paediatric Defibrillation

An Automatic External Defibrillator (AED) should now be present in every UK dental practice. AEDs are safe, reliable and easy to use. They are capable of identifying arrhythmias accurately in children and are extremely unlikely to deliver a shock erroneously. If an AED is to be used on a child, there are specific pads and programs that need to be used. These purpose-made paediatric pads or programmes, typically attenuate the output delivering a shock of only 50-75 Joules.[4]

AEDs with the ability to attenuate their output are recommended for children between 1 and 8 years.

If no such system or manually adjustable machine is available, an unmodified adult AED may be used.

Although shockable rhythms are extremely unusual in infants, there are rare case reports of the successful use of AEDs in this age group. For an infant in a shockable rhythm, the risk: benefit ratio favours the use of an AED (ideally with an attenuator) if a manually adjustable model is not available.

The following illustration is the UK Resuscitation Council Paediatric Defibrillation Algorithm and this is available online from:

file:///C:/Users/Owner/Downloads/Paediatric_ALS.pdf

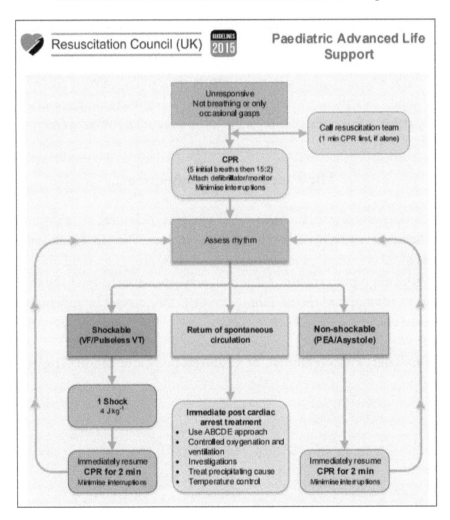

On one hand, paediatric defibrillation falls into the domain of advanced life support and so is not within the scope of practice for dental professionals outside of a hospital environment. Summoning a paediatric rapid response team or a medical emergency team is critical to ensure the best possible outcome for your child patient. The attending team should include a paediatric specialist and one specialised nurse who can expertly evaluate the critically ill child to give them the best possible cardiac care and the best chance of survival.[5]

On the other hand, use of an AED is now an integral part of basic life support, especially when collapse in a child is sudden, the residual electrical activity may respond to immediate defibrillation within 3 minutes of collapse.

So, whenever necessary, you must be prepared to use an AED on a child, regardless of the administrative schemes from professional regulators, who allocate defibrillation into a basic or an advanced criterion.

The Paediatric AED Sequence

Place one defibrillator pad on the chest just below the right clavicle. The second pad is placed in the mid-axillary line. The pads for children are 8 - 12 cms in diameter, and for infants, they are 4.5 cms in diameter. With both infants and small children, it may be better to apply the pads to the front and to the back of the chest if they cannot be attached as noted above.

Paediatric Pad Placement for Children (left) and Infants (right).

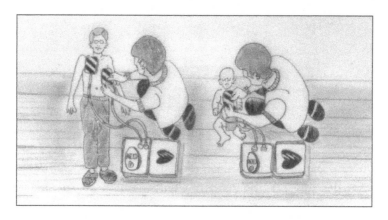

Note the location of the pads, on the left: For a child, they match the adult positions, whereas on the right: For an infant the antero-posterior positioning is perhaps more beneficial, giving the best defibrillatory arc across the infant's heart. The AED will assess existing cardiac rhythm, determine the nature of residual electrical activity and deliver a shock if necessary.

I.   Non-shockable Asystole or Pulseless Electrical Activity. (PEA) Is more common in children.
II. Shockable ventricular fibrillation or ventricular tachycardia. Is more common in adults.

If using an AED for a child over 8 years, an adult shock can be given.

If using an AED for a child of less than 8 years old, an attenuated shock will be given.

Resuming and continuing CPR

Without reassessing the rhythm or feeling for a pulse, resume CPR immediately, starting with the chest compressions. Continue CPR for 2 minutes and then pause, while the AED checks if the patient is still in Ventricular Fibrillation (VF) or Ventricular Tachycardia. (VT). As the patient still has the defibrillator pads attached, the AED will detect any residual electrical activity and deliver another appropriate shock. If necessary, a second shock will be given. Following this shock, resume CPR immediately for another 2 minutes. If your patient is still in VF/VT, a third shock will be delivered. Once more, return to CPR, starting again with chest compressions.

This sequence will continue for up to 20 minutes, until the medical emergency responders arrive and you can handover the care of your paediatric patient to them.

In addition to the above sequence of CPR, you need to continually look for "signs of life" and these are:

I.   Responsiveness: Monitor the **AVPU** level of the patient
II.   Coughing.
III. Normal breathing.
IV.   Monitor the **NEWS** of the patient.

CPR must be administered throughout this procedure. The patient is ventilated with oxygen at 15 litres per minute, with 15 X Chest Compressions to 2 X Ventilations or Breaths. A rate of 100 X to 120 X per minute chest compressions will be given.

In children, the outcome from cardiopulmonary arrests is still poorer than in adults.[6] In any paediatric emergency, especially those of a cardiac nature, it is essential that you recognize the clinical signs indicating those stages leading to the medical emergency and make every attempt to stop a medical emergency from developing further. Should you find yourself managing a paediatric medical emergency, then despite a poorer prognosis, you must aim for Return Of Spontaneous Circulation (ROSC). To achieve this goal, you must maintain the patients:

A B C: Airway Breathing Circulation

Then:

MOVE the patient as follows:

Monitor: The A B C Continually throughout the CPR.

Oxygen: Continue at 15 litres per minute

Verify: The emergency medical responders have been notified and are aware of the nature of the emergency.

Emergency: Actions: Investigate and treat the causes of the cardiac emergency, controlling the temperature of the child, preventing hyper or hypothermia.

Further notes to Paediatric CPR and Defibrillation

Residual shockable rhythms are unusual in children. Therefore, the focus of your management of paediatric cardiac emergencies must be on good quality CPR, before considering the use of an AED. Most people who initially manage a paediatric medical emergency will not be specialists, because of this; the measures detailed in this section will be both simple and effective. However, these techniques do require training. Regular revision of this training is essential, as your skill in delivering effective CPR will decrease in the weeks and months following your attendance in a medical emergencies CPD course.[7,8]

Decrease in skill levels in managing paediatric medical emergencies has been noted in as little as six weeks following attendance on CPR courses. This problem has been known and documented in the scientific literature for some two decades, with various methods being used to mitigate the loss of CPR skills in nursing staff.[9] The following strategies to improve CPR skill retention have been acknowledged to be useful:

I. Regular training in CPR, using manikins, revising the signs and symptoms of cardiac arrest.

II. Instructor assessment on compression depth and rate with feedback at the time of training.

III. Training in the use of AEDs, with frequent access to AED and training literature for all staff.

IV. Formal assessment with instructor feedback on AED use and pad placement on manikins.

V. Provision of remedial training as often as necessary.

In addition to these five strategies, the use of video self-instruction for all dental staff to improve skill acquisition and skill retention is beneficial. The internet has a wealth of data on CPR and the video sharing web sites have many training videos, some with real life documentary on CPR and AED use in both adult and paediatric medical emergencies.

Although not performed on a paediatric patient, there is a short documentary film available online from:

https://www.youtube.com/watch?v=w32PUDL2lb8

This short film clearly demonstrates the successful outcome from the use of an AED and CPR by professional health care workers on one of their colleagues!

References to Paediatric CPR and Defibrillation

1. Nolan P, Hazinski MF, Billi JE. et al International Consensus on Cardiopulmonary Resuscitation and Emergency Cardiovascular Care Science with Treatment Recommendations Part 1: Executive Summary. Resuscitation 2010; 81: 1219-1276.

2. UK Resuscitation Council Chapter 9: Paediatric Basic Life Support in Resuscitation Council UK 2010 Resuscitation Guidelines. London. 91-105.

3. Babbs CF, Nadkarni V. Optimizing chest compression to rescue ventilation ratios during one-rescuer CPR by professionals and lay persons: children are not just little adults. Resuscitation 2004; 61:173-81.

4. Tang W, Weil MH, Jorgenson D, et al. Fixed-energy biphasic waveform defibrillation in a pediatric model of cardiac arrest and resuscitation. Crit Care Med 2002; 30:2736-41.

5. Tibballs J, Kinney S. Reduction of hospital mortality and of preventable cardiac arrest and death on introduction of a paediatric medical emergency team. Pediatr. Crit. Care Med 2009; 10:306-1

6. Kitamura T, Iwami T, Kawamura T, et al. Conventional and chest-compression only cardiopulmonary resuscitation by bystanders for children who have out-ofhospital cardiac arrests: a prospective, nationwide, population-based cohort study. Lancet 2010; 375: 1347-54.

7. Mokhtari Nori J, Saghafinia M, Kalantar Motamedi MH, Khademol Hosseini SM. CPR Training for Nurses: How often Is It Necessary? Iranian Red Crescent Medical Journal 2012; 14(2):104-107.

8. West H Basic infant life support: retention of knowledge and skill. Paediatr Nurs. 2000 Feb;12(1):34-7

9. Hamilton R. Nurses knowledge and skill retention following cardiopulmonary resuscitation training: a review of the literature. Jnl. Adv. Nurs. 2005 Aug; 51(3):288-97.

Medical Emergencies
Enhanced CPD Questions

The first 20 questions will deal with basic approaches to the ten medical emergencies considered in this chapter.

1. **The most common medical emergency is the Vaso-Vagal syncope or faint, this is caused by:**
   A. Fear of the dentist and needle phobia.
   B. Clothing being too tight especially around the neck.
   C. Patient having low blood sugar due to missing a meal before a dental appointment.
   D. The patient has poor physical health, doesn't look after themselves and has become breathless after running to the surgery.
   E. A neurally mediated interruption in adequate blood flow to the brain resulting in loss of cerebral perfusion causing a temporary loss of consciousness. Some factors such as those above can make a patient more likely to faint.

2. **Fainting can be prevented by:**
   A. Giving the patient a stern warning about their previous lack of dental attendance and tell them to arrive on time and not run if they are going to be late for an appointment.
   B. Empathically advising the patient they are in complete control. Don't do any operative dentistry, but give them oral hygiene instruction and tooth brushing advice.
   C. Loosening the patient's clothing, raising their legs and giving them a cold glass of water to drink after which you can carry on

with any surgical dentistry eg: administering local anaesthetic with no complications.

D. Referring the patient to another dentist where they can have IV or RA sedation because fainting will always occur and they can't be helped in general practice, specialist dental care is needed.

E. Taking a full series of histories from the patient including their social, medical and medication history; then avoiding any triggering factors. When treating the patient, unless they are cardiovascularly compromised; treat them in the supine position ie: flat on their back.

3. **You know a patient is asthmatic from their medical history, the clinical warning signs are:**

A. Difficulty breathing in with an over-inflated chest and a productive cough.

B. Decreased chest movements with difficulty breathing out but no productive cough.

C. Fever and chest pains, the patient cannot breathe in or out.

D. Difficulty in exhaling but inspiration seems easier for them; the patient's chest is over-inflated on both sides.

E. All of the above clinical signs can be seen.

4. **The patient above is in respiratory distress; they are having an asthma attack you would:**

A. Tell the patient to calm themselves and place their hands over their mouth to slow their breathing down and then get emergency oxygen.

B. Stop what you are doing and call for an ambulance immediately.

C. Administer Oxygen at 10 to 15 litres per minute and wait until the patient recovers.

D. Use the patient's inhaler either: blue, brown or purple and give them 2 puffs immediately.

E. Stay with the patient and instruct your nurse to collect and then for you to use the Blue (Salbutamol) inhaler from the dental practice drug box. Give two puffs via a spacer and be prepared to use Oxygen if necessary and monitor the patient until they recover.

5. **You have been called to help an orthodontic colleague who is treating a nervous child who has asthma. When you arrive, the child is sitting up in the dental chair, coughing and gasping for breath, they are clutching at their throat. Your colleague looks shocked. You would:**

A. Tell them to sort out the problem as you aren't an orthodontist, perhaps the child is playing up and you don't want to get involved.

B. After a quick assessment of the situation you would call for an ambulance as you aren't sure what the problem is as you are neither an orthodontist nor a paediatric dental specialist.

C. Approach the child, check their airway, as you use the blue inhaler from the emergency drug box.

D. The child is coughing, you would encourage them to keep coughing. Ask your colleague if something is stuck in their throat and encourage them to keep coughing until the object is dislodged. Attempt to look in their mouth to see if an arch-wire or bracket has been dislodged.

E. As answer D but keep monitoring the situation, until the signs improve, if not be prepared to give back slaps and abdominal thrusts and to give salbutamol and oxygen and to call for an ambulance.

6. **While working in the clinic just before lunchtime you can hear shouting and a banging noise from the surgery next door. After a few minutes of this, you get up to see what is going on. The patient is lying flat in the chair, but kicking with both legs. Your colleague is sitting, holding a dental drill over the patient while repeatedly telling them to calm down, the nurse is standing holding the suction, she looks confused, and then she faints. You would:**

A. Ask what is going on, call the manageress to help the nurse while your colleague sorts out their patient, shut the surgery door so other patients in the waiting room can't hear and let them get on with it.

B. Ask your colleague if there is anything in the patient's medical history. Move all equipment aside, ask for the emergency oxygen be prepared to give this to the patient.

C. Take control immediately, alert others: ask for help for the nurse. If necessary get your colleague out of the way and approach the patient if safe to do so. Tell your colleague to re-check the patient's medical history, while repositioning the patient in a safe place if necessary to prevent injury. You can give Oxygen at 10 to 15 litres per minute and continue to assess and monitor while the medical history is being given to you and help is being given to the dental nurse.

D. Tell your colleague to get out of the way while you help the nurse (she has banged her head) and your colleague can carry on telling the patient to calm themselves.

E. Leave the room and call an ambulance immediately for the nurse and the patient.

7. **Anaphylaxis is:**

   A. Very rare, an all or nothing event commonly caused by Penicillin and can take several hours or days to develop into a life threatening incident.

   B. An immune reaction to certain common or naturally occurring substances, the onset is immediate and can rapidly become a threat to the life of a patient if not managed rapidly, effectively and correctly.

   C. Nothing to worry about as the patient's medical history will reveal any allergies and you don't give antibiotics to patients due to the antibiotic stewardship guidelines that are now being followed.

   D. Easy to distinguish from asthma as the two are entirely separate medical conditions that have no clinical overlap

E. Never treated with adrenaline as this can cause rapid broncho-constriction leading to an irreversible loss of the patient's airway.

8. A patient who attends and has chest pain:

A. Is at risk of having a heart attack as heart attacks are always preceded by chest pains.

B. Should be monitored and the pain assessed. You need to be prepared to deal with an emergency such as angina or myocardial infarct occurring. It should be borne in mind there are non-cardiac causes of chest pain too.

C. As above and the patient must have their medical and medication history updated. While the patient is in pain, it would be inadvisable to proceed with any dental treatment. In addition: The patient's GP needs to be informed of your concerns.

D. Should be sat upright and given oxygen at 10 to 15 litres per minute until the pain passes.

E. Should be told to go to hospital to the Accident and Emergency Department.

9. A patient complains of a sudden severe acute crushing band like pain in the chest while at rest, they are perspiring and don't look well at all with a grey pallor. This is most likely to be:

A. Indigestion caused by too much food rapidly eaten before the patient attends with you.

B. Radiating pain from a periodontal abscess in the lower jaw the hygienist is treating. Remember: Oral pain commonly spreads to the chest via the Vagus Nerve (CN X) mimicking something more serious.

C. If the pain is relieved by GTN spray it is a myocardial infarct. Aspirin should be given.

D. Stable angina that should pass in time, an aspirin is sufficient to treat the problem.

E. Unstable angina if the pain is rapidly relieved with GTN spray, if not then the patient could b in the process of suffering a myocardial infarct. The patient's vital signs must be monitored, oxygen given and an ambulance called.

10. Angina is:
  A. A common and benign problem all in men and women older than 55 who smoke, drink and have periodontal disease.
  B. Can be stable at rest or unstable on exertion it is caused when the blood supply to the heart muscle is compromised usually by an atherosclerotic plaque.
  C. Whether stable or unstable Angina can be relieved with GTN spray at 400 ugms per dose.
  D. If there is no relief from GTN spray the patient could have a myocardial infarct and the patient needs to be laid out flat immediately and you must start CPR, do not wait until they lose consciousness.
  E. As answer C but the patient needs to be kept in the seated or Fowler's position to assist in oxygenation and decrease their breathlessness. Patient monitoring is essential. If there are no contra-indications consider Aspirin 300 mgs if there is a risk of a further cardiac emergency occurring.

11. A healthy and physically active patient attends for treatment with his wife who is a medical nurse. This is their first visit, you do not have a medical history. While chatting the patient becomes less responsive, after a few minutes, he seems to faint. You lower the patient until supine, raise their legs this has no effect. The patient is drowsy, but conscious. You would:
  A. Consider the patient hasn't fainted something else is going on you ask his wife.
  B. As the wife is a nurse you feel she might get in the way and ask her to leave the room so you can think about what to do next, possibly using oxygen or adrenaline.
  C. Do nothing; wait until the patient should eventually recover. The patient has simply fainted, tell the wife you have the situation completely under control and not to worry as fainting

is a common condition, especially in fit young men who are scared of the dentist.

D. As for answer A and then go through the A B C with the wife attending to the patient who is still conscious but disorientated.

E. Get oxygen immediately and attach a pulse oximeter until you can find out what is going on from the wife.

12. **The wife tells you her husband has a history of: Thyroid disease, Coeliac disease and Type I IDDM, all of these were treated and the patient self administers insulin. The patient above is:**

A. Is Hyperglyceamic.

B. Is Hypoglycaemic.

C. Has simply fainted.

D. Is in a steroid crisis.

E. Possibly B and C but not A or D.

13. **In an emergency in the conscious dental patient with Diabetes, hyperglycaemia is more common than Hypoglycaemia.**

A. False

B. True

C. Hyperglycaemia will not be treated with insulin whereas hypoglycaemia will be treated with glucagon if the patient is unconscious.

D. Hyperglycaemia is untreated and hypoglycaemia is treated with a glucose drink or glucose tablet if the patient is conscious and responsive.

E. Answers A, C and D are true.

14. **A patient who has collapsed must be immediately approached and attended to:**

A. True

B. False

C. You need to protect yourself first and make sure there is no danger to yourself or others from your actions.

D. You must assess the situation first and if there is no clear danger as a registered health care professional in the UK: You have a duty to respond and to assist if you can do so.

E. You must not get involved if the event occurs outside of a dental surgery and if harm comes from your actions then the GDC will become involved risking your registration.

15. A patient who is in cardio-respiratory arrest will be:

A. Most at risk in hospital, in a doctor's or in a dentist's surgery due to the stress and drugs. These events rarely if ever occur outside of a health care environment.

B. The most common form of cardiac arrest is from atrial fibrillation or AF.

C. Most commonly a VF or ventricular fibrillation leads to a cardiac arrest but this is a non-shockable rythm from which the patient will eventually succumb.

D. Cardiac Arrest needs urgent attention it is most commonly a result of VF caused by ischaemic heart disease in older patients, acute asthma, drug abuse especially; recreational drugs, shock from blood or fluid loss or hypothermia in younger patients.

E. The patient's medical history will determine whether or not your efforts with CPR should commence and if the patient will benefit from CPR. Essentially, as a dentist, before you commence CPR or use a defibrillator: Check the patient's medical history first.

16. When a patient suddenly collapses you would:

A. Either freeze or panic but try to get as far away from the patient as possible. There could be a danger to yourself by staying where you are, the patient may have been electrocuted. Your safety must come first.

B. Don't call or ask for help as a dental professional you can deal with this, the others will only get in the way and slow down the process of your dealing with the patient.

C. Immediately call for help, assess both the situation and the location and if it is safe to do so; attend to the patient. Go through the routine of A B C and place the patient in a supine position, if they have fainted they will recover. If not, then administer Oxygen and with your dental team, if there is no pulse then commence CPR. Attach the practice AED and react to the voice prompts, continue as guided until the ambulance arrives.

D. Assess the patient, immediately administer Oxygen regardless of the clinical signs and suspected causes. Attach a pulse oximeter and take a series of vital signs for NEWS grading and if necessary MOVE the patient and proceed as answer C only if necessary.

E. As answer C and be prepared to deal with the patient recovering or developing another medical emergency while you stay with them and wait for an ambulance crew to attend. If you can then take AVPU and NEWS scores that can be passed to the emergency responders on patient hand-over.

17. **The clinical signs of anaphylaxis:**
   A. Are seldom confused with acute asthma, anaphylaxis rarely involves the airways asthma always does.
   B. Anaphylaxis may be accompanied by angio- oedema, there can be facial swelling and flushing, itching, wheezing, nausea, loss of circulation to the limb extremities, abdominal pain and the skin becomes cold and clammy.
   C. Will resolve in a short while and you need do nothing more than lay the patient flat to prevent them from losing consciousness, you might give them oxygen if the patient starts to hyperventilate.
   D. As answer B and there could be extreme pallor, the pulse become weak, thin and thready with a risk of loss of consciousness.
   E. Is most likely to be caused by a patient reacting to adrenaline that is contained in some dental local anaesthetics.

18. A patient suddenly develops a facial weakness and cannot understand what you are saying to them, they cannot raise their arms. From these signs you firmly believe they are having a stroke, you would:

A. Give them 300mgs Aspirin from the dental practice emergency drug box.

B. Assess their A B C and if necessary administer Oxygen but nothing else by mouth and urgently call an ambulance dialling 999. Immediately continue by AVPU and NEWS monitoring and be prepared for patient hand-over with as much information as possible.

C. Observe and assess the patient but do nothing more as giving oxygen could increase the blood flow to the brain with a risk of further or permanent brain damage from oxygen.

D. Phone the patient's relative explain what you think has happened and get them to make an appointment to see a doctor in a week or so as most strokes are quite minor and the patient should recover in time.

E. As C and after hand-over write up the patient's notes and document any drugs that have been given or administered as the risk of drug interaction with a hospital therapeutic regimen is possible.

19. For a child with a suspected cardiac arrest you must:

A. Do nothing as a child having a cardiac arrest is such a rare occurrence, basic or even advanced life support is unlikely to work and if it does there is a grave risk of the child having severe brain damage if they survive.

B. Make an immediate assessment of their A B C, then within 10 seconds: Deliver 5 rescue breaths and 15 chest compressions and call for help: Dial 999 and ask for an ambulance. Stay with the child until help arrives and you can use an AED with a set of attenuated or paediatric pads. The child should be kept in the supine position as you attend to them.

C. Immediately leave the child, find an AED in the practice, request an ambulance.

D. Give oxygen with adrenaline in accordance with their age (< 6 years: 150 μgms, 6 to 12 years: 300 μgms and >12 years: 500 μgms).

E. Assess the A B C and then sit the child upright to deliver the oxygen and use a pulse oximeter to assess oxygenation levels, if you cannot resuscitate the child consider calling an ambulance.

20. **An adult patient has just collapsed in the surgery.** When you arrive your nurse tells you before collapsing the patient complained of feeling dizzy and had vomited. The patient does have a pulse but this is both weak and irregular. Your nurse has helpfully placed the patient in the recovery position with their mouth open and airway clear. The patient is cold and clammy to the touch but they are breathing; there are no chest sounds and their airway is clear Their medical history stated they have had a long history of hay fever with nasal obstruction and have been irregularly self-medicating with nasal Fluticasone spray and other tablets to reduce the swelling in their sinuses, but the patient stopped taking these a week or so before attending with you.

Taking these clinical signs into consideration, the most likely cause of the patient's collapse is:

A. Myocardial infarct.
B. Asthma.
C. Adrenal insufficiency or crisis.
D. Anaphylaxis
E. Syncope

You proceed to treat the patient by:

A. Dialling 999, laying the patient flat and following: ABC, AVPU NEWS and MOVE and give Oxygen at 15 litres per minute, stay with the patient and monitor them be prepared to hand them over.

B. Monitor their ABC and sit the patient upright giving them salbutamol inhaler. Dial 999.

C. Give GTN and Aspirin 300mgs crushed and placed sublingually with Oxygen at 15 litres per minute. Dial 999

D. Dial 999 and administer Adrenaline 500 µgms intramuscularly.

E. Option A and also consider IV access for 500mgs hydrocortisone.

The following 20 questions will deal with Immediate Life Support

21. **Effective communication and team work are of safety critical importance when managing the deteriorating patient. Working according to SBAR (Situation Background Assessment Recommendation) and RSVP (Reason Story Vital-signs Plan) can reduce which percentage of problems due to poor communication in the dental team?**
    A. Under 20%
    B. 30%
    C. 50%
    D. 60%
    E. Over 80%

22. **Which of the following clinical signs may be seen before a cardiac arrest?**
    A. Hypothermia
    B. Hyperthermia
    C. Hypoxia
    D. Hypotension
    E. Hypertension

23. **The Acute Coronary Syndrome (ACS) is the presentation of chest pain or extreme discomfort from myocardial ischaemia**

or myocardial injury, which of the following methods are appropriate to treat this condition?

A. 300mgs Aspirin orally crushed or chewed as soon as possible.
B. Sublingual Glyceryl Trinitrate.
C. Controlled oxygen to a defined saturation of 94- 98%.
D. High flow oxygen at 15 litres per minute.
E. Pain relief with Intravenous opiates titrated to a specific concentration dependent on the patient response.

24. A patient with COPD or type 2 respiratory failure who also has the ACS should be given:

A. High flow oxygen at 10 litres per minute.
B. High flow oxygen at 15 litres per minute.
C. Oxygen through a nasal cannula at 2 litres per minute and no more.
D. Oxygen with a Venturi face mask at 28% and 4 to 5 litres per minute.
E. Oxygen at 4 Litres/minute with a 24% to 28% Venturi face mask and Pulse oximeter monitoring to achieve a target saturation of 88%- 92%.

25. A NEWS score of 5 or 6 or a 3 in any one NEWS area will demand which clinical response?

A. A minimum observation frequency of 12 hours and routine NEWS monitoring
B. A minimum observation frequency of 4-6 hours and nurse led assessment and more frequent NEWS monitoring
C. A minimum observation frequency of 2 hours with registered nurse assessment and accelerated NEWS monitoring
D. A minimum observation frequency of 1 hour with medical team and urgent care assessment of NEWS by an acute care medical clinician in a monitored environment.
E. Continuous medical monitoring and observation of NEWS status with the patient being transferred to a CCU or high dependency unit.

26. **Pulse oximetry is a useful non-invasive measurement of which of the following?**
    A. Adequacy of venous oxygenation saturation or Sv O_2
    B. Adequacy of arterial oxygenation saturation or SpO_2
    C. Ventilation efficiency of the patient and thus blood gas exchange.
    D. Oxygen saturation and content and thus tissue perfusion.
    E. All of the above can be achieved with simple pulse oximetry.

27. **The most common initial cardiac arrest rhythm is the Ventricular Fibrillation or VF, which of the following can cause VF?**
    A. Acute Coronary Syndrome
    B. Hypertension, valve defects, inherited cardiac conditions or other defect in the heart.
    C. Drug use or abuse such as Tricyclic Antidepressants or Cardiac glycosides such as Digoxin.
    D. Acidosis, electrolyte imbalance or abnormal electrolyte concentrations.
    E. All of the above can initiate ventricular fibrillation.

28. **Secondary heart problems may follow from which of the following conditions?**
    A. Asphyxia,
    B. Apnoea
    C. Anaemia
    D. All of the above
    E. None of the above.

29. **The heart can also be affected by which of the following changes in the body?**
    A. Hypoxia
    B. Hypotension
    C. Hypothermia
    D. All of the above
    E. None of the above

30. Which of the following physiological imbalances and pathological conditions could also lead to secondary heart problems and sudden cardiac arrest or death?
    A. Hyperkalaemia or Hypokalaemia
    B. Hypocalcaemia, acidaemia or other metabolite imbalance.
    C. Hypoglycaemia
    D. All of the above
    E. None of the above.

31. The normal respiratory rate is what?
    A. 5-10 breaths per minute
    B. 10-20 breaths per minute
    C. 20-30 breaths per minute
    D. 30-40 breaths per minute
    E. 40-50 breaths per minute

32. With regard to chest sounds which of the following statements are correct?
    A. A rattling sound indicates the presence of secretions in the airways.
    B. Stridor can be heard on inspiration only and is a normal sound
    C. Stridor can be heard on expiration only and is a normal sound
    D. Stridor can be heard on inspiration or expiration and is a particularly worrying sound as it indicates a partial but significant lung obstruction.
    E. Wheezing can only be heard on inspiration in asthmatics.

33. For chest sounds which of the following statements are correct?
    A. Dullness in the chest indicates pneumothorax.
    B. An absence of sounds or reduced sounds indicates pneumothorax.
    C. A dullness in the chest indicates consolidation or the presence of fluid.
    D. An absence of sounds or hyper-resonance indicates the presence of fluids.
    E. Crepitus indicates surgical emphysema or pneumothorax.

34. **Hypovolaemia is a common cause of shock, the Capillary Refill Time (CRT) after squeezing the finger for 5 seconds should be:**
    A. Less than 1 second.
    B. No more than 2 seconds.
    C. 4 seconds.
    D. 6 seconds.
    E. More than 10 seconds.

35. **Gas exchange can be impaired by:**
    A. Pneumothorax but not Haemothorax
    B. Pneumothorax and Haemothorax
    C. Haemothorax but not Pneumothorax.
    D. Tension pneumothorax reducing the venous return with a decrease in blood pressure.
    E. Pulmonary embolus, acute respiratory distress or chronic obstructive pulmonary disease.

36. **Which of the following statements is correct for a patient in shock?**
    A. The blood pressure will always be low.
    B. The blood pressure could be within the normal range due to physiological compensation.
    C. Peripheral vasodilation is a helpful physiological response to hypovolaemia.
    D. Low diastolic blood pressure is indicative of arterial vasodilation.
    E. A narrowed pulse pressure (a difference between systolic and diastolic) of less than 35 mmHg is indicative of arterial vasoconstriction following cardiogenic shock or hypovolaemia.

37. **The assessment of the patient to LOOK LISTEN and FEEL for breathing or determine if they are in cardiac arrest should take how long?**
    A. Less than 5 seconds.
    B. No more than 10 seconds.
    C. Up to 15 seconds.

D. No more than 20 seconds.

E. Up to 30 seconds to be certain before you need to consider asking for help.

38. Which of the following statements are correct for respiratory arrest?

A. There is a pulse but the patient is not breathing.

B. There is no pulse but the patient is breathing.

C. There is no pulse and the patient is not breathing.

D. All patients in respiratory arrest unless corrected will develop cardiac arrest very quickly.

E. Not all patients in respiratory arrest will develop cardiac arrest the two are unconnected.

39. A patient in the dental surgery has collapsed and there is no pulse.... which of the following procedures would you initiate?

A. First check the medical history, then check for signs of danger before calling for an ambulance and advising the patient's relative there is a problem, after which you can consider CPR.

B. If there are no signs of life and there is no danger then start CPR immediately, you would do this by first giving up to 5 breaths and then about 10 or may be 20 or so chest compressions, but you might give a few more rescue breaths first.

C. If there are no signs of life and there is no danger then start CPR immediately, you would do this by first delivering 30 chest compressions and 20 breaths and shout for help.

D. After giving this first round of CPR, you or a colleague would apply the automatic defibrillator and another colleague would have called for an ambulance.

E. You would then continue with chest compressions and bag-valve ventilation while being prompted to do so by the automatic defibrillator, but you would not stop until help arrives.

40. A patient has collapsed; there is a pulse but they are not breathing which answers are correct?
   A. Placing the patient in the recovery position is all that is required.
   B. Monitor the patient and go through ABCDE and then ventilate the patient with Bag-Valve-Facemask further pulse monitoring more than taking a radial pulse not needed.
   C. Monitor the patient and go through ABCDE and then ventilate the patient with Bag-Valve-Facemask further pulse monitoring with a pulse oximeter is needed and you should be prepared to give chest compressions and use a defibrillator if necessary.
   D. As answer C and an ambulance must be called.
   E. A patient who has collapsed with a pulse but is not breathing could be in respiratory arrest if not managed correctly and promptly respiratory arrest leads to cardiac arrest.

The following 20 questions will deal with paediatric immediate life support.

41. With paediatric cardiopulmonary resuscitation, how many rescue breaths should be given?
   A. One
   B. Two
   C. Three
   D. Four
   E. Five

42. A child is gasping for air, it is clear there is agonal or non-effective breathing, what must be done?
   A. Do nothing other than call the resuscitation team and let them deal with the situation.
   B. Give chest compressions first then call the resuscitation team.
   C. Give the correct number of rescue breaths.
   D. As answer C and continue to monitor the patient's Airway Breathing and Circulation an ambulance will be called and the

patient will be supported and monitored until the emergency services attend and the patient recovers.

E. All of the above are incorrect, irregular noisy infrequent gasps are normal for children and so nothing needs to be done.

43. Ideally, where should chest compressions be given?

A. In the upper part of the sternum
B. Over the the middle part of the sternum
C. In the lower part of the sternum.
D. It doesn't matter where they are given
E. Chest compressions must never be delivered to a child as there is a risk of rib fracture and tension pneumothorax.

44. A cardiac arrest in a child is mostly:

A. Due to a conduction defect between the Sino-Atrial and Atrio-Ventricular Nodes.
B. Preceded by bradycardia which deteriorate into pulseless electrical activity then asystole.
C. Due to a congenital cardiac defect.
D. A very sudden event.
E. Associated with morbidity and mortality from damage to vital organs caused by tissue hypoxia.

45. For paediatric breathing which of the following are correct?

A. A child's tongue is relatively smaller than that of an adult with respect to their mouth.
B. Children seldom if ever use their diaphragm for breathing.
C. A child's rib cage is relatively inflexible when compared to that of an adult.
D. During inspiration the diaphragm will ascend generating positive pressure.
E. During inspiration the diaphragm descends into the abdomen creating negative pressure.

46. **Match the following rates of breathing to the age groups:**
    (i) <1year, (ii) 1-2 years, (iii) 2-5 years, (iv) 5 -12 years, (v) >12 years.
    A. 12-20 Breaths/minute
    B. 30-40 Breaths/minute
    C. 26-34 Breaths/minute
    D. 24-30 Breaths/minute
    E. 20-24 Breaths/minute

47. **For circulating blood volumes which of the following are correct values?**
    A. In a newborn the circulating blood volume is 30ml/Kg body weight, this increases to 80/90ml/Kg in adulthood, therefore even a small loss of blood can be critical.
    B. In a newborn the circulating blood volume is 30ml/Kg body weight, this decreases to 10/20ml/Kg in adulthood, therefore even a small loss of blood can be critical.
    C. In a newborn the circulating blood volume is 80ml/Kg body weight, this decreases to 60/70ml/Kg in adulthood, therefore even a small loss of blood can be critical.
    D. In a newborn the circulating blood volume is 80ml/Kg body weight, this remains the same in adulthood, physiological compensation means that very large losses of blood can be tolerated.
    E. In a newborn the circulating blood volume is 120ml/Kg body weight, this decreases to 60/70ml/Kg in adulthood, therefore while small losses of blood are critical in adults in children there are significant physiological reserves to tolerate such losses.

48. **Cardiac output is the product of Stroke Volume X Heart Rate, a child's heart rate is:**
    A. Very slow compared to an adult.
    B. Much higher than an adult.
    C. The same as an adult.

D. The determinant of cardiac output, as the stroke volume is less variable in a child.

E. Not a critical factor in determining an adequacy of cardiac output as the stroke volume is variable.

49. **The lower limit for systolic blood pressure can be calculated by which rule of thumb?**
   A. 10 + 2 X Age in Years
   B. 30 + 2 X Age in Years.
   C. 50 + 2 X Age in Years
   D. 70 + 2 X Age in Years.
   E. 90 + 20 X Age in Years.

50. **In paediatric basic life support the recommended sequence of events to follow is:**
   A. Safety (personal), Stimulate (patient), Shout (help), Airway, Breathing, Circulation, Finish.
   B. Shout (help), Stimulate (patient), Safety (personal), Stimulate (patient again), Shout (again), Airway, Breathing, Circulation, Shout (for help if none is arriving)
   C. Safety (personal), Stimulate (patient), Shout (help), Airway, Breathing, Circulation, Reassess and Repeat; ABCDE until first emergency response arrives.
   D. Stimulate (patient), Shout (help), Safety (personal), Airway Breathing Circulation finish.
   E. Any order is acceptable as long as the child patient is being attended to.

51. **Which of the following statements are correct for the use of oro-pharyngeal airways?**
   A. The correct size of airway when placed on the side of the face extends from the incisors to the angle of the mandible.
   B. The correct size of airway when placed on the side of the face extends from the incisors to the Cricoid cartilage.

C. The correct size of airway when placed on the side of the face extends from the incisors to the eminence of the Thyroid cartilage or Adam's Apple.

D. If an incorrect size is used then trauma will result with laryngospasm and further airway obstruction.

E. With any type of oropharyngeal airway device there is always a risk of trauma to any part of the patient's airway from the palate to the pharynx with an incorrect introduction technique.

52. Which of the following statements are correct?

A. In paediatric resuscitation, airway obstruction is a common occurrence.

B. Due to the flexibility and elasticity in a child's airway obstruction is rarely if ever seen.

C. To improve airway opening in a child, appropriate head positioning is important.

D. Due to the flexibility and elasticity in a child, head positioning is less critical than in adults.

E. Bag mask ventilation is not as important for children as it is for adults.

53. In <u>basic</u> paediatric resuscitation and ventilation which of the following are appropriate measures and techniques for all health care professionals working with children?

A. Tracheal intubation.

B. Open ended bag mask ventilation with gas source achieving positive expiratory pressure.

C. The delivery of a high concentration of oxygen.

D. Correctly performed bag mask ventilation.

E. All of the above are essential skills for all health care professionals working with children.

54. **Which of the following statements are correct for airway sounds?**
    A. A high pitched inspiratory noise or stridor is characteristic of an upper airway extra-thoracic obstruction.
    B. A high pitched inspiratory noise or stridor is characteristic of a lower airway intra-thoracic obstruction.
    C. In a severe obstruction a less pronounced stridor can be heard on expiration this is biphasic stridor.
    D. Stridor is never heard on expiration.
    E. Wheezing is an expiratory sound as a result of lower intra-thoracic airway narrowing at the bronchiolar level.

55. **Respiratory failure can be recognized by:**
    A. Tachypnoea: an increase in the rate of breathing.
    B. Recessions or retractions in the sternal, intercostals and subcostal musculature.
    C. A head-bobbing motion as the accessory muscles of respiration are used.
    D. A see-saw respiratory motion with diaphragmatic contraction as the thorax contracts and the abdomen expands.
    E. All of the above clinical signs can be seen.

56. **While the clinical signs of respiratory distress and failure can be seen, which of the following may contribute to an absence of such signs:**
    A. Exhaustion.
    B. Neuro-muscular diseases.
    C. Depression of the Central Nervous System
    D. All of the above.
    E. None of the above.

57. **For pulse oximetry in children which of the following statements are true?**
    A. A pulse oximeter should be used on any child at risk of respiratory failure.

B. A peripheral arterial oxygen saturation ($Sp\,O_2$) of less than 90% in air or less than 95% with supplemental oxygen is indicative of respiratory failure.

C. A peripheral arterial oxygen saturation ($Sp\,O_2$) of less than 95% in air or less than 99% with supplemental oxygen is indicative of respiratory failure.

D. The use of a pulse oximeter is unreliable in children with poor peripheral circulation.

E. If the $Sp\,O_2$ is less than 70% then pulse oximetry becomes unreliable.

58. With respect to heart rate and respiratory failure which of these statements are true?

A. Initial hypoxia can result in tachycardia.

B. Initial hypoxia can result in bradycardia.

C. Prolonged hypoxia can result in tachycardia.

D. Prolonged hypoxia can result in bradycardia.

E. In a severely hypoxic child bradycardia is a pre-terminal sign.

59. Which of the following causes of the clinical signs are correct?

A. Hypoxia produces vasoconstriction and skin pallor.

B. Hypoxia produces vasodilation resulting in skin mottling

C. Cyanosis around the lips and mouth are a result of hypoxia.

D. Cyanosis is a very reliable indicator of the degree of hypoxia.

E. Cyanosis is not a reliable indicator of the degree of hypoxia.

60. Which of the following statements concerning circulation are correct?

A. The capillary refill time in a healthy child is less than 2 seconds.

B. If skin perfusion is decreased the capillary refill time is prolonged.

C. If the skin perfusion is decreased the capillary refill time is reduced.

D. Cyanosis due to circulatory failure is initially peripheral.

E. Hypoxaemia due to respiratory failure causes central cyanosis.

The following 20 questions will deal with post resuscitation care

61. **Which of the following steps can minimize the risk of secondary brain injury?**
    A. Stabilizing the blood pressure.
    B. Preventing secondary seizures.
    C. Maintaining normal blood gasses
    D. Correcting electrolyte imbalances.
    E. All of the above.

62. **To determine the prognosis for the patient's brain function, which of the following should be noted both during and immediately after resuscitation?**
    A. The level of consciousness either AVPU or Glasgow Coma Scales.
    B. Pupillary response to light stimulus.
    C. A full medical examination including any head injuries or suspicious rashes such as those associated with meningitis!!
    D. All of the above are important clinical observations to take and record.
    E. None of the above can meaningfully contribute to determining the post resuscitation prognosis.

63. **Post-resuscitation investigations are essential, which of the following might be usefully requested in the immediate period after resuscitation?**
    A. Arterial blood gasses and lactate, to ensure adequate tissue perfusion and ventilation.
    B. Biochemistry to assess liver and kidney function from electrolyte and blood glucose levels.
    C. Full blood screen and count.
    D. Radiography of the chest, abdomen and any other area.
    E. All of the above can be usefully requested to support the post-resuscitation care.

64. Which of the following statements are correct for the immediate post-resuscitation period?

A. Maintaining the body temperature at precisely 37° Centigrade is absolutely critical

B. Mild hyperthermia is beneficial

C. Mild hypothermia has been shown to be beneficial in adults in suppressing the chemical reactions associated with reperfusion injuries.

D. Hypothermia in children is harmful.

E. Mild hypothermia of 32°C to 34°C is well tolerated in children and should be considered beneficial.

65. Up to 48 hours post resuscitation what phenomena are commonly seen?

A. Hyperpyrexia.

B. Hypopyrexia.

C. Poor neurological outcomes with hyperpyrexia.

D. Poor neurological outcomes with hypopyrexia.

E. Any of the above phenomena can be seen in the immediate post-resuscitation period.

66. With post-resuscitation oxygen use, which of the following statements are correct?

A. Prolonged exposure to a high concentration of oxygen is beneficial.

B. Prolonged exposure to a high concentration of oxygen is harmful.

C. The process of reaching target oxygen saturation is achieved gradually by titration.

D. Inspired oxygen should be at a target range of 94% to 98%.

E. In those patients with anaemia and in cases of airway obstruction the dissolved oxygen concentration is more important than the concentration being inspired.

67. **The post-cardiac arrest syndrome comprises which of the following pathologies?**
   A. Myocardial dysfunction.
   B. Brain injury.
   C. Systemic ischaemia.
   D. Inappropriate reperfusion response.
   E. All of the above can be seen with the post-cardiac arrest syndrome.

68. **The severity of the post-cardiac arrest syndrome can be made worse by which of the following?**
   A. A cardiac arrest that is prolonged and complicated.
   B. Poor overall health of the patient.
   C. Activation of coagulation and immunological pathways that could initiate organ failure.
   D. Any underlying infection that could lead to sepsis.
   E. All of the above.

69. **Following a cardiac arrest both heart rate and rhythm are likely to be unstable, which of the following statements are true?**
   A. Continuous monitoring of an ECG either 12 lead or 10 lead is essential.
   B. If the neck veins are grossly distended with the patient sitting upright then the right ventricle could be failing.
   C. If the neck veins are grossly distended with the patient sitting upright then the left ventricle could be failing.
   D. If there are fine inspiratory crackles and pink frothy sputum, the left ventricle is failing.
   E. If there are fine inspiratory crackles and pink frothy sputum, the right ventricle is failing.

70. **Following resuscitation a chest radiograph is essential to reveal which of the following?**
   A. The position of a tracheal tube, supraglottic airway, gastric tube or venous catheter.

B. Pulmonary oedema.

C. Pulmonary aspiration or presence and location of foreign bodies.

D. The presence and extent of pneumothorax.

E. The contour of the heart and pericardium.

71. **Post resuscitation cardiac care can involve which of the following measures?**

    A. Assessment with echocardiography to determine the extent of myocardial dysfunction.

    B. Treatment with fluids to counteract hypotension.

    C. Treatment with inotropic drugs to control the force of cardiac muscle contraction.

    D. Treatment with vasopressors to increase blood pressure through vasoconstriction.

    E. All of the above are appropriate measures to reduce post myocardial dysfunction.

72. **In post-resuscitation care which of the following target values are aimed for?**

    A. Systolic blood pressure of 70mm Hg and urine output of 0.7mg/Kg body weight.

    B. Systolic blood pressure of 90mm Hg and urine output of 0.9mg/Kg body weight.

    C. Systolic blood pressure of 100mm Hg and urine output of 1mg/Kg body weight.

    D. Systolic blood pressure of 120mm Hg and urine output of 1.2mg/Kg body weight.

    E. Systolic blood pressure of 140mm Hg and urine output of 1.4mg/Kg body weight.

73. **Following the return of spontaneous circulation blood flow to the brain is characterised by:**

    A. A decrease in cerebral blood flow

    B. An increase in cerebral blood flow

    C. A loss of cerebral blood flow auto-regulation

D. Answers A and C are correct

E. Answers B and C are correct.

74. In post resuscitation care the greatest risk leading to mortality comes from:

A. Further myocardial infarcts

B. Hospital acquired infections

C. Neurological injuries

D. Undiagnosed injuries such as broken ribs sustained during CPR.

E. Airway obstruction from reaction to airway adjuncts or drugs used in resuscitation.

75. The ideal post resuscitation temperature can be achieved by:

A. Rapidly cooling the patient using wet towels and ice packs.

B. Slow and controlled cooling of the patient with blankets, pads and monitoring.

C. Recognizing that a target temperature is not the same as normothermia

D. Recognizing that normothermia must be achieved.

E. By using IV infusion of cold fluids and temperature monitoring.

76. The post resuscitation depletion in intravascular volume and vasodilation can be caused by:

A. Sepsis without a rise in temperature.

B. Sepsis but only if there is an accompanying rise in temperature.

C. The post-cardiac arrest syndrome.

D. Normal physiological reaction to a cardiac arrest.

E. None of the above, it would be caused by blood loss and shock.

77. In those patients who have been successfully resuscitated which of the following could be considered appropriate?

A. Simple discharge from hospital after 24 hours with a patient information leaflet on what to do if there are further problems.

B. Continued monitoring and then discharge when the heart rate has stabilized.

C. Referral to a cardiologist in a critical care unit for further investigations and the possibility of placing an implantable cardioverter defibrillator.
D. Referral to the patient's general medical practitioner so they might alter any medications, referral to a cardiologist or into critical care is seldom required and has survived.
E. The patient should be kept in hospital for several weeks or months until a care package is arranged with the social work department.

78. **After resuscitation from cardiac arrest, blood glucose should be maintained in which range?**
A. Between 2.0 mmol/L and 14.0 mmol/L
B. Between 3.0 mmol/L and 12.0 mmol/L
C. Above 4.0 mmol/L and up to 10.0 mmol/L
D. Between 5.0 mmol/L and 8.0 mmol/L
E. Between 6.0 mmol/L and 8.0 mmol/L

79. **With return to spontaneous circulation following cardiac resuscitation there is a risk of seizure, which of the following statements are correct?**
A. Seizures although noted are an incredibly rare event.
B. Seizures are a common event occurring in up to 1/3rd of all adult patients being resuscitated.
C. Seizures have a very limited effect on the cerebral metabolism.
D. Seizures have a profound effect increasing the cerebral metabolism by a factor of 3X and may result in cerebral injury.
E. Post anoxic seizures can be difficult to treat with phenytoin being particularly ineffective; drugs such as clonazepam, sodium valproate and levetiracetam are more successful.

80. **In the period following resuscitation which of the following statement s are correct?**
A. For most cardiac arrest survivors the neurological outcome is very good.

B. For a significant number of patients surviving a cardiac arrest cognitive and emotional problems with fatigue are common.
C. In over half of those who survive a cardiac arrest memory loss and cognitive deficit are seen and patients can benefit from a formal program of rehabilitation.
D. For those patients who do not survive a cardiac arrest organ donation should be considered and the relatives must be made aware of such an opportunity.
E. All of the above are correct.

Answers to Questions in Medical Emergencies

The Basic Approaches to Medical Emergencies:

1. E	6. C	11. D	16. E
2. E	7. B	12. E	17. D
3. B	8. C	13. E	18. B
4. E	9. E	14. D	19. B
5. E	10. E	15. D	20. (i) C 20. (ii) A

Immediate Life Support:

21. E	26. B	31. B	36. B D E
22. C D	27. E	32. A D	37. B
23. A B C E	28. D	33. B C E	38. A D
24. E	29. D	34. B	39. C D E
25. D	30. D	35. B D E	40. D E

Paediatric Immediate Life Support:

41. E	46. A (v)	47. C	52. A C
42. D	46. B (i)	48. B D	53. C D
43. C	46. C (ii)	49. D	54. A C E
44. C D E	46. D (iii)	50. C	55. E
45. E	46. E (iv)	51. A D E	56. D
57. A B D E	58. A D E	59. A C E	60. A B D E

Post Resuscitation Care:

61. E	66. B C D E	71. E	76. B C
62. D	67. E	72. C	77. C
63. E	68. E	73. E	78. C
64. C E	69. A B D	74. C	79. B D E
65. A C	70. A B C D E	75. B C E	80. E

Certificate of Enhanced CPD in Medical Emergencies

C U S P I D
Clinically Useful Safety Procedures In Dentistry

CPD Topic:	Medical Emergencies
Focussed subject:	

Enhanced CPD Record and Certificate for:

Name:	
GDC Number:	
Professional Role:	

Pages accessed:	
For the CPD Period:	
MCQ Questions answered:	
Enhanced CPD hours claimed:	

Signed: Date:	
Counter signed: Date:	
Name + GDC number:	

Please copy to add further focussed subject areas as required.

CUSPID Log sheet for Enhanced CPD in Medical Emergencies

Date and venue	Method eg: self study or training sessions	Topic(s) Covered	Pages studied:	MCQs used:	Reflection and areas for improvement? If so what?	CPD Hours	Signed

(Copy as necessary to add further CPD).

Total hours this page

Evaluation and Self Satisfaction Survey

CUSPID E-CPD in Medical Emergencies

Name:	
Date:	
Venue:	

Section A. Please consider the following statements and decide if they reflect your views.

Please score each statement from: 1 - Strongly Disagree to: 5 - Strongly Agree

1	This CPD has improved my knowledge of the subject.	1 2 3 4 5
2	This CPD has confirmed my perception of current best practise.	1 2 3 4 5
3	As a result of this CPD,701 I plan to make changes to my practice.	1 2 3 4 5
4	The learning aims and objectives for this CPD were appropriate.	1 2 3 4 5
5	The learning aims and objectives for this CPD were met.	1 2 3 4 5
6	I was given enough background information about this CPD.	1 2 3 4 5
7	I was satisfied with the educational standard of this chapter.	1 2 3 4 5
8	The CPD organisation and delivery was excellent.	1 2 3 4 5
9	The venue was appropriate and conducive to learning.	1 2 3 4 5
10	I would recommend this CPD to my colleagues.	1 2 3 4 5

Section B. Please answer each of the following questions:

1.	Is there any part of the CPD activity that you felt was particularly successful?
2.	Is there any part of the CPD activity that you felt needed improvement?
3.	If so, how would you like to see it improved?
4.	Do you have any other comments or suggestions relating to this CPD?

(For CPD to be verifiable the GDC state the opportunity to give feedback should be provided.)

Section C.
Please add your further notes and updates

Professional and Personal Development
in Medical Emergencies

CUSPID – Medical Emergencies Reflective Notes

Name:	
Date:	
Topic:	Medical Emergencies
Subject:	

The Main Points I have learned from this CPD activity:

1.	
2.	
3.	

Do these points have a relevance to my work?

Yes	
Possibly	
No	

The possible changes to improve safety for my patients and my profession:

1.	
2.	
3.	

On review the actual changes to my practise of dentistry were:

1.	
2.	
3.	

Verifiable Enhanced CPD Hours claimed for:

Preparation	
Activity	
Reflection	
Review	
Total hours:	

Name, GDC NumberSigned.	
Dated.	
Name, GDC Number Countersigned.	
Dated.	

223

CHAPTER TWO

Medicine and Drug Safety

CONTENTS

INTRODUCTION

This chapter will deal with those drugs you commonly use in the dental clinic and those you might frequently prescribe for your patient's use outside the clinic. Additionally, the actions of medicines your patient may be taking and the potential for their interactions with drugs you either administer or prescribe will be discussed in this chapter.

Even though, at the time of writing, the subject of drug safety and drug interaction does not form part of the core for your Enhanced Continuing Professional Development (CPD) for the General Dental Council (GDC), in the past, in practice; it has proven to be a safety critical subject. As such, it is important that you keep up to date with the latest guidelines and those regulations governing your administration of drugs. As the intensity of GDC interest in our clinical activity increases, from now onwards it would be prudent to maintain and retain records of how you continually improve your working knowledge in drug safety and drug interaction.

So that you are practicing to the best of your abilities and to the highest standards your patients deserve and your colleagues demand from you, your knowledge and skills in this subject must be:

I.   Maintained through frequent collegiate discussion, peer review and attendance on courses.
II. Updated regularly with those developments in this area affecting your clinical work.
III. Developed effectively in accordance with your professional associations and regulator.

As stated above, the General Dental Council has not yet stipulated that training in drug safety or drug interactions are either mandatory or need to be demonstrably undertaken within your five-year Enhanced CPD cycle either for Dentists or for Dental Care Professionals.

However, despite this omission, there remains a professional, an ethical and a regulatory responsibility to protect your patients from the adverse outcomes that could follow from inappropriate drug administration. With the absence of any legal or professional framework governing this subject, the accepted knowledge and guidelines that determine the drugs we can use and the quantities we can use them in will form the framework for this chapter.

You can therefore utilize such a framework to:

I. **Maintain.**
II. **Update**   } **Your working knowledge of this safety critical subject.**
III. **Develop**

By following the above, you will be able to demonstrate your enhanced continuing professional development ensuring your patients will have the best dental treatment in the safest possible clinical environment that you and your colleagues can provide.

In this chapter, the drugs most commonly used in general dental practice will be discussed, as will the drugs used in specialist sedation centres. There will be times when you, or your colleagues will refer patients for sedation and it is important that you know something of the sedative regimens and the framework of consent that determines the treatment options for your patients.

If you are practicing outside the UK or the EU, you should make yourself aware of the specific requirements for drug administration or prescription that your governing body or professional associations will demand from you. The professional practising standards outside the UK may well be different from those expected of you in the UK, by the GDC, the NHS and the Dental Faculties of the Royal Colleges of Surgeons or the Royal College of Anaesthetists.

Outside the UK, in Europe, the Commonwealth Countries and in North America, certain prescribing protocols and standards might well be collectively accepted as they are based on the firm clinical or epidemiological evidence that has been gathered in those jurisdictions and as a result they could differ and justifiably so; from those conclusions in prescribing practises we have arrived at in the UK.

With antimicrobial prophylaxis against bacterial endocarditis, the rest of the world differs from the UK. Whereas (for the UK) the most recent National Institute for Health and Care Excellence (NICE) guideline (CG 64 2008 updated in 2015) maintains the accepted position of there being absolutely no need for antimicrobial prophylaxis for adults and children with either structural cardiac defects or prosthetic valve replacement[1.] In contrast, in 2007, The American Dental Association (ADA), firmly supported by the American Heart Association (AHA) assured their members and their patients that in some cases antimicrobial prophylaxis should still be used[2].

Even with a dogmatic approach to drug administration and prescribing, this area of clinical practice is far from being universally accepted, or static. A recent survey of 5,500 dentists in the USA revealed that while over 75% of the respondents (and their patients) agreed with the recommendations of the ADA and AHA, some 70% of dental patients still took antibiotics even though the guidelines no longer recommended their doing so[3]. Adding another layer of complexity to the confusion, many of the antimicrobial drugs for antimicrobial prophylaxis were never approved for such use by the US Federal Drugs Administration (FDA) in the first place![4].

Some years after NICE blanket banned antimicrobial prophylaxis for infective endocardits in the UK, NICE announced a call for research on the subject[1]. Two years after the NICE guidelines were published, a "before and after" study into Infective Endocarditis (IE) noted no significant increase in IE cases. This reassuring result seemed to support the cessation of antimicrobial prophylaxis[5]. However, by 2015 there were increases in IE cases noted in Holland, where notably there is no absolute cessation of antimicrobial prophylaxis[6]. Following this finding, one French paper asked: Whether the discontinuation of prophylaxis in England was to blame?[7].

Placing the complexities of BREXIT and the European Community to one side, the most recent evidence seems to suggest there has been a significant increase in infective endocarditis cases in the UK, but it is still difficult (and perhaps too early) to establish whether there is a causal association of this finding with the 2008 NICE guideline (NICE as in NIHCE- UK, not NICE as in Nice- France)[8].

As our knowledge of the complex interaction of drug pharmacology, human physiology and microbial pathology continues to evolve, the evidence from clinical outcomes will ultimately determine those policies that will be rejected from those that will be implemented; that not so much influence but will adversely impact on the very ways and means with which we practice clinical dentistry.

As the example of antimicrobial prophylaxis has shown, there will be regional and administrative variations in research outcomes upon which guidelines are based that will add strength to those discussions we have with our patients, as we inform and recommend appropriate treatment plans to which they might consent.

We have a professional responsibility to contribute to the meetings and discussions from which the standards of dentistry in general and standards for drug use in particular will be created. This responsibility can only be maintained if we safeguard our right to actively participate in those advisory committees shaping clinical policy that will ultimately affect patient safety.

Another way in which we can uphold our professional responsibilities with drug safety is by keeping up to date with the latest developments in this subject, while anticipating those changes that will affect how we deliver care to our patients. With drug safety we have to accept; where needed and reject; where necessary those external influences of policy, administration and management that intrude daily into our clinical lives if we feel they are inappropriate to either the reasonable requests of our patients or the requirements of our profession. However, we can only act in this way if we are doing so from a position of informed professionalism and that position comes from the most up to date knowledge we can access.

By reading this chapter, together with the latest published guidelines and taking into account the administrative framework in your dental clinic, you will add further support to your already safe and effective work with your patients with regard to demonstrating your adherence to drug safety in dental practise.

Everyone who works in a clinical team should by now, either be trained and qualified or undergoing an approved training program leading to qualification and registration. At appropriate intervals after qualification and registration in the CPD cycle, all dental team members must undergo refresher training to maintain a comprehensive and contemporary working knowledge of the drugs we can administer and prescribe, together with those medicines our patients are taking, either by prescription, or self medication; be that for alleviation, recreation or addiction.

With drug administration, there are certain tasks that need to be learned and then carried out repeatedly, such as checking batch numbers of anaesthetics and their expiry dates or the potential for adverse action or interaction with a patient.

Such tasks are your responsibility, but they are only one essential part of a clinical skill-set in drug safety; a skill-set that you should continually adhere to, but additionally seek to improve upon. Ultimately, your understanding of drug safety, their actions and their interactions are for the protection of your dental patients, your colleagues and yourself.

By reading this chapter, together with the relevant and required regulations, you will build on the knowledge that you qualified with to maintain a safety critical approach for drug safety in your dental practice and in your practise of dentistry.

As a reminder, the GDC at the time of writing; still do not recommend within your 5 year enhanced CPD cycle that there should be any verifiable continuing education or professional development in this subject. Despite this, the Surgical Royal Colleges, and the Post Graduate Dental Deaneries in the UK do recommend training in this core clinical subject should be undertaken on a regular basis. Given the dynamic nature of developments in the pharmaceutical industry, combined with the rapidity of policies arising and being implemented, you should frequently visit and revisit this subject throughout your CPD cycle to keep up to date with the latest developments.

As mentioned in the previous section, if you choose to undertake ECPD in this area (although not yet mandatory) you must not cram all of your studying into one frenzied session before printing off a certificate to post off to the GDC. Acquiring information, especially if it forms the basis for your working knowledge in a clinical activity, particularly one that is so safety critical, such as medicines handling, dose calculations and drug administration, must be achieved in a methodical and timely manner.

It is a certainty that within every five-year cycle of CPD, frequent updates and new developments in drug safety contributing to the current best-accepted standard of care will take place. It remains your professional duty to your patients and to your colleagues that you keep up to date with those announcements in medicine safety, such as those issued from the Medicines and Healthcare products Regulatory Agency (MHRA) and the Department of Health (DOH), as they are made and to implement required changes in your practice in a timely manner.

By not following such an approach, your patients could be at risk from unwitting breaches in drug safety. In this regard, ignorance cannot be offered as a defence either to the GDC in their regulatory or disciplinary processes, even though paradoxically, the GDC have clearly stated by their own bizarre omission that drug safety is not (yet) a mandatory core CPD subject.

With respect to this issue, despite the GDC being clearly remiss in their duty, we remain fortunate in the UK, that it has been several years since an adverse event occurred in a dental practice arising from inappropriate drug administration. The most noteworthy example we must not forget and continue to learn from is the 1998 case of Darren Denholm. In this fatality, not only were drugs given inappropriately, there proved to be an inability of the attending medical and dental staff to work as a coherent team managing the physiological distress endured by a 10 year old boy due to the cardiac arrhythmias induced by a combination of halothane and adrenaline.

Darren Denholm died on the 9th October 1998 in a high street dental practice in Edinburgh, in part because of the failings of a GMC registered doctor to deliver a general anaesthetic correctly, together with the inability of a GDC registered dentist to recognize the signs of cardiac arrest. Neither doctor nor dentist fully appreciated the criticality of the situation facing them. During Darren's procedure, even though the dental nurse had correctly identified that a cardiac arrest was imminent because of inappropriate drug administration, neither the attending doctor nor the dentist correctly managed Darren's medical emergency and so an entirely avoidable but tragic outcome followed.

It would be easy to suggest this tragedy was a result of a failure to respond to an emergency and a lack of teamwork, but that is too easy. We should remember at that time, the other contributory parts. At that time, there was neither compulsory registration for dental nurses, nor a requirement to demonstrate that doctor, dentist or dental nurse had undertaken verifiable CPD for medical emergencies. However, not least in the 1990's in the UK, there was not the slightest concept of a dental team or even team training.

Rather, the failings go beyond the events that occurred in a dental clinic and they extend to the maladministration of two professionals by their professional regulators of medicine and of dentistry. The employing dentist had neither verified the adequacy of qualification, nor the currency of training that the anaesthetizing doctor had undertaken. He came from an agency that was similarly inattentive to these critical details. The profession's failure of Darren Denholm extends from the dental clinic in Edinburgh, where he suffered an agonizing death, all the way to London to the GMC and to the GDC. These two health care regulators, despite participating in a series of reports and recommendations into the safety of general anaesthesia and sedation (Poswillo in 1990, then Jackson in 1993) subsequently did little if anything to ensure their professionals involved in these activities would follow the recommendations of these two reports... until it was too late.

Following GMC and GDC disciplinary hearings, the doctor and dentists involved in this tragedy were erased and with that outcome, something of the dental profession's indifference towards the recommendations of earlier reports came to light.

Nearly three decades ago in 1990, the report of the Expert Working Party into General Anaesthesia, Sedation and Resuscitation in Dentistry was published that made some 50 recommendations aimed at reducing the risk of death, or of adverse health effects during dental treatment, including treatment under general anaesthesia[9]. This report was named after its chairman, Professor David Poswillo (1927- 2003).

Among the recommendations specifically aimed at dental practices were that: Standards should be set for dental anaesthetic practise, standards were to be set for equipment, for the facilities and for training. In addition, practice inspections and registrations were to take place. In the years following the Poswillo report, it became clear that implementation of the recommendations was neither comprehensive nor consistent. In three consecutive years in the 1990s (1993-1995) there were no deaths in primary dental care, which seemingly suggested the professional's acceptance of Poswillo. Then with a truly appalling disparity, the four subsequent years (1996–1999), saw eight deaths in primary dental care of which five were children[10].

Investigations into these deaths were critical of the care provided. There was little preoperative assessment and incorrect monitoring of electrical heart activity, blood pressure, oxygen and carbon dioxide levels, while resuscitation and specialist care transfer was delayed, with no formal or mandatory training in drug use.

A review at the time was striking, only a handful of dentists accounted for the majority of General Anaesthetic (GA) use in primary dental care. In the period from July to September 1999, just 45 dentists provided 69% of all GA's used in NHS general dental practice[10]. By today's standards, the numbers were astounding. Some 57,000 GA's were administered in dental practices from July to September 1998. One year later, following the death of Darren Denholm, an intervention from the Chief Medical and Dental Officers, coupled to the GDC issuing guidance in November 1998, resulted in the numbers of GA's falling to 12,000 (for the same quarter). Further recommendations from the GDC required the use of an appropriately trained medically qualified anaesthetist, with the development of protocols for transferring patients to a critical care facility in the event of an emergency[11].

Although Darren Denholm died on the 9th October 1998, the time limit by which all dental practices were to cease providing GA's would be 31st December 2001. In the three years following the 1998 GDC directive three more children died. These deaths were associated with lapses of standards in availability, maintenance and application of equipment of skills, or the administration of drugs[10].

Medical practitioners provided the anaesthesia in all of these cases (the dentist being the second appropriate person in accordance with Poswillo). However, it is unclear whether the Royal College of Anaesthetists' guidelines were followed. Manslaughter charges were brought by the police in one case with a practitioner being found guilty and being imprisoned.

From this brief introduction, you can see the profound importance of drug safety in the dental clinic. Adverse incidents are rare, the tragedy of (an avoidable) death in a dental surgery, rarer still. As we approach two decades since the last death from an adverse drug reaction in a dental clinic, dentistry has moved away from GA into safer multi-drug sedation regimens.

With the latest Standards for Conscious Sedation in Provision of Dental Care (2015) report of the Intercollegiate Advisory Committee for Sedation in Dentistry, we will be moving into an era of single drug and inhalation sedation treatments.

Indeed, we will be moving towards a future practicing culture that seeks to implement many more of David Poswillo's unfulfilled recommendations made some thirty years ago.

It is quite incredible to reflect on the £20 Million of NHS funds invested in 1990 to achieve safer practices in dentistry. Very few of the recommendations made then were ever put into practice in a timely manner. As a result, children continued to die in dental surgeries from a lack of training in drug safety.

Setting these events to one side and returning to today's practise of dentistry. If you work in the UK, your dental clinic will be Care Quality Commission (CQC) registered. As such, your workplace will comply with the CQC Safety Standard. This standard should extend to medicine handling and drug safety. However, in common with an absence of any clear GDC guidelines covering this subject, there might well be no training schedule ensuring that you or members of your dental team undergo regular revision of drug safety or administration.

Notwithstanding this, there should be sufficient time within your working day so that every week you should be able to set aside a few minutes for revision of this subject working through the framework provided by this chapter. By doing so, the subject matter can be covered well within your 5-year CPD time limit while attending to your other professional commitments.

The educational aims, objectives and outcomes in this chapter

Maintain, update and develop your active working knowledge of drug safety with their actions and interactions as they apply to your work in clinical dentistry. By using the data in this chapter and the reference sources cited you should be up to date with the latest information in this field. There are clear aims and outcomes listed below. The CPD you complete in this chapter will comply with the GDC's requirements for verifiable and enhanced, but not yet mandatory continuing professional development in drug safety.

The CPD that you undertake in this chapter should also focus on those subjects you have identified as learning requirements from your Professional Development Plan (PDP). These could be the administration of drugs and prescribing medicines in general practice or delivery of those drugs used in specialist or referral practices, such as those used in: Conscious; IV or RA (Inhalation) Sedation.

The aim

The educational aim in completing this chapter, will allow you to broaden your knowledge, and understanding, enhancing your clinical safety skills in drug use.

The objective

The objective of this chapter is to provide you with both a core of knowledge and an understanding of drug safety in the clinical environment. By undertaking CPD in this subject, your working knowledge of the actions and interactions of medicines and drugs commonly used in clinical practise will be enhanced. Acquiring such knowledge should lessen the risk of drug related incidents or accidents occurring.

While undertaking your CPD, you will be adhering to those fundamental standards determined by two regulators, the CQC (Safety) and the GDC Principle One: Put patient's interests first and Standard 1.5.4: The recording of all patient safety incidents, reporting them promptly to the appropriate national body. Together with GDC Principle Eight: To raise concerns of patients at risk and Standard 8.1: Putting patients' safety first.[12]

A further objective is to develop your knowledge of the reporting systems to the Medicines and Health Care Regulatory Products Authority (MHRA), or the National Patient Safety Agency (NPSA), should an adverse incident related to drug use occur. Alternatively, where appropriate, you should seek advice and guidance from your professional associations such as the BDA or BADN if there should be any concerns about performance or practice in relation to medicine handling or drug safety in your clinical workplace.

The theoretical knowledge gained in completing this chapter should be combined with practical work-based experience and training. By doing this, you will gain the most benefit from theoretical but still verifiable CPD, together with the practical drug safety and medicine handling tasks that you undertake with your dental team members.

In addition to the professional and educational benefits for yourself and your team members, in completing this chapter, you will be able to attain and maintain an improved level of service, providing your patients with dentistry that is both safe and up to date.

The outcomes

The outcomes of this chapter are for you to revise and update where necessary, the following:

I.   Enhance your working knowledge of medicine handling and drug safety.
II. Revise your understanding of the best-accepted practices for the drugs you use.
III. Know the importance of drug actions.
IV. Revise your knowledge of the types of drug interactions.
V.   Appreciate and understand the actions to take in the event of adverse interactions.

Further expected outcomes in this chapter

Actively read this chapter, making notes and revisions, updating your knowledge where necessary. To be aware of the latest guidelines on drug safety contained in the British National Formulary (BNF), your professional associations (BDA or BADN) and the post graduate Dental Faculties in the Royal Surgical Colleges.

Correctly answer all the questions at the end of this chapter to demonstrate that you have read and understood the principles of drug safety, their actions and interactions in the dental surgery.

Demonstrate your participation in regular group training exercises, with other members of your dental team to demonstrate your knowledge and practical skills can be maintained to an appropriate level.

Quality Control

If the questions you answer are marked by a third party, with your regular training in drug safety being logged and the results from your performance in these exercises being audited, together with documented training by an appropriately qualified trainer, then working through this chapter will count towards your verifiable and enhanced CPD.

The information in this chapter should be discussed in your regular dental practice meetings. By doing so and with your personal reading, this chapter should also count towards your personal development plan in this safety critical area of clinical practise.

References: Introduction to Medicine and Drug Safety

1. NICE Prophylaxis against infective endocarditis: antimicrobial prophylaxis against infective endocarditis in adults and children undergoing interventional procedures. NICE Guidelines (CG64) Published March 2008 Updated 2015. Available online: http://www.nice.org.uk/guidance/cg64
    Accessed October 2015.

2. Wilson W, Taubert KA, Gewitz M, Lockhart PB, Baddour LM et al. Prevention of infective endocarditis: guidelines from the American Heart Association: a guideline from the American Heart Association Rheumatic Fever, Endocarditis and Kawasaki Disease Committee, Council on Cardiovascular Disease in the Young, and the Council on Clinical Cardiology, Council on Cardiovascular Surgery and Anesthesia, and the Quality of Care and Outcomes Research Interdisciplinary Working Group. JADA 2008 Jan; 139 Suppl:3S-24S. Available Online:
    http://jada.ada.org/article/S0002-8177(14)62745-8/pdf
    Accessed October 2015.

3. Lockhart PB, Hanson NB, Ristic H, Menezes AR and Baddour L. Acceptance among and impact on dental practitioners and patients of American Heart Association recommendations for antibiotic prophylaxis. J Am Dent Assoc. 2013 Sep; 144 (9):1030-5.

4. Enzler MJ, Berbari E and Osmon DR. Antimicrobial Prophylaxis in Adults. Mayo Clinic Proceedings. 2011; 86(7):686-701. Available online: http://www.ncbi.nlm.nih.gov/pmc/articles/PMC3127564/
    Accessed October 2015.

5. Thornhill MH, Dayer MJ, Forde JM, et al. Impact of the NICE guideline recommending cessation of antibiotic prophylaxis for prevention of infective endocarditis: before and after study. BMJ. 2011; 342:d2392. Available online from:
    http://www.ncbi.nlm.nih.gov/pmc/articles/PMC3086390/
    Accessed October 2015.

6. Krul MMG, Vonk ABA, Cornel JH. Trends in incidence of infective endocarditis at the Medical Center of Alkmaar. Neth Heart J. 2015;

23:xx. doi: 10.1007/s12471-015-0743-0. Available online from: http://www.ncbi.nlm.nih.gov/pmc/articles/PMC4608930/ Accessed October 2015.

7. Botelho-Nevers E. Increase of infective endocarditis incidence: Is the discontinuation of prophylaxis in England to blame? Med Mal Infect. 2015 Jun; 45 (6):241.

8. Dayer MJ, Jones S, Prendergast B, Baddour LM, Lockhart PB and Thornhill MH. Incidence of infective endocarditis in England, 2000-13: a secular trend, interrupted time-series analysis. Lancet. 2015 Mar 28; 385 (9974):1219-28.

9. General Anaesthesia, Sedation and Resuscitation in Dentistry – Report of an Expert Working Party prepared for the Standing Dental Advisory Committee. (March 1990)

10. A Conscious Decision. A Report of an expert group chaired by the Chief Medical and Dental Officer. Department of Health. July 2000. Available online from: http://webarchive.nationalarchives.gov.uk/20130107105354/ http://www.dh.gov.uk/prod_consum_dh/groups/dh_digitalassets/ @dh/@en/documents/digitalasset/dh_4019200.pdf Accessed October 2015.

11. Maintaining Standards. Guidance to Dentists on Professional and Personal Conduct. General Dental Council. London (November 1998 and May 1999).

12. General Dental Council. Standards for the dental team. London: GDC, 2013.

The Basics of Drug Safety

Volumes weights and measures

In your dental surgery, all drugs that you might:

I.   Prescribe orally, the antimicrobials, antibiotics or fluorides
II. Apply topically, the proprietary eutectic mixes of local anaesthetics.
III. Inject through the oral mucosa to infiltrate or block nerves to achieve anaesthesia.
IV. Inject intravenously or spray intranasally to deliver a drug for sedation
V.   Or deliver as a gas via nasal mask; Nitrous Oxide for inhalation sedation.

Will have both volume and weight noted in the metric system using SI units.

At all times when treating your patients you should be attentive to the measures of any drug you administer or prescribe, together with an awareness of those doses and routes of administration of the drugs your patients have been taking from their doctor.

The units of volume are the:
Litre (**L**) and millilitre (**mL**)
1 Litre = 1,000ml

While the units of weight are the:
Gram (**g**), the milligram (**mg**), the microgram (**μg**) and the nanogram (**ng**)
1 Gram = 1,000mg, 1mg = 1,000ug and 1 ug = 1,000ng.

Many of the drugs you will administer or prescribe to patients will have their dose expressed in volume or weight in mgs, µgm or mls and others you will see in specialist practice or hospital departments will be measured in terms of their pharmacological properties.

The **International Unit or IU**, is commonly used to measure the power or action of many drugs our patients take, therefore in dental practice we should be aware of the IU. The volume or weight of an International Unit will vary from drug to drug.

For example, it is possible to measure the bactericidal effect of an antibiotic in IU's as well as mgs or mls. As an example: In a test aimed at eliminating a pre-determined bacterial species: If one antibiotic is mixed so that 5ml contains 100,000 IU and another antibiotic is mixed so that 5 mL contains 300,000 IU, the second drug is then 3X more potent than the first drug in our assay. <u>Even though their weight and their volume are the same.</u>

Commonly prescribed drugs such as Insulin, Heparin and Penicillin all of which we have seen in the dental clinic, either through our own prescribing or that from our medical colleagues can be measured both in IU's or in mgs/ mls. In addition, International Units can be applied to Vitamins, Hormones, and Blood Clotting Factors too. However, it is very important to note that the **volume, weight or unit of one drug is usually different** from another. While 1 mL of an antibacterial drug may contain 100 IU's, 1 ml of an antiviral may contain 100,000 IU's.

When dealing with, or handling any drug, it is important to both carefully and clearly note four further types of measure we may frequently see in clinical practice:

1. The Ratio. Concentrations expressed as ratios are most commonly used with local anaesthetics identifying the amount of adrenaline or other active agent they contain. These ratios are predetermined by the manufacturer. However, we do need to know what this ratio actually means in terms of the safe concentrations or the maximum number of local anaesthetic cartridges we can use for all our patients. We shall return to this in detail in the subsequent section on local anaesthetics.

2. The Percentage. Concentrations expressed in percentages are the number of grams dissolved in 100mls. 1% w/v = 1 gram in 100ml. In the dental clinic, the most common use of such measurements will be in those medications we use for endodontic disinfection. Chemical irrigation with Sodium Hypochlorite in a concentration range of 0.5% to 5.0% has proven to be a useful adjunct to mechanical debridement of the root canal system[1]. A great variety of chlorine bleaches are available worldwide, being produced in different strengths. Standard or general-purpose household bleach may vary between 5% and 15% active chlorine content or base strength[2,3].

One essential task of the dental nurse is to dilute Sodium hypochlorite with sterilized distilled water to give the required concentration for intracanal applications (or for surgery disinfection). With this simple addition-dilution the following reaction occurs:

$$Na\ OCl + H_2O => HO\ Cl + Na\ OH$$

While concentrations of between 0.5% and 5.0% Na OCl are used for intracanal endodontic debridement, sodium hypochlorite concentrations of 0.5% and 0.05% (wet contact for 10 minutes) are recommended for disinfecting contaminated clinical surfaces[2].

Concentrations of 0.5% are equal to 5,000 Parts Per Million (PPM) Free Active Chlorine (FAC) and 5.0 % is equivalent to 50,000 PPM FAC respectively. Assuming the starting concentration of the bleach is 5.0%, the 0.5% solution is achieved by the dental nurse diluting in a ratio of 1:9, bleach to water. With other concentrations to achieve the required application, the following simple formula can be used by the dental nurse:

$$\text{Total Parts Water} = \left[\frac{\text{\% Bleach Concentration}}{\text{Desired \% Dilution}} \right] - 1$$

In the UK, a common proprietary brand of 1% Na OCl and 16.5% NaCl is used in dilutions of 1:4 for wound management; this has 0.25% w/v Cl or 2,500 PPM FAC.

3. Parts Per Million (PPMs) we most frequently see this with any medication containing Fluoride. You and your patients will have used Fluoride in topical applications eg: toothpastes, varnishes, tablets or mouthwash, most usually:

I.   Proprietary toothpastes can contain Fluoride from 500 PPM to 1,500 PPM (0.05% to 0.15%).

II.   Prescription toothpastes can contain 2,800 to 5,000PPM Na F (= 0.619% and 1.1%) Fluoride.

III.   Topical Fluoride Varnish ranges from 8,000 to 56,300 PPM (0.8% to 5.6%) Fluoride.

IV.   Sodium Fluoride Tablets can be 1.1 mgs /500 ugm or 2.2mgs/1.0ugm Fluoride.

V.   Sodium Fluoride Mouthwashes can be 0.2% or 2.0% applied for 1 minute only[4].

With both sodium hypochlorite and fluoride, a good working knowledge of the concentrations used and what this actually means in terms of clinical effectiveness is crucial. The dental literature contains a considerable number of reports of tissue damage and injuries caused by concentrated hypochlorite being inadvertently injected into the peri-radicular spaces during root canal procedures[5,6]. Although rare and seldom life threatening, destruction of intraoral soft tissues, periradicular vasculature and cancellous bone can result from extremely low concentrations of sodium hypochlorite[7,8,9]. In greater concentrations, a severe inflammatory response with significant morbidity serves as a warning that the correct dilution of hypochlorite must be applied with an appropriate technique at all times. The results of a survey of 314 Endodontic specialists in the USA, was revealing. Over 1/3 reported hypochlorite accidents. This finding serves as a reminder of the importance of using the correct operative techniques, but also the need to ensure the correct concentration of hypochlorite is used to begin with[10].

With topical fluoride applications and prescriptions; should excessive quantities of fluoride be ingested it is important to note the possibility of toxicity or poisoning. The most common cause of this relatively rare problem, (3,000 cases per year in the USA[11]) is the unsupervised young child who eats their toothpaste, their resulting gastro intestinal distress being a sign of fluoride toxicity.

While the application of fluoride remains a valid dental public health measure, cases of fluoride toxicity are nevertheless still possible. In order to reduce the incidence from low risk to no risk, your administration of the correct and appropriate doses of fluoride-containing prescriptions should be carefully considered for all patients and by all members of the dental team.

4. Drug Dose and Volume. Not so much in clinical dentistry, often in clinical medicine, and always in paediatric dentistry, you will need to prescribe an amount of drug that is determined by the child's body weight. (We will return to this concept in the next part of this section). Paediatric doses are usually expressed as:

Mg/Kg or ug/Kg.

As with local anaesthetic cartridges, the concentration of the commonly used medications is predetermined, so calculating the dose required is simple multiplication. In the interests of good practice your calculations should be present in the notes.

There are certain medications where the dose required is a fraction of the concentration stated on the label. Once the dose has been calculated the volume required needs to be worked out. Don't panic (as with diluting concentrations of hypochlorite) the formula for doing so is straightforward:

$$\text{Volume needed} = \left[\frac{\text{Concentration Required}}{\text{Concentration Presented}}\right] \times \text{Volume Present}$$

Another set of measurements we should be aware of but not necessarily have an everyday working knowledge of are concentrations expressed in molarity. A mole is the unit of measurement for a substance, the concentration of a solution is then expressed as its molarity.

5. The Molar concentration is a measure of the <u>concentration</u> of a <u>solute</u> in a <u>solution</u>. The commonly used unit for clinical applications is the millimole, this being 1/1,000 of a mole in 1 Litre of water.

6. Electrolyte concentrations for intravenous fluids are expressed in Millimoles per Litre. The following table is useful:

Intravenous Infusion	Concentration in Millimoles per Litre				
	Na^+	K^+	$HCO3^-$	Cl^-	Ca^{2+}
Normal Plasma Values	142	4.5	26	103	2.5
Normal Saline Sodium Chloride Values	150			150	

In clinical dentistry, we will most commonly see molarity being used with Normal Saline. Normal Saline is used for wound irrigation whereas Sterile Saline is used for Intravenous applications. Both have concentration of 9 gms of NaCl dissolved in 1 Litre of sterile H_2O. From Chemistry principles:

I.   The molecular weight of Na Cl is 58.5 gms/ mole => 1 Mole of Na Cl weighs 58. 5 gms.

II. 1 Litre of Normal Saline contains 9 gms of NaCl. So: 9/58.5 => 0.154 moles/litre of NaCl

III. Na Cl + H20 => Na+ + Cl- is 2 osmolar.

IV. Normal Saline contains 154 millimoles/Litre of Na+ and 154 millimoles/Litre of Cl-

V.   Normal Saline at 0.9% therefore contains 308 millimoles/Litre of NaCl.

At every dental appointment, the updating of your patient's first medical history will uncover not only those drugs, both prescribed or acquired they may have taken between dental visits, but those changes in established medications or the start of new ones, will alert you to variations in the progression or regression of diseases or conditions your patients present with.

With your enquiries delivered professionally, you will become acutely aware of the chronic state of health or illness of your patient. In addition, your questions about your patients medications, is one of the most effective ways that your patients will communicate their innermost medical matters to you. Very often, when asking if a patient has any heart, chest or lung, troubles, an often heard (and in some cases, an undeserved) retort from the patient is:

"What's that got to do with my mouth? I've only come to get measured for a new set of dentures"

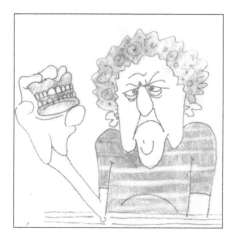

Whereas asking about their medication has the desired effect of revealing drugs that are being taken for heart, chest or lung troubles. The side effects of these may result in a dry mouth, the dentures being poorly retained and the request for new ones to be made.

Far less common than the patient who is cardiovascularly compromised are those who are immuno- compromised. In such cases, you need to be aware of the risk of drug interactions causing a complex of problems for the patient's medical teams to resolve.

The patients will neither thank you, nor think much of your clinical skills if you engage in reckless polypharmacy by prescribing for localized dental conditions while not considering the impact of your prescribing on the bigger medical and systemic picture.

In those patients with immune related illnesses, strongly associated with or arising from HIV and AIDS, tactful professional enquiries into medications being taken, without asking:

"Why are these drugs being taken?"

Often reveal much more than open questions on whether your patient has Hepatitis B, C or HIV, to which a refusal to answer such questions is the inevitable, perhaps justifiable, but regrettable response, to your: "Why?"

No matter how well meant, your: Why? Nearly always sounds like a reproach, leaving you in the dark, your nurse in the lurch and your patients with the hump.

Drug administration and the administration of drugs

In your work, you can administer medicines to your patients either internally or externally. Surprisingly the most common route of drug application in dentistry is the external application. Of course it is, when we consider; the sheer quantity of toothpaste, mouthwash and gels we prescribe adding to the mass of drugs our patients take.

Even tooth bleaching is an externally applied process, although it exerts an internal influence in teeth! Other frequent external drug applications in dentistry include the antifungal and antiviral preparations and the commonly used obtundant dressings containing Zinc Oxide Eugenol or Iodine, Butamben and Eugenol. All of these are delivered externally albeit in close proximity to the tooth pulp or the alveolar bone of a dry socket.

Following this route, are the internal deliveries of medicines. These can be anything from the oral prescription to injections given either intra orally or intravenously and the inhalation or intranasal delivery of sedative agents.

With both routes of drug delivery, there are defined safety parameters that must be followed.

SOPs CQC and the GDC!

From your undergraduate (dentist) or pre-registration (dental nurse) teaching and after a good length of time in practice, it will feel like these Standard Operating Procedures (SOPs) have been welded into your brain-box and not only can you complete them with your eyes shut, you will, after many years still be doing so correctly albeit with your eyes open.

In many cases, these SOPs are common sense and second nature; *eg*: looking for damaged or open packaging, checking your drugs are in date and <u>perhaps:</u> clearly writing into the patient records, both batch number and expiry date for the medicines and drugs you will be using along with noting down any change in the patient's medication at every visit.

You will also be aware of the importance in not deviating from your learned SOPs but such adherence must not be blind. If you believe your procedures could be improved upon, or you have the slightest nagging doubt about a bad habit that has somehow crept unseen into your work ....

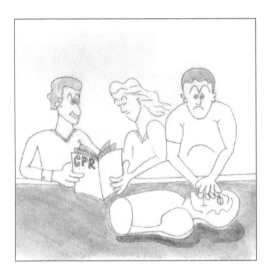

If you have questions, doubts or fears; then raising concerns where necessary with your colleagues, their respecting your unease and for them to act accordingly is a professional duty expected by both the GDC and the CQC.

In turn, we would expect the GDC and CQC to respect those who approach them with concerns too...

Your observance of drug safety begins with your purchase, storage and administration (covering the prescription and dispensing) of drugs in your dental surgery, it also extends to the local pharmacy (chemist in the UK), where your patient will collect their prescriptions.

The clear legal requirements and restrictions for drug purchasing, storage, delivery, use and disposal are overseen by both the GDC and the CQC in the standards they have laid down.

In your dental team, only the dentist registered with the GDC is legally entitled to prescribe anything from the British National Formulary (BNF: www.bnf.org)[12].

However, if you work within the National Health Service (NHS), dental prescribing is restricted to those drugs contained within the List of Dental Preparations in the Dental Practitioners' Formulary section (DPF) of the BNF, which is updated every six months.

The latest prescribing information is accessible from this source, both online and in print. In addition to the BNF there is a BNF C (Children's) formulary providing essential practical information for all who are involved with paediatric prescribing. The BNF C is updated annually[13].

In the UK, a dentist can prescribe additional drugs listed within the BNF, however the responsible duty is for the dentist to follow the guidance from colleagues in local pharmacy committees together with updates from the NICE Supplements and at all times, only prescribe within a range of competencies as applied to the clinical practice of dentistry.

If you feel the urge to prescribe out-with these parameters, then 37 Wimpole Street will provide a salutary lesson. The filing cabinets there are overflowing with their never-ending cases, now online for us to inspect.

The lamentable outcomes of the GDC's Fitness to Practice Hearings should give you an indication of what invariably happens to those who indulge in recreational prescribing.

Whenever we need to consult the BNF, we should use the most recent edition. We need to be aware that prescribing for some patient groups, including the elderly, patients who are pregnant and nursing mothers will most likely differ from the fit, well and healthy patients we safely treated in dental schools and the time we were sheltered throughout our Vocational Training.

The BNF is suitable for informing almost all dental practitioners of their needs in the primary care sector. The data it contains, applies to all patients, including adults, children and those with special needs whom we might treat in general practice.

However, those dental specialists in secondary care with their clinical expertise often prescribe a wider range of drugs in a broader variation of regimens than their colleagues in primary care and often do so with unlicensed and off-label applications. In such cases, the BNF provides the basis but not the authority for a clinician's work.

In secondary hospital care, the balance of risk v benefit when prescribing for patients with complex conditions is not weighed up in the same way as a dentist who operates alone in general practice, but rather such tasks are undertaken in consultation with a team of medical and surgical specialists. Such prescribing is often for patients who are at best in critical states of health or at worst approaching the end of a life limiting disease process or in palliative care. In dental practice, we should be cautiously aware of our patients with complex drug regimens and observe the following three principles:

I. **We must not alter the prescription a medical colleague has authorized for a patient.**

II. **Nothing we prescribe should interfere with a medical colleague's prescription.**

III. **However there may be times when we need to treat the patient and not the diagnosis and placing the patient first could mean altering a doctor's prescription.**

Although the third principle is incredibly rare, above all else it is the patient, who must ALWAYS come first, neither the doctor, nor the nurse and certainly not a set of local rules.

As a dental professional while you might not be medically qualified, you are surgically qualified and clinically experienced and this should never be forgotten.

While the drug interaction borne of ignorance is at worst negligent or at best forgivable, altering an established drug regimen is at best considered the illegal practice of medicine, while at worst, discourteous. While your medical colleagues will forgive you for many things, including (possibly) illegally practicing their profession, they will seldom, if ever forgive or forget your discourtesy in attempting to do things better than them, even if you are successful in doing so.

The first two principles will apply to almost all medical specialists and most hospital dentists, while the third principle must be used judiciously and only in an emergency; in those circumstances where doing nothing would place the patient at risk of harm or death.

Antibiotic use or antibiotic misuse?

For our general medical practitioner colleagues, with their uninhibited enthusiasm (un)helpfully prescribing antibiotics for tooth aches, the root cause often remaining unknown, before getting them around to the subject of antibiotic stewardship, we might consider the following:

In 2008/9 the UK press began reporting the findings of surveillance reviews into antibiotic prescribing patterns[14]. Among the headline grabbing news, the following could be deduced:

I.   More antibiotics were prescribed in Britain than in nearly half of the other EC states.
II. The UK has one of the highest rates of antibiotic resistance among European countries.
III. In 2008, 38 Million prescriptions were written in England alone.
IV. Resulting in a cost to the NHS of some £175 Million.
V.   In 2008 on average, one prescription was issued every 1.2 seconds!

Such data followed from statistical reporting from the European Centre for Disease Prevention and Control (ECDC). Their first pan-European report of 2010; Surveillance of Antimicrobial Consumption in

Europe, comprehensively demonstrated the patterns of those providing and receiving, not only antibiotics, but the full range of antimicrobials including antiviral and antifungal medication too.

From this report (updated in 2013) the following results are interesting. Whereas most countries such as Lithuania now report a decreasing consumption in antibiotics from 19.7 Defined Daily Doses (DDD) per 1,000 patients/day in 2009, to 12.7 DDD in 2010.

In contrast, the UK displays the largest increase in community use of antibiotics with 18.6 DDD per 1,000 patients/day in 2010, compared to 17.3 DDD per 1,000 patients/day reported for 2009. In the hospital setting, antibiotic use was in the order of 10 magnitudes lower than community use. While Penicillin remains the most commonly (mis) used antibiotic in the EC, the UK is among the highest consumer for Tetracyclines and Sulfonamide antibiotics in the EC[15]. By 2013/14 the figures for antibiotic use in the UK had increased to 41.6 Million prescriptions with a reported cost to the UK NHS of £192 Million. It was estimated that ¼ of those prescriptions, some 10 Million were unnecessary[16].

These unsafe habits are not limited to general medical practice alone. In dentistry, every year some 3 Million prescriptions for antibiotics are handed over to demanding patients. This represents just under 10% of the total number of all prescriptions. At best, these antibiotics are given in the absence of any clear indications for doing so, at worst, in clear breach of guidelines or best clinical practice. Such prescribing patterns have undoubtedly influenced the emergence of a 10 fold increase in Penicillin resistant strains in dental abscesses (5% to 55% in one decade), contributing in a small but significant way to the deaths occurring at least once a month in UK hospitals from the unsuccessful management of dento-facial infections[17].

In view of these developments, if we choose to treat a patient medically, rather than surgically, *ie:* prescription rather than incision, then we must consider all factors relative to the patient, followed by all factors relative to the species of infective organism we wish to eliminate or control. The drug options available depend firstly on the information from the medical history taken for each patient at every visit and secondly from the results of laboratory testing of microbiological samples taken from the patient. The first of these is almost always done, the second of these is almost always never done and so our start point for appropriate prescribing is less than ideal. This isn't necessarily game-over, but we must bear this in mind when working out the doses and duration of the drug we intend to prescribe.

The following are important medical factors we must consider and the questions we ought to ask from the patient at each visit:

I.   Is there a history of susceptibility to infection?
II. Are there documented allergies?
III. Is there impairment of the hepatic or renal system?
IV. If so, is there an impact on the cardiovascular system from pathology or medication?
V.   Is the patient male or female, underweight or overweight?

From this list, you can see the need for not only standardizing the measurement of drugs we give but for standardizing the measurements for the patient we give them too. Additionally if female:

I.   Is the patient taking an Oral Contraceptive?
II. Is the patient at present; pregnant?
III. Or breast feeding?

In addition for all patients:

IV. Is there any inability to take a medication orally or through another route?
V.   Is the patient otherwise fit, well and healthy?

Once the medical history is completed, we can then turn to the matter of what do we know about the likely organism and its antibiotic sensitivity? (Assuming it is bacterial). In all likelihood, with most dento-facial infections, in the absence of bacteriological testing, we will know very little of the nature of the infecting organism. If we are to prescribe an antibiotic in favour of incision and drainage, there has to be a defined need to do this. Such a need could be mandated by a clinical microbiologist issuing their recommendations on the basis of culture tests on clinical samples sent to them.

Blind antibiotic prescribing is no longer acceptable

In any event, local policies will be in force to limit the drugs we can use, in an attempt to reduce or limit the emergence of resistant bacterial strains, while attempting to achieve control of our clinical cases in the most economical, efficient and expeditious way possible for patient, practitioner and provider (the NHS if in the UK).

To commence antibiotic treatment we need to:

I.   Eliminate the chance that a viral or fungal infection is the causative organism.
II. Obtain the results of culture tests from clinical samples
III. Use specific doses of narrow-spectrum, rather than broad-spectrum antibiotics.
IV. Both dose and duration are calculated from measurements of the patient eg: weight or BMI.
V.   The route of administration, either IV or Oral will depend on the severity of the infection.

Only when all of the above have been considered should we then go ahead and prescribe antibiotics for the dental patient. Once a prescription has been issued, the story does not end there and we must follow up the patient to ensure the infection is responding to the dose of antibiotic given for the next 48 hours. In dental practice, this means recall and review in 2 days. If there is no change in either the symptoms the patient reports, or the clinical signs we observe and compare in the notes, then further bacteriological testing is required to investigate any causes, complications and co-factors, such as:

I. Was there an incorrect diagnosis?

> It frequently happens especially if medical microbiology were not consulted.

II. Is there poor host resistance or impaired immunity?

> Sometimes these are known to have been overlooked.

III. Is there poor compliance?

> Patients are great at complaining, then not taking the medicines we give them.

IV. Is there a need to combine antibiotics?

> Grouping Penicillin with Metronidazole results in a powerful bactericidal synergy.

V. The need for incision and drainage?

> This should always have been considered before antibiotics are prescribed.

The rise of antibiotic resistance

In 1945, Alexander Fleming forewarned that exposing bacteria to sub-optimal doses of Penicillin could lead to their developing resistance. In the 70 years following the discovery of antibiotics, this phenomenon is now recognized and well established. As antimicrobial resistance continues to rise, the discovery of new treatments to deal with it falls. Despite Fleming's warning and our growing understanding of resistance, dealing with this problem has proved elusive. Convenience, laziness, and perverse financial incentives from the pharmaceutical companies all conspire to nullify attempts to stop the emergence of bacterial resistance[18].

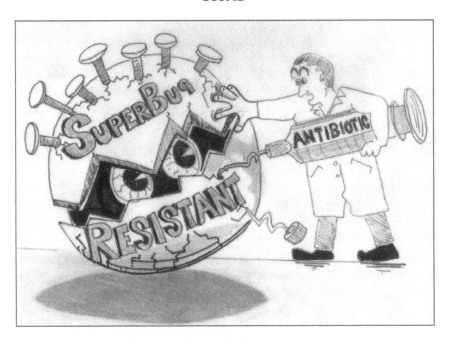

In response to the relentless increase in bacterial resistance, against a downward development rate of new antibiotics, novel methods with which existing medications can be used effectively must now be implemented. Every day, patients continue to suffer lingering morbidity frequently ending in mortality, from bacterial infections, against which there is no longer an effective treatment. In response, existing antibiotics should only be deployed against those infections a patient demonstrably has and never against those, either they think, or we think they might have.

<u>If we are not involved in creating new drugs, then we must be involved in conserving existing ones.</u>

In contrast to our medical colleagues cleaning out their clinics by waiving pads filled with antibiotic prescriptions at waiting rooms full of hypochondriacs, (some 50% of hospital prescriptions for antibiotics are unnecessary[19]), in dentistry we must be more effective in dealing with our case-work and we must do so with more respect for our patients than our medical colleagues seem to have for theirs. Which, given the ratio of prescriptions issued for doctors to dentists, versus their relative numbers, is something that is perhaps already happening.

In the USA, tens of thousands of patients are dying every year from infections caused by antibiotic resistant microorganisms. In the past 2 decades, only 2 new antibiotics have been approved for use. The Infectious Disease Society of America has now called for 10 new antibiotics to be in use by 2020 and for a global commitment to support this goal[20]. Our part in this global commitment to clinical safety is the upkeep of our measured use of antibiotics. There are now several programs under an Umbrella of Antibiotic Stewardship. This has been defined as:

I.   The optimal selection, dosage, and duration of antimicrobial treatment.
II. Resulting in the best clinical outcome for the treatment.
III. Or where necessary the prevention of infection.
IV. This should have minimal toxicity to the patient.
V.   Together with minimal impact on subsequent bacterial resistance[21].

Applying these principles to safe antibiotic prescribing in dentistry, we might take the proposals of Joseph and Rodvold and who wrote about the 4 D's of optimal antimicrobial therapy: Right Drug, Right Dose, De-escalation to pathogen-directed therapy, and Right Duration of therapy[22] and apply these, to form our own 5D approach to Dental Antibiotic Stewardship:

The 5 D's of Dental Prescribing

I. Deduce	Is the condition actually caused by a bacterium? Alternatively, is there another reason for the infection against which antibiotics are ineffective? If so then we do not use antibiotics
II. Define	If we are certain that a bacterial infection is present, then medical microbiology must be involved in the selection of a specific narrow spectrum antibiotic they will consider for our patient.
III. Direct	With the results of medical microbiology, might a surgical intervention directed locally, still be more effective than the ineffective use of systemic antibiotics, with risks of side effects? Incision and drainage of an abscess rather than prescription
IV. Diminish	If we need an antibiotic, then prescribe with regard to medical microbiology recommending the optimum dose for the minimum duration and we do so with respect to the patient's Body Mass Index (BMI) if this is applicable for the drug of choice.
V. Deliver	Clear unambiguous instructions on how the patient is to take the drug must be given. Any surplus drugs must be disposed of. You must review the effectiveness of any drug you give at the end of treatment.

Antibiotic stewardship

If antibiotic stewardship is to work in dentistry, then the dentist and patient need to work together to prevent antibiotics from being misused either through the patient's inappropriate demands, or through the prescriber's over reliance on an unsuitable antibiotic. Following such an accord, for a patient who needs (not wants) an antibiotic, then the most effective one should be used in a regimen measured specifically for that patient. By achieving these aims, we might well be on the way towards a significant reduction in the development of bacterial resistance.

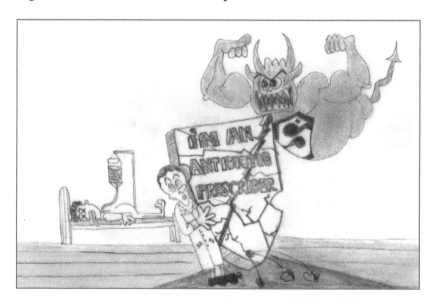

In our dental clinics, we might further secure antibiotic stewardship by appointing a member of the dental team to be the dedicated antibiotic steward. Their role would be to sanction, before treatment, all antibiotic prescriptions written by the dentists and then review after treatment, the outcomes of their prescription. The completion of a patient questionnaire asking about improvement in symptoms of pain and swelling or any untoward effects could be used effectively to provide data fulfilling this outcome.

In such a way, not only will inappropriate antibiotic prescribing be prevented, the monitoring of the patient for 48 hours post prescription, provides the necessary period of focus, whereby doses can be reduced or a non-effective regimen stopped and further tests started immediately.

There is now considerable evidence suggesting in those hospital settings where antibiotic stewardship has been successfully implemented; not only was there reduced drug consumption and thus expenditure, there was an increase in practitioner and patient satisfaction from improved treatment outcomes[23,24,25 26].

Drug timing, DDD(s) and DOT(s)

In addition to those measurements outlined previously, we can add another dimension to our measurement of drug administration and that is: Time.

The duration for which a drug should be taken and the rate or frequency at which it will be taken, are two particularly important parameters we must note in the patient records, duplicating that data written on the prescription.

The frequency of administration of each drug is generally given as X times daily, the duration being for a specified number of days. Patients must be informed of the need to regularly take their medicine at equal intervals throughout their day.

If, after giving a prescription, we need to review our patients, the duration and rate of medication taken can provide valuable information on drug consumption. The two most common methods used to evaluate drug consumption are DDD(s) or DOT(s):

I.	The DDD are the Defined Daily Doses. Or the total number of grams of antimicrobial agent used, divided by the number of grams in an average daily dose[27].
II.	The DOTs are the Days of Therapy. Expressed as the administration of a single agent on a given day regardless of the number of doses administered or dosage strength prescribed.

The DDD has the advantage of an ability to compare standardized doses among different clinical disciplines eg: the efficacy of an antibiotic given in a hospital maxillofacial unit can be compared with the same dose, same antibiotic given to an outpatient in general dental practice.

The disadvantage is that the DDD does not account for alternative dosing regimens due to hepatic or renal deficiencies, extremes of age or other confounding medical factors.

Therefore, in many cases the administered dose could be different from the DDD recommended by the BNF DPF or other authority. This can result in either over-estimation or under-estimation of the patient's consumption of an antibiotic or other drug.

The alternative measurement is the number of DOTs[28] . The advantage is that DOTs are not affected by changes in dosing regimens. However, the DOTs will not reflect actual doses and may not adequately represent antibiotics that are commonly administered multiple times daily.

On one hand, the DDD is useful in assessing many dental practices with respect to their use of a drug or the effectiveness of a drug regimen. While on the other, DOTs may be more applicable to compare the effectiveness of many different antibiotics being used by one practice or a defined group of practitioners across several episodes of treatment.

While DDDs and DOTS are really only useful for research and review, the SI units upon which such activity is based are always used to quantify every drug in dentistry and are the units of choice for prescribing those medicines listed in the BNF. As such, we will use the SI unit on a daily basis in our clinical work.

Reducing errors: Drug conventions and the BNF

To ensure errors in prescribing are reduced or at best removed, the following conventions should always be used:

I. Drug strength or quantity is noted in milligrams, millilitres, grams or litres. Whole numbers are used and the decimal point is to be avoided.

II. Quantities of Grams are written as 1 g. Quantities less than 1 Gram are written as 1 mg.

III. Quantities less than 1 mg are never abbreviated. These are written as: 1 microgram, 1 nanogram or 1 Unit.

IV. If we need to use the decimal this is always preceded by 0.

V. For liquid preparations, multiples of 5 ml are used wherever possible. If not then an oral syringe is to be requested with clear dose volume measurements[12,29].

For all routine medicine requests, after writing the patient's name, address, date of birth and age, the following data must be written legibly on the prescription:

I. The Name of the drug to be used.

II. The Dose of drug: The concentration or the weight requested.

III. The Quantity of the drug with doses in whole numbers.

IV. The Frequency in doses per day.

V. For prescriptions to be taken as required: A minimum dose and totals are specified.

In the UK NHS, the legal responsibility for prescribing rests with the practitioner who signs the prescription. The BNF contains advice on completing prescription forms with specific details of the data you need to enter into the prescription forms; FP10 in England, the WP10 D in Wales, the GP 14 in Scotland or the HS 47 in Northern Ireland.[12,29].

As previously mentioned, the BNF DPF is your definitive authority for prescribing in general dental practice, the latest print or online editions should be readily accessible for you to consult before you write out a prescription.

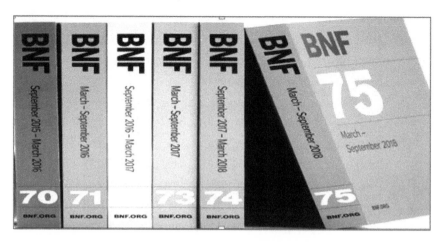

Every drug in the BNF will have its own monograph. Following the drug name, the arrangement of the following sections is almost universally accepted, being found in the formularies of most countries in the Commonwealth, the EC and North America too:

i.	**Indications**	*Details of the clinical uses*
ii.	**Cautions**	*Restrictions or monitoring required*
iii.	**Contra-indications**	*The patients in which to avoid a drug*
iv.	**Hepatic impairment**	*Advice on dose changes in liver disease*
v.	**Renal impairment**	*Advice on dose changes in kidney disease*
vi.	**Pregnancy**	*Whether or not the drug can safely be used*
vii.	**Breast-feeding**	*Whether or not the drug can safely be used.*
viii.	**Side-effects**	*The frequency of occurrence from Very common: >1/10, Common: 1/10 to 1/100. Less common: 1/100 to 1/1000, Rare: 1/1000 to 1/10,000 and Very rarely: < 1/10,000*
ix.	**Dose**	*In SI units for Adults and Children.*
x.	**Approved name**	*The generic or non proprietary name*
xi.	**Proprietary name**	*The manufacturer's name for their product*

With children, we should refer to the BNF C. When prescribing for children who are up to one-year young, we should consult with a paediatrician. Always deferring to their advice, we must be mindful that doses calculated are with regard to the child's health and body weight. As the child grows, there are five broad age/ weight/ dose ranges they "fit into" with respect to prescribing:

I.	**Birth to 1 Year**	Mean wt: **5** to **10**kgs	¼ Adult dose
II.	**From 1 to 3 Years**	Mean wt: **10** to **15**kgs	1/3 Adult dose
III.	**From 3 to 6 Years**	Mean Wt: **15** to **20**kgs	**2/5** to ½ Adult dose
IV.	**From 6 to 12 Years**	Mean Wt: **20** to **40**kgs	½ to ¾ Adult dose
V.	**From 12 to 18 Years**	Mean Wt: **40** to **70**kgs	¾ to Total Adult dose

The table above is based on the percentage method for calculating drug doses[31,32].

Although definitive doses are not indicated, the table provides an indication for paediatric dental prescribing. After calculating a paediatric drug concentration or drug dose, if the amount we end up with falls outside the range from:

Drug Dose or Volume X Mean Range of Body Weight

Then our result should give rise to concern.

Too low and the drug could be ineffective, too high and there could be drug toxicity or an adverse drug interaction.

With such a result, our calculations must be reviewed, revised if necessary and if the doubt remains, refer our prescription to a paediatrician or a pharmacist. Although not yet a requirement in the UK for critical paediatric prescribing, our dose calculations might be provided on the prescription form for the pharmacist to check.

With such transparency, should an error in prescribing occur, the dispensing pharmacist can act as a safety-check-point, before an administrative error results in clinical consequences.

The same safety measures should apply not only to our geriatric patients, to those in extremes of health (especially; in renal and hepatic disease or pregnancy), but generally to all of our patients in general dental practice. With hospital dental prescribing, the same principles apply to drugs that are usually dispensed in the following ways:

I. A suggestion is offered for medication that can be purchased (OCM) see below.
II. A prescription is provided for medicine that can be collected from a high street chemist.
III. A prescription is issued for a drug that is dispensed by the hospital pharmacy.
IV. A medicine is administered directly to the patient.
V. A controlled drug is prescribed by a specialist, *e.g.* a liaison consultant psychiatrist.

Drug classification

Those drugs we commonly use in the clinic and prescribe for our patients can be classified in many ways. Perhaps the most straightforward way is to organise them according to their therapeutic effect, however to give one example: Aspirin, being both analgesic and anti-inflammatory, can be placed in the first two of the following categories:

I.   Analgesic
II. Anti-inflammatory (and co-analgesic) Steroidal or Non Steroidal Drugs (NSAIDs)
III. Antidepressant
IV. Anxiolytic
V.   Antimicrobial: Antibiotic, Antiviral or Antifungal

I. Analgesic drugs can act on the peripheral nervous system or the central nervous system to relieve pain. Acetaminophen (Paracetomol) is the most common and well-known example of a peripherally acting analgesic, while it has no anti-inflammatory properties, it is moderately antipyretic. We have to be aware of the risk of liver toxicity from doses in excess of 4 gms/ 24hours in adults.

The Opioids are the most common and well known of the centrally acting analgesics, they have no anti-inflammatory properties. Codeine phosphate can be used for moderate short-term analgesia and Morphine can be administered long-term for pain relief, being particularly valuable in terminal care. While both drugs are incredibly useful, their administration to patients who have cranial injuries, can depress an injured patient's CNS respiratory function and specialist advice must be sought or their use guarded. Noted side effects are reduced GI tract motility, bladder retention and nausea.

II. Anti-inflammatory drugs can be non-steroidal (NSAID), or steroidal. The most widely recognized and used NSAID is Aspirin (Salycilic acid). In addition to being anti-inflammatory and analgesic, it is antipyretic too, being useful for alleviating mild to moderate pain. However, it cannot be used in children under 12 years old, due to the increased risk of developing Reye's syndrome. This is a rapidly progressing post-viral encephalopathy arising from metabolic mitochondrial dysfunction. A fatty liver, cerebral oedema, brain damage and fatality are seen in nearly one third of cases[32]. Nor should Aspirin be used in patients who are being medicated for coagulation disorders, stomach or intestinal bleeding or allergies to other NSAIDs. Other than these established restrictions, its use is routine and acceptable.

Steroidal anti-inflammatory drugs are derived from the glucocorticoid hormones, cortisol being the most important of these. It regulates metabolic, homeostatic immune and cardiovascular functions. Steroidal anti-inflammatory drugs work in relatively high concentrations (pharmacological versus physiological doses) by negative feedback reducing the effects of inflammatory processes, many of these arising from exaggerated immune responses. Steroids can be administered via topical, oral, intralesional or parenteral routes. Perhaps the most common steroid we use in dentistry is Triamcinolone acetonide (mixed with Di-methyl chlortetracycline in that familiar green paste we spin into root canals!) For those of us who have an aversion to endodontics or an affinity with oral medicine, then we will be more familiar with Betamethasone phosphate or Prednisolone mouthwash useful for alleviating, but not curative of the painful symptoms of Recurrent Aphthous Stomatitis (RAS)

Despite their clinical value, there can be some striking dose-dependent side effects from steroids. In low doses, inhaled steroids control asthma, but they can cause hoarseness and painful oral ulcers. Both the higher acute doses and the lower chronic doses of steroids, delivered and absorbed systemically will be responsible for bruising and weight gain, while long term; osteoporosis, diabetes, cataracts, immune-suppression and oedema of lower limbs impacting on mobility are all seen.

III. Antidepressant medication is frequently prescribed for conditions impacting on dentistry such as Atypical Facial Pain (AFP) and Tempero-Mandibular Joint Pain Dysfunction Syndrome (TMJ PDS). The effect exerted by these drugs is one of sedation with co-analgesia. At the time of writing, no such drugs can be prescribed from the BNF DPF, such medication being firmly within the domain of the hospital medical specialist. Perhaps with good reason too, although they are being administered for TMJ PDS[33], there is no firm evidence to support the effectiveness of their use[34]. For your information the following important classes of antidepressants are in current and widespread use:

i.	Selective Serotonin Reuptake Inhibitors (SSRIs),
ii.	Serotonin–Norepinephrine Reuptake Inhibitors(SNRIs),
iii.	Tricyclic Antidepressants (TCAs),
iv.	Monoamine Oxidase Inhibitors(MAOIs),
v.	Reversible Monoamine Oxidase A inhibitors (rMAO-A inhibitors),
vi.	Tetracyclic Antidepressants (TeCAs),
vii.	Noradrenergic and Specific Serotonergic Antidepressant (NaSSAs)
viii.	St John's wort

In our clinical work we should be aware of our patient's use of antidepressants for two reasons:

1. Despite an unfavourable risk to benefit ratio and the National Institute for Health and Care Excellence (NICE) 2009 guidelines stating antidepressants should not be used to treat mild depression[35], more than a few of our medical colleagues in general practice continue to ensure their use is widespread and established. In the UK, there was a doubling of antidepressant use from 2000 to 2010, while in the USA antidepressants are the most widely prescribed medication[36,37 38].

2. In dentistry, even though we do not prescribe antidepressants, from the above, it is clear that a significant number of our patients will

be taking them and therefore the risk of antidepressant side effect and drug interactions with medications we can prescribe will be present. Among the safety critical side effects and interactions we must be aware of are:

i. Mania and age dependent suicidal ideation and risk actualization.[39,40].

ii. Of note is the interaction between MAOI and Tyramine with the risk for a potentially fatal hypertensive crisis developing. Although there seems to be no risk of inducing this with adrenaline containing dental local anaesthetics.

IV. Anxiolytic drugs provide an important means whereby the acute fear experienced by many of our patients can be brought under effective control for short periods, so they might tolerate dental treatment. Benzodiazepines are perhaps the best-known anxiolytic, with midazolam being the most frequently used example, due to its water solubility, powerful action and rapid recovery time when administered intravenously.

Benzodiazepines exert their influence by selectively binding to a specific allosteric protein complex contained within the trans-membrane cell receptors located in neural tissues in the CNS (Central Nervous System), in the PNS (Peripheral Nervous System) and in some non-neural tissues too. (GABA sites are located throughout the body). Some sites respond to benzodiazepines and some do not, while others respond to ethanol[41].

From your undergraduate studies, you will remember these as the $GABA_A$ receptors (Gamma Amino Butyric Acid A); $GABA_A$ being the endogenous ligand for this receptor and the main inhibitory neurotransmitter in the CNS. When benzodiazepine binds to a distinct site in the $GABA_A$ receptor, the entire receptor becomes activated. A trans-membrane channel opens and Chloride ions flow into the cell.

Hyper-polarization of the neurone results from inward Chloride ion flow. An inhibitory effect on neurotransmission results as the cell cannot generate an action potential. In this way, benzodiazepines facilitate the inhibitory effect of $GABA_A$ on post-synaptic receptors[42].

Any exogenous agonist attaching to $GABA_A$ receptors do so in a highly conformative way, enhancing the effect of $GABA_A$. Such binding causes more chloride channels to be open, more frequently and for longer than if $GABA_A$ alone was bound.

Consequently, any neurone involved in fear or inhibitory behaviours will shut down until the benzodiazepine is metabolized and the binding sites are freed and recovery from sedation occurs.

While this short summary explains why benzodiazepines influence your patients, because $GABA_A$ sites are to be found throughout the body, it also explains the throbbing hangover dental students get after celebrating their exam successes. In the same way benzodiazepines exert anxiolysis and anterograde amnesia, after a celebratory night out; the students apparently enjoyed themselves but on specific questioning, they cannot remember where they did so.

If you haven't fallen asleep by now, this short revision will have stimulated the neural matter in your cerebral hemispheres to read further into the subject.

Just before you do, as with almost all drugs, although they are regarded as safe, benzodiazepines do have some untoward side effects. Therapeutic sedation extends to prolonged impairment of reasoning and cognition, (hence the need for a chaperone and for supervision for 24 to 48 hours post procedure). Profound disinhibition in patients can paradoxically lead to agitation, panic and aggression while sedated even during a procedure[43]. Infrequent short-term exposures for dental treatment carry little if any risk; however, with long term frequent use there can be psychological, then physical dependence and adverse behavioural effects upon withdrawal.

With any anxiolytic, we should be particularly cautious when treating those patients who may be pregnant or breast-feeding. The developing foetus can be at risk from teratogenic injury eg: cleft lip and palate and behavioural problems in later childhood. More acutely, but just as critical, are unintended sedation and CNS suppression in the unborn, with clear risks of overdose, brain damage, developmental impairment and/or permanent mental retardation to the unborn child. If we must use any anxiolytic, then using the lowest effective dose for the shortest period; minimizes the risks to the mother and to either the unborn and/or the newborn[44].

The same principles apply to our elderly patients where the effects of benzodiazepines can exacerbate those signs of pre and peri-dementia. The symptoms then reported by a geriatric patient given benzodiazepines, can so easily be confused with those signs associated with the age related dementing processes themselves[45].

V. Antimicrobial medication as stated above, can be antibacterial, antiviral or antifungal. The principles of protected prescribing in antibiotic stewardship have already been outlined in the previous section. If after considering these, we are still confident that prescribing an antimicrobial will benefit the patient, then we must give due consideration to the patient's state of health. After this, we should turn our attention to the questions of; what is the most likely organism responsible for the problem? Once those two questions have been answered, we must finally ask which antimicrobial will give the greatest benefit with the least possible risk?

When considering any antimicrobial treatment, three essential questions are asked in this order:

I.   Which patient?
II. For which pathogen?
III. With what prescription?

I. The Patient.

In the dental clinic our patients present in the extremes of age or health, or often both. Dental patients frequently have impaired renal or hepatic functions, present with allergies to the medication we wish to prescribe, or they are either immuno-suppressed or immuno-compromised.

Our patients may be receiving medication from their doctor for conditions they have listed in their medical histories. It is so important to inquire about such medications, together with their dose and duration. Even if the patient will benefit from antimicrobial treatment for a dental problem, we must ensure it will not interact with an ongoing medical treatment. Another consideration that is obvious in (actually but not literally) our female patients is pregnancy. Less obvious might be the use of oral contraceptives, or breast-feeding. Asking about these two issues is no less important than congratulating the soon to be mother, but questions about these issues must be asked sensitively and sensibly, *i.e.* the relevance of their medication with respect to our potential prescribing must be made clear to our patient.

II. The Pathogen.

Ideally, the infecting organism will have been isolated and identified with a report from medical microbiology being received before we even think about reaching for the prescription pad. In the UK in the NHS, in general dental practice, that is not going to happen; we rarely if ever consult medical microbiology. Our prescribing patterns using antibacterial drugs are seldom narrow spectrum and species-specific intimacies; invariably they end up being broad-spectrum affairs. While the former would be the choice attained by the idealist in academia, the latter is more easily aspired to and achieved by the realist in practice!

III. The Prescription.

In contrast to our rather raggy reputation for antibacterial prescribing, we seem to do a lot better when it comes to the common clinical problems caused by viruses. A good example is the cold sore on the lip as it arrives in our surgery with its patient closely behind it. Having correctly identified that cold sores arise following reactivation of the HSV (Herpes Simplex Virus; commonly Type 1), we could prescribe an antiviral drug such as acyclovir, but frequently do not prescribe anything (if only we could do the same for the patient with toothache and abscesses). Instead, we do the honourable thing, refusing to treat the cold sore until the patient goes away!

Although the aim of antiviral treatment is to interrupt viral replication, enabling an easing of symptoms and faster healing of the lesions, there are good reasons for neither prescribing, nor treating patients with active herpes labialis. Following the prodromal phase, once the lesions are clinically established, antiviral medication is of little benefit to alleviate symptoms, or arrest the condition, as the natural healing process begins after the viral titre reaches its peak in less than 24 hours from onset of symptoms[46,47]. If you decide to treat a patient with active herpes labialis, consideration should be given to the ease with which cold sores rupture, releasing active viral particles into the dental surgery environment, exposing dental clinic personnel and patients to the risk of infection. In addition to remembering that the lesions of herpes *labialis* are contagious; we must not forget the dental patient who attends an appointment while suffering with these painful lesions might be fractious, being neither agreeable to examination nor amenable to receiving dental treatment.

Nevertheless, Herpes *labialis* provides a good example of what are essentially the two choices we have, not only for antiviral but for all dental antimicrobial prescribing and that is either the topical or the oral route. The former are easily and rapidly obtained by the patient as Over Counter Medicines (OCM), while the latter being Prescription Only Medicines (POMs) first require an appointment with a doctor or dentist, then an examination, or consultation, within a framework of guidelines and finally; the Prescription is given.

You can see there are advantages and disadvantages to both routes.

POMs and OCMs

At this point, we should remember in the UK; all antibiotics and every systemic antiviral drug are only available as POMs and not as OCMs. There are however other jurisdictions; within the EU, in Australasia and North America; where the public (and not patients) can easily obtain more medications and do so without the need for a prescription than in the UK.

While the clinical evidence indicates that systemic antiviral treatment that is delivered orally is more effective than that which is topically applied[48], such therapeutic direct access for our patients is not yet an option in the UK. With respect to drug safety, efficacy, patient monitoring and the possibility of drug resistance; if we can move the responsibility for prescribing out of the surgery and into the pharmacy, such a move could result in effective treatment that is achieved more rapidly for our patients.

Certainly, for HSV antiviral medication, there is little risk to the patient and the oral route of drug administration is highly effective. Given the nature of the condition, patients are unlikely not to medicate, nor indeed to overdose. In stark contrast to the predicament of antibiotic resistance we are facing, for HSV, at least, there seems to be little evidence of significant drug resistance. Thankfully, this appears to be the case for both our immuno-competent and our immuno-compromised patients[49].

Despite the advantages in moving responsibility for prescribing away from the surgery and into the pharmacy, not much is known about how often people obtain prescription drugs from unregulated resources such as online pharmacies. A substantial number of patients appear willing to accept the considerable risks from off-label use to gain greater access to medication[50][51].

The potential for the accidental, or the deliberate misuse of any drug across a wider range of clinical conditions needs to be addressed and monitored before we embrace a world of OCM rather than POM, or somewhere between the two.

Emergency Drugs

To finish this section with a reminder that advice on drugs used to manage medical emergencies is also provided in both the BNF and the BNF C. This follows the guidance published by the Resuscitation Council UK. However, consulting the BNF during an actual emergency is not advised. This is perhaps one section of the BNF where those drugs, their concentrations and routes of delivery need to be recalled at a moment's notice should a medical emergency develop in your dental practice. To assist in your learning and enhanced CPD, this information is reproduced below and summarises the information from the previous chapter:

Dental Practice Emergency Drugs

The current recommended drugs for medical emergencies are:

1) Adrenaline, 1-ml ampoules of 1:1000 solution for intramuscular injection.
2) Aspirin, 300 mg dispersible tablets.
3) Glucagon, for intramuscular injection of 1 mg
4) Glyceryl trinitrate (GTN) spray, 400 µg per dose
5) Midazolam buccal liquid, 10 mg/ml for topical buccal administration.
6) Oral glucose, glucose gel, powdered glucose or sugar lumps.
7) Salbutamol inhaler: 100 µg per actuation.
8) Oxygen cylinder, two size D or two size CD or one size E (see below)

Oxygen Cylinders

The Oxygen cylinders must allow an adequate flow rate of: 10 to 15 litres/minute until the ambulance arrives or the patient recovers fully.

1. The D cylinder contains nominally 340 litres of oxygen = 30 minutes supply.
2. The CD cylinder contains nominally 460 litres of oxygen = 45 minutes supply.
3. The E cylinder contains nominally 680 litres of oxygen = 60 minutes supply[52].

References: Basics of Drug Safety

1. Zehnder M. Root canal irrigants. J Endod 2006; 32: 389-98.
2. Johnson WT, Noblett WC. Cleaning and Shaping in: Endodontics: Principles and Practice. 4th ed. Saunders, Philadelphia, PA, 2009.
3. WHO, Manual, Infection and Prevention Control Policies and Guidelines, Section VII: Disinfection and Sterilization, May 2003.
4. Public Health England. Delivering Better Oral Health, an evidence based toolkit for prevention Third Edition London 2014 PHE DOH. Available online from:
   https://www.gov.uk/government/uploads/system/uploads/attachment_data/file/367563/DBOHv32014OCT MainDocument_3.pdf
   Accessed October 2015.
5. Zhu W, Gyamfi J, Niu L, et al. Anatomy of Sodium Hypochlorite Accidents Involving Facial Ecchymosis – A Review. Journal of dentistry. 2013;41(11):10.1016 Available online from:
   http://www.ncbi.nlm.nih.gov/pmc/articles/PMC3824250/
   Accessed October 2015.
6. Mehdipour O, Kleier DJ and Averbach RE. Anatomy of sodium hypochlorite accidents. Compend Contin Educ Dent. 2007 Oct; 28(10):544-6, 548, 550.
7. Ingram TA. 3rd Response of the human eye to accidental exposure to sodium hypochlorite. Journal of Endodontics. 1990; 16:235–238.
8. Serper A, Ozbek M, Calt S. Accidental sodium hypochlorite-induced skin injury during endodontic treatment. Journal of Endodontics. 2004; 30:180–181.
9. Heling I, Rotstein I, Dinur T, Szwec-Levine Y and Steinberg D. Bactericidal and cytotoxic effects of sodium hypochlorite and sodium dichloroisocyanurate solutions in vitro. Journal of Endodontics. 2001; 27:278–280
10. Kleier DJ, Averbach RE and Mehdipour O. The sodium hypochlorite accident: experience of diplomates of the American Board of Endodontics. Journal of Endodontics. 2008; 34: 1346–135.

11. Whitford GM. Acute toxicity of ingested fluoride. Monogr Oral Sci. 2011; 22:66-80.

12. Joint Formulary Committee. British National Formulary, Edn. 69, London. British Medical Association and Royal Pharmaceutical Society of Great Britain (2015) (www.bnf.org)

13. Paediatric Formulary Committee. BNF for Children, London. British Medical Association, Royal Pharmaceutical Society of Great Britain, Royal College of Paediatrics and Child Health, and Neonatal and Paediatric Pharmacists Group (2015) (www.bnfc.org)

14. Ryan Kisiel 2009 Available online from: DailyMail: http://www.dailymail.co.uk/health/article-1226270/Doctors-told-stop-prescribing-antibiotics-coughs-colds-ensure-infections-dont-resistant-them.html#ixzz3qSa3BP9I
Accessed October 2015

15. European Centre for Disease Prevention and Control. Surveillance of antimicrobial consumption in Europe, 2010. Stockholm: ECDC; 2013

16. James Meikle. Doctors write 10 Million needless antibiotics prescriptions a year says Nice. 18th August 2015 London. The Guardian Newspaper. Available online from:
http://www.theguardian.com/society/2015/aug/18/soft-touch-doctors-write-10m-needless-prescriptions-a-year-says-nice
Accessed October 2015.

17. Lewis M. Opinion: Why we must reduce dental prescription of antibiotics: European Union Antibiotic Awareness Day. British Dental Journal 2008 205, 537 – 538.

18. The Economist. Resistance to Antibiotics. The Spread of Superbugs. What can be done about the rising risk of antibiotic resistance? The Economist London 31.3. 2011. Online:
http://www.economist.com/node/18483671 Accessed Ocotber 2015.

19. Dellit TH, Owens RC, McGowan JE Jr, Gerding DN, Weinstein RA, et al. Infectious Diseases Society of America, Society for Healthcare Epidemiology of America Clin Infect Dis. 2007 Jan 15; 44(2):159-77

20. Doron S, Davidson LE. Antimicrobial Stewardship. *Mayo Clinic Proceedings*. 2011; 86(11):1113-1123. Available online from: http://www.ncbi.nlm.nih.gov/pmc/articles/PMC3203003/ Accessed October 2015.

21. Gerding DN. The search for good antimicrobial stewardship. Jt. Comm. J. Qual. Improv. 2001 Aug; 27(8): 403-4

22. Joseph J and Rodvold KA. The role of carbapenems in the treatment of severe nosocomial respiratory tract infections. *Expert Opin Pharmacother*. 2008; 9(4): 561-575

23. Seligman SJ. Reduction in antibiotic costs by restricting use of an oral cephalosporin. *Am J Med*. 1981; 71(6): 941-944

24. Britton HL, Schwinghammer TL and Romano MJ. Cost containment through restriction of cephalosporins. *Am J Hosp Pharm*. 1981; 38(12):1897-1900

25. Hayman JN and Sbravati EC. Controlling cephalosporin and aminoglycoside costs through pharmacy and therapeutics committee restrictions. *Am J Hosp Pharm*. 1985; 42 (6): 1343-1347

26. Fraser GL, Stogsdill P, Dickens JD, Jr, Wennberg DE, Smith RP and Prato BS. Antibiotic optimization: an evaluation of patient safety and economic outcomes. *Arch Intern Med*. 1997; 157 (15): 1689-1694

27. WHO Collaborating Centre for Drug Statistics Methodology Definitions and general considerations. Available online: http://www.whocc.no/ddd/definition_and_general_considera/ Accessed October 2015.

28. Polk RE, Fox C, Mahoney A, Letcavage J and MacDougall C. Measurement of adult antibacterial drug use in 130 US hospitals: Comparison of defined daily dose and days of therapy. *Clin Infect Dis*. 2007; 44(5): 664-670.

29. The Joint Formulary Committee. British National Formulary, Edn. 68, September 2014 – March 2015. Prescription Writing pp4-5. London. British Medical Association and Royal Pharmaceutical Society of Great Britain (2015) (www.bnf.org)

30. Joint Formulary Committee. British National Formulary, pp 11-12. Edn. 47, March 2004. London. British Medical Association and Royal Pharmaceutical Society of Great Britain.

31. Roberts GJ and Hosey MT Chapter 4, Pharmacological management of pain and anxiety pp66- 67 in Welbury RR, Duggal MS and Hosey MT. Paediatric Dentistry Third Edition Oxford University Press 2005.

32. Gosalakkal JA, Kamoji V Reye syndrome and Reye-like syndrome. Pediatric Neurology 39 (3): September 2008. 198–200.

33. Marbach JJ. Temperomandibular Pain Dysfunction Syndrome. History, physical examination and treatment. Rheum. Dis. Clin. North. Am. 22 (3): 477- 498 1996.

34. Mujakperuo HR, Watson M, Morrison R, Macfarlane TV. Pharmacological interventions for pain in patients with temporomandibular disorders. Cochrane Database Syst Rev. Oct 6; (10) 2010.

35. NICE UK. Depression in adults: The treatment and management of depression in adults Recognition and Management. NICE guidelines: CG90. National Institute for Health and Care Excellence (UK). October 2009. Available online from:
http://www.nice.org.uk/guidance/cg90/chapter/key-priorities-for-implementation
Accessed October 2015

36. Olfson M, Marcus SC. National patterns in antidepressant medication treatment. Arch. Gen. Psychiatry. 2009;66: 848–856.

37. Reid S and Barbui C. Long term treatment of depression with selective serotonin reuptake inhibitors and newer antidepressants. BMJ. 2010; 340: 1468

38. Davis, Rowenna. Antidepressant Use Rises as Recession Feeds Wave of Worry 11 June 2010. The Guardian London Available online from:
http://www.theguardian.com/society/2010/jun/11/antidepressant-prescriptions-rise-nhs-recession
Accessed October 2015.

39. Cox GR, Callaghan P, Churchill R, Hunot V, Merry SN et al. Psychological Therapies versus antidepressant medication alone and in combination for depression in children and adolescents. Cochrane Database Systemic Review Number 11. 2012.

40. Stone M, Laughren T, Jones ML, et al. Risk of suicidality in clinical trials of antidepressants in adults: analysis of proprietary data submitted to US Food and Drug Administration. BMJ : British Medical Journal. 2009; 339: b2880 Available online from: https://www.ncbi.nlm.nih.gov/pmc/articles/PMC2725270/ Accessed October 2015.

41. Sigel E and Lüscher BP. A closer look at the high affinity benzodiazepine binding site on GABAA receptors. Curr Top Med Chem. 2011; 11(2): 241-6.

42. Haefely W. The biological basis of benzodiazepine actions. Journal of Psychoactive Drugs. 15:19. 1983.

43. Lader M, Tylee A and Donoghue J. Withdrawing benzodiazepines in primary care. CNS Drugs. 2009; 23 (1):19-34.

44. Iqbal MM, Sobhan T and Ryals T Effects of commonly used benzodiazepines on the fetus, the neonate, and the nursing infant. Psychiatr Serv. 2002 Jan; 53 (1): 39-49.

45. Madhusoodanan S and Bogunovic OJ. Safety of benzodiazepines in the geriatric population. Expert Opinions on Drug Safety. 2004 Sep; 3(5):485-93.

46. Spruance SL, Overall JC Jr, Kern ER, Krueger GG, Pliam V and Miller W. The natural history of recurrent herpes simplex labialis: implications for antiviral therapy. N Engl J Med. 1977 Jul 14; 297(2):69-75

47. Fatahzadeh M and Schwartz RA. Human herpes simplex virus infections: epidemiology, pathogenesis, symptomatology, diagnosis, and management. J Am Acad Dermatol. 2007 Nov; 57(5): 737-63.

48. Worrall G. Herpes labialis. BMJ Clinical Evidence. 2009; 2009: 1704. Available online from: http://www.ncbi.nlm.nih.gov/pmc/articles/PMC2907798/ Accessed November 2015.

49. Piret J and Boivin G. Resistance of herpes simplex viruses to nucleoside analogues: mechanisms, prevalence and management. Antimicrob Agents Chemother. 2011; 55: 459–72. Available online from: http://www.ncbi.nlm.nih.gov/pmc/articles/PMC3028810/
Accessed November 2015.

50. Nielsen S and Barratt MJ. Prescription drug misuse: is technology a friend or foe? Drug Alcohol Rev.2009; 28:81–6

51. Cunningham A, Griffiths P, Leone P. et al. Current management and recommendations for access to antiviral therapy of herpes labialis. Journal of clinical virology : the official publication of the Pan American Society for Clinical Virology. 2012; 53 (1): 6-11.
Available online from: http://www.ncbi.nlm.nih.gov/pmc/articles/PMC3423903/#R47
Accessed November 2015.

52. Medical Emergencies and Resuscitation. Standards for Clinical Practice and Training for Dental Practitioners and Dental Care Professionals in General Dental Practice. Resuscitation Council (UK) (2006, revised and updated 2011) (www.resus.org.uk/pages/MEdental.pdf)

Medicine and Drug Safety: Drug Actions

Pharmacology is so rapidly advancing that the BNF has to be updated every 6 months[1]. When you think about it, this is hardly a revelation, but what might be a surprise is Professor RA Cawson wrote this a quarter of a century ago. Since then, there has been no let up in pharmaceutical growth. A further 50 editions of the BNF, together with numerous reports into medicine safety and dental prescribing, have all conspired to characterise the way we have and the way we will continue to prescribe in practice. With this, there is both bad news and good news. The bad news is there will be even more regulation and with that, comes even more restriction; with less drugs to use and choose from in various fields of dentistry such as sedation. The good news is while we will have fewer drugs at our disposal; those remaining should give less cause for concern, fewer adverse reactions and less risk of drug interactions. Additionally, although this is hardly good news for the conscientious knowledge hungry young dental professional as there will be less to learn, in contrast to this, for the older more experienced dentists, the good news is: there will be more to forget.

Today our patients are living longer, one reason for this has to be the wider choice and greater availability of medicines and especially those drugs used to treat age related conditions[2]. Of note, some ¾ of our patients over 55 years old are now taking medication to support the functioning of their vital organs[3]. Through regulation and restriction, the number of drugs we use in dentistry will be decreasing, however, with the increase in medical treatment, the chance of drug interactions will be increasing and so we should be vigilant to this risk with our dental patients.

Despite all of this, those essential concepts of drug actions we learned as students remain unchanged. If we can maintain a working knowledge of pharmacology as it applies to the drugs we prescribe, then for sure, by mastering drug actions, the only challenge we face, will be to consider drug interactions; those relationships between two or more medicines our patients are taking. Before we consider that, we should now begin by revising the basic concepts of pharmacology we learned as students.

I add me: Pharmacokinetics

The way in which our patient's body deals with the drugs we give them is important, essentially drugs can be:

I.   Introduced....................
II. Absorbed......................
III. Distributed/ Dispersed..   **These are the Pharmacokinetic**
IV. Metabolized..................   **Factors.**
V.   Excreted......................

**Pharmacokinetics are what our patient's bodies
will do to the drugs they are taking.**

Pharmacokinetics follow a time dependent relationship with the above factors. We can remember the pharmacokinetic factors and their order by the acronym: **I ADD ME**:

Introduce, then; Absorb, Distribute, Disperse, Metabolize and lastly: Excrete. -Precisely what our patients do with the drugs we give them and what happens when we give them any drug.

A patient can be introduced to drugs in many ways, the simplest being topical application. With this method, drugs are passively absorbed through the cells of skin or mucosa by diffusion down a concentration gradient, two frequently used examples are:

i.   Benzocaine, the ethyl ester of Para Amino Benzoic Acid (PABA) achieves local anaesthesia in the oral and pharyngeal mucosal tissues of our patients[4]. Especially those suffering from: sore throats, cold sores, mouth ulcers, toothache, sore gums or trauma from the poorly adjusted new dentures that have reportedly been fitted satisfactorily. Unlike such dentures, benzocaine is well tolerated and non-problematic when used as directed. However, from a safety point, excessive intra-oral use can suppress the gag reflex and the risk of accidental inhalation-aspiration (FBAO) increases. In children and pensioners, the use of benzocaine use has been associated with methaemoglobinaemia[5] (a reduced ability for haemoglobin to transport oxygen due to more $Fe3+$ and less $Fe2+$ being bound (the normal value of $Fe3+$ is 1%))

ii. Eutectic Mix of Local Anaesthetic (EMLA) cream, used prior to intravenous cannulation for dental sedation contains a non-crystalline, liquid emulsion of two amide anaesthetics: lidocaine (2.5%) and prilocaine (2.5%) in equal parts. Both anaesthetics are passively absorbed through the stratum corneum to achieve dermal analgesia. Such topically applied amide anaesthetics are released into the deeper dermal layers of the skin, accumulating around pain receptors and nerve endings, where neuronal membranes are stabilized through inhibition of the Na^+ ion flows required to initiate action potentials. The conduction of impulses is then blocked and the feeling of numbness soon follows.

In addition to these two commonly used drugs in dentistry, we should also consider the contents of our emergency drugs box. Specifically: Glyceryl Trinitrate, topically sprayed it is absorbed to a significant level from the sublingual vasculature, entering the venous circulation and thus bypassing the hepato-portal system. Within seconds, it can exert a powerful effect on the heart of our patient experiencing the cardiogenic pain of angina pectoris. From this one example, the value of topical drug application should not be underestimated.

Following our consideration of topical drug application, the oral administration of drugs is the method most preferred by dental patients. Think of all those patients who hate the "needle" and just want but do not necessarily need an antibiotic from you. However, despite the many drugs administered orally, this is far from the ideal method. Absorption into the blood stream is slow, the notable exceptions being that well known psychoactive Central Nervous System (CNS) depressant: ethanol, which can readily be absorbed from the stomach wall. Some 24 hours later if one has taken too much ethanol, acetylsalicylic acid is just as easily absorbed through the same route to deal with the symptoms of excessive alcohol intake (the student hangover). We have already considered the risk of Reye's syndrome in children when given aspirin, in adults, the adverse effect comes from the risk of gastro intestinal bleeding and liver damage, especially so if aspirin follows alcohol[6].

Most drugs taken orally are absorbed through the upper part of the small intestine. Perhaps the most commonly absorbed drug is that well known CNS stimulant of the methylxanthine class: caffeine. So well known, that if you take a walk down many city high streets you will see five coffee shops to one dental practice. Except central London, where you can frequently see five dental practices to one coffee shop or fast food outlet. One dentist in London infamously offered dental treatment in a coffee shop (among other places), while another offered coffee (among other things) to their patients, waiting patiently...

If we leave our colleagues in coffee shops and return to pharmacokinetics, the hepato-portal circulation takes drugs from the small intestine through the portal vein into the liver before reaching the rest of the body.

Hepatocytic enzymes are able to metabolize certain drugs to such an extent that only a small amount of the active drug will emerge from the liver into the systemic circulatory system. This is the basis of first-pass metabolism, whereby the concentration of a drug taken orally is greatly reduced before reaching the systemic circulation[7,8]. The amount of drug loss during the passage to a drug's target tissue is related to enzyme action in both the gastro-intestinal tract and the liver. One drug used in dentistry that is significantly reduced by the first-pass effect is midazolam, hence the need for this drug to be administered intravenously.

First-pass through the liver diminishes the bioavailability of drugs. Bioavailability is a subcategory of absorption, it is the fraction of the introduced and administered dose of a drug that remains unchanged to reach the patient's systemic circulation. In other words, bioavailability is a measure of the rate and extent to which a drug can reach its target tissue.

<u>**There are five factors governing bioavailability:**</u>

I.   **Drug Chemical properties:** Whether acid, base, hydrophilic or hydrophobic, and solubility.

II. **Drug Physical properties**: Whether immediate, delayed or modified release, or encapsulated.

III. **Patient's Gastro intestinal tract:** The emptying rate, dependent on the GI tract motility.

IV. **Patient's age and health** of the hepatic and renal system and their enzymatic metabolites.

V.   **The Interaction** with other drugs and certain foods too.

The routes of drug administration

While these five factors alter the bioavailability of a drug introduced and administered either orally or mucosally, by definition, any drug injected intravenously, will have a 100% bioavailability. Bioavailability follows a time dependent curve; the diagram below demonstrates drug bioavailability following oral and intravenous routes of administration:

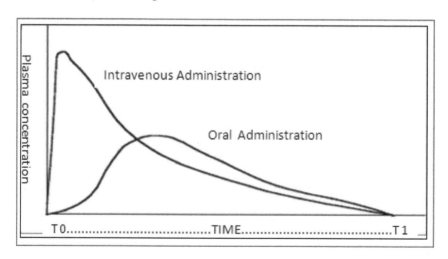

From the previous diagram, although patients and practitioners prefer the oral route of drug administration, you can see the advantages in intravenous injection. Not only are the complexities of hepatic and GI tract enzyme action avoided, the drug works faster, being available almost immediately and large doses can be given in a short time period.

In addition to the intravenous injection, when applied intra orally, injected local anaesthetics will act precisely where needed. However, when injecting any drug by any route, there are five important risk factors we need to consider:

I.   Sharps or inoculation injuries are always present for the practitioner and staff.
II. With intravenous administration, infective bacteria can enter the bloodstream.
III. Your knowledge of intra-oral and regional anatomy must be excellent for accurate injections.
IV. Unsightly and painful haematomas from torn veins are caused by poor technique.
V.   There is a risk of patient allergy to the solvent or vehicle with which a drug is injected.

In dentistry, we seldom inject subcutaneously and rarely, if ever, inject intra-muscularly. The only examples you will recall from the previous chapter being the emergency use of Glucagon and Adrenaline, both being injected intramuscularly for hypoglycaemia and anaphylaxis respectively and in these matters the consideration of risk to benefit, carries far less weight than for the everyday practical procedures in a dental clinic.

Whereas by the oral route, although providing lower and slower drug availability, the therapeutic effect can be of a greater duration as the drug remains in the patient's body tissues for longer.

Building on the previous diagram, we might also consider the following with respect to the therapeutic window of drugs administered by different routes:

A. Intravascularly, particularly the inadvertent intra arterial delivery of a drug.
B. Orally
C. Subcutaneously

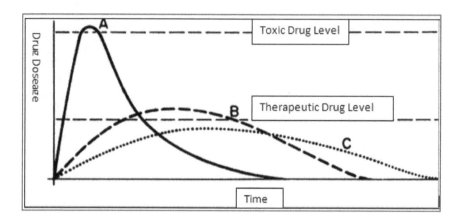

From the previous diagram, you can see the importance of using the correct route of drug administration. With A and C the inappropriate route of drug delivery can be at best: ineffective or at worst: dangerous.

1. Toxic drug level

From the previous diagram, if we first consider A:

Particular care must be taken when injecting local anaesthetics to ensure arterial injection does not occur. There has been one case report of permanent blindness following accidental intra-arterial injection of a dental local anaesthetic[9].

In other cases, following an Inferior Dental (ID) Nerve Block, temporary ocular disturbances resulted; it was proven that accidental intra-arterial injection of the inferior alveolar artery had occurred. The local anaesthetic passed into the internal maxillary artery, then the middle meningeal artery and finally, into the lacrimal and ophthalmic arteries, diplopia, and amaurosis (transient loss of vision) resulted[10,11].

The toxic level of drug had been attained, not through an increase in dose, but by the right dose being in the wrong place. We will return to consider these problems in greater detail in the following sections of this chapter.

2. Suboptimal drug level

From the previous diagram if we next consider C:

If an inadvertent subcutaneous rather than intentional intramuscular drug delivery is performed, the drug of choice will enter into a layer of fatty adipose tissue and either not achieve its desired effect within a reasonable time or not achieve its effect at all.

A good example of this can be demonstrated by injecting a vaccine into the layer of subcutaneous fat, the poor vascularisation of this tissue produces poor antigen processing with vaccine failure.[12] With relevance to our safety in dentistry, the hepatitis B vaccine will not work as well if injected into subcutaneous fatty tissues if compared to intramuscular delivery[13,14].

The subcutaneous injection of hepatitis B vaccine leading to significantly lower seroconversion rates and more rapid decay of antibody response. For patients in many regions of the world, where many zoonoses are endemic, the same principle applies for the administraton of many drugs such as the vaccine used to prevent rabies.[15.] This is an example of the therapeutic level not being attained, not from an insufficient drug dose, but rather, once more, the right dose but in the wrong place.

3. Therapeutic drug level

From the previous diagram if we finally consider B:

The oral route of drug administration; although the dose barely achieves the therapeutic level, it does so in a safe, prolonged and predictable way, hence the popularity of this method of drug delivery.

Most drugs administered orally are molecularly small and lipophillic. These properties are also essential for any centrally acting drug that needs to cross the blood-brain barrier (including those delivered intravenously).

You can ignore this...its only small print!

Most things in clinical dentistry can be classified according to five main characteristics; this applies to the pharmacology of oral drugs too. The Lipinski rule of fives determines those qualities that go towards the ideal oral drug[16]:

> i. No more than 5 Hydrogen bond donors in the drug's N_2, H and O_2 bonds.
>
> ii. No more than 2 x 5 Hydrogen bond acceptors in N_2 and O_2 in the drug's structure.
>
> iii. A <u>molecular mass</u> up to 5X 100 Daltons.
>
> iv. An octanol-water <u>partition coefficient</u> log P not greater than 5.
>
> v. Rule 5: Oral drugs should not breach more than one of the above rules.

You are probably asking....

THAT REALLY IS: SMALL PRINT...WHY IS THIS IN A BOOK ON CLINICAL SAFETY?

But you can't ignore this!

Well, given that most drugs our patients take are via the oral route and the chance of drug interaction is increasing [2,3], we should know as much about the medicines our patients are taking as we can. Beginning with our knowledge and understanding of the basic chemistry of a drug, we might then understand the pharmacology behind the increasing risk of drug interaction.

While a little learning is a dangerous thing (Alexander Pope 1709), more learning is certainly not. We need to bear this in mind, when considering patient safety, if we accept that the more we learn the less we know, we might then proceed cautiously, albeit safely with our own drug prescribing.

While the first-pass enzymes diminish a drug's concentration and degrade its effectiveness, the process can be harnessed to helpfully convert a pro-drug to an active drug. Although this is of little consequence for clinical dentistry, we need to be aware of this process, as far as those oral drugs we prescribe could disrupt the conversion of a pro-drug to an active drug.

One habitually cited example being the theoretical reduction in effectiveness of the Combined Oral Contraceptive Pill (COCP). Our frequent and oftentimes inappropriate dental prescribing of Amoxycillin could possibly eliminate the resident bacteria in the gastro-intestinal tract of our patients. Of note in this example is that the first-pass metabolism is not altered and there is no drug interaction, oestrogen still being conjugated with glucoronic acid in the liver then excreted from the bile duct into the GI tract. However, due to the bactericidal effect of Amoxycillin, the ensuing paucity of active GI flora, will mean this conjugate (in theory) cannot then be hydrolysed.

Upon molecular splitting, oestrogen is released to suppress ovulation. Potentially, oral contraceptive (COCP) failure might be seen because of the potential inability to split or hydrolyse the conjugated COCP molecule. (We will return to consider this interaction in greater detail in the next section).

This is an example of an indirect pharmacokinetic action. In the next section, we will consider the pharmacodynamics of drug interactions in detail, as contraceptives steroids may exert a pharmacodynamic influence on lipid lowering drugs, antidiabetics and anti-hypertensives. The focus of this section will remain with pharmacokinetic actions and effects.

Another means of drug introduction is via pulmonary absorption. Sedative gases used in dentistry, (ie: nitrous oxide (N_2O) in ratios up to 70% N_2O: 30% O_2) are absorbed through the membranes of the alveoli. From here, passage into the pulmonary, then systemic circulation to cross the blood-brain barrier occurs. An anxiolytic and analgesic effect results, by an as-yet undefined influence on several different types of ligand gated ion channels present in CNS neurones[17]. Other drugs can be absorbed through alveolar membranes such as the aerosol of the short acting B_2 Adrenergic receptor agonist Salbutamol (in your emergency drug box). Unlike N_2O, systemic spread is extremely limited and a high local concentration develops to maintain and exert an influence on the smooth muscles of the bronchioles.

Protein binding, bioavailability and age

Following drug absorption, distribution from the upper gastro-intestinal tract into the hepato-portal and systemic circulation with further drug dispersal occurs. Drugs can either dissolve in the plasma fraction of blood, or can be bound to plasma proteins such as:

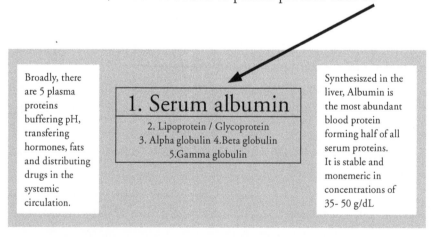

Broadly, there are 5 plasma proteins buffering pH, transfering hormones, fats and distributing drugs in the systemic circulation.

1. Serum albumin
2. Lipoprotein / Glycoprotein
3. Alpha globulin 4.Beta globulin
5.Gamma globulin

Synthesiszed in the liver, Albumin is the most abundant blood protein forming half of all serum proteins. It is stable and monemeric in concentrations of 35- 50 g/dL

The extent of drug binding is inversely proportional to the pharmacological activity of a drug, only the unbound drug being active. Plasma protein binding hinders the extent to which a drug can join into a cell surface receptor or pass through a cell's membrane and thus exert the desired medical effect. We should remember that with certain diseases, the plasma protein profile will be distorted and it follows that not only will drug binding be altered, but the effect of a drug can be altered too[18.] It is therefore of considerable importance at every dental visit that we are aware of:

The state of health or the stage of illness our patients are in.

Updating our patient's medical history with their medications is important to remove (at best) or to reduce (at worst) the risk of any drug interaction. Drugs with an acidic or neutral pH will preferentially bind to serum albumin as it is basic. As albumin binding reaches saturation, in turn the other plasma proteins will display drug binding. However, as stated with certain disease processes, the plasma protein profile of our patients will be altered.

In clinical dentistry, we must be aware of frequent occurrences of lower albumin levels (hypoalbuminaemia) in our patients, the most common causes being:

I. Liver disease (Cirrhosis; commonly chronic alcoholism and/or the end stages of viral Hepatitis)
II. Kidney disease (The nephrotic syndrome)
III. Pregnancy (from temporary redistribution and haemodilution)
IV. Gastro-Intestinal Pathology (the loss of absorption or the loss of functional bowel *e.g*: Coeliac Disease or Crohn's Disease)
V. Malnutrition (in the Western clinical settings this could be from Anorexia or from Bulaemia)

Infrequently, there may be hyperalbuminaemia. We may occasionally see this in our patient who has become acutely dehydrated. The endurance athlete who has over-trained is one example and the strength athlete taking food supplements is another, both causes giving rise to hyperalbuminaemia[19].

Not only do extremes of health produce variations in plasma protein levels, with extremes of age, we can see differences in drug handling that is attributable to a variation in plasma protein composition. The neonate's body composition differs from that of the adult with greater susceptibility to the action of drugs[20]. In children up to the age of 10 years old, drug absorption and metabolism takes place at a much slower rate compared to that of an adult. In the neonate and very young child, the time to reach the maximum plasma concentrations is even longer[21].

The volume of intra and extra-cellular fluid, when corrected for body mass is higher in neonates, infants and children, when compared to adults and so their albumin and alpha glycoprotein concentrations will be correspondingly lower. In essence, this means free drugs not bound to plasma protein will be present to a greater degree in children than in adults[22].

Despite such differences, the most important physiological variation between children and adults is in their elimination of drugs. Drug metabolism develops with age, children having lower and more immature pathways when compared to adults[23][24]. The activity of metabolic enzymes in children is 1/5th to 3/4 of an adult's with drug elimination also being far slower[23][24]. The glomerular filtration rate (GFR) in neonates is 1/3rd to ½ of the adult level[25]. The GFR increases rapidly during the first 2 weeks of life, due to an increase in renal blood flow combined with a postnatal drop in renal vascular resistance. The GFR then rises rapidly until the adult values are reached at only 8 to 12 months of age[25].

We must be vigilant to the effect of drugs in our older patients too. Ageing can be thought of as a predictable but a progressive loss in the function and capacity of multiple organs to resist physiological stresses. These processes will result in a lowered drug handling ability, adding to this, the medical profession's attempts to halt the onset of natural degenerative and dementing conditions result in our dental patients being prescribed with complex and multiple arrays of drug regimens.

Against this background, our elderly patients also have a decreased hepatic and renal mass with lowered enzyme functioning and when all things are considered, it is little wonder that the bioavailability of some drugs can be strikingly increased in the elderly[26].

Significant changes in body composition occur with advancing age and we often find a diametric opposition of body tissue composition. As lean muscle mass decreases, adipose layers increase. Thus, the distribution, relative concentration and half-life of lipophilic drugs increase, while the same parameters will correspondingly decrease for aqueous drugs in the elderly patient.

Hepatic drug clearance of some drugs can be reduced by up to 1/3rd in the elderly and renal drug excretion can fall by ½ in the majority of our elderly patients[26,27].

While we understand some of the changes that ageing brings to drug absorption, there is still much to learn about GI tract enzymes, drug transport systems and the changes throughout a patient's life[28]. Other afflictions are associated with advancing age such as coronary heart disease and hypertension. While they may confound the clinical picture further, they do predictably impact on renal function decreasing it even more[28].

Age related physiological and pharmacokinetic changes as well as the presence of comorbidity and polypharmacy will complicate drug therapy in the elderly, while in the younger patient, undeveloped metabolic pathways and a dynamic composition of body tissue could result in unpredictable reactions to those drugs we routinely prescribe.

Putting all the small print and detail to one side:

When we either administer or prescribe drugs for patients in either extremes of age, or indeed anyone, we should apply the axiom:

START LOW + GO SLOW

One feature of drug binding is that the more it occurs; the duration of the drug action will be longer. Only the free drug can act, become metabolized and then be excreted in urine.

A second more troubling feature is the higher degree with which a drug is bound to plasma proteins, then there will be a greater risk of another drug interaction.

Some interesting clinical inconveniences can be seen with such pharmacokinetic interactions:

Warfarin

The best-known example of a drug with a high plasma protein binding (of some 97% to 99%) is the orally administered anticoagulant: **Warfarin**.

(This was name was given after the development work of the **W**isconsin **A**lumni **R**esearch **F**oundation into coum**arin** derived from spoiled sweet clover in animal feeds, (so now you know))

Warfarin is the most commonly administered oral anticoagulant used for the prevention and treatment of thrombo-embolic diseases and cardiovascular conditions. In the UK, at least 1% of the whole population and 8% of those aged over 80 years are taking warfarin[32][33].

The increase in warfarin in the past 10 years is due to its clinically proven effectiveness in dealing with the following conditions[34].

I.   Atrial fibrillation.

II. Ischaemic heart disease.

III. Heart valve incompetence, defects or replacements.

IV. Deep vein thromboses with a risk of Cerebro-vascular Accidents.

V.   Pulmonary embolism.

Warfarin inhibits the Vitamin K dependent enzyme: epoxide reductase. This enzyme is responsible for recycling and reducing Vitamin K, after it becomes oxidized when it carboxylates the glutamic acid residues on the precursors of the Calcium dependent clotting factors: **II, VII, IX** and **X**, together with the regulatory proteins **C, S** and **Z**.

In the main, warfarin acts to reduce clotting factor **II.** By depleting the levels of active Vitamin K, the clotting factor subunits cannot bind to phospholipid receptors found on cell of the vascular endothelium and blood clots will not form. Once administered, the anticoagulation effect of warfarin will take several days to become clinically evident as the patient's active clotting factors are replaced with non-active under-carboxylated or non-carboxylated factors[33][34].

Warfarin effects begin at 8 to 12 hours, are maximal around 36 hours and persist for 72 hours. Such a pattern fits well within the dose: time curve plot for orally administered drugs that we have seen in the preceding pages (curve B). Our dental patients on warfarin will have an International Normalised Ratio (INR) above 1.0 indicating a prolonged Prothrombin time or an increase in clotting time.

The safe clinical management of our patient on warfarin must take into account any underlying medical condition, not only the reason for their taking warfarin in the first place, but their hepatic and renal health too. Following this, we must consider the INR together with the dental procedure, but above all else, we must consider the medication the patient has taken together with those drugs we might consider using in our dental treatment.

The clinical effect of warfarin can be altered by many drugs. Principally, an altered effect is realized when the highly bound inactive warfarin is displaced from plasma protein receptors to become free and pharmacologically active.

A drug such as warfarin with 99% to 97% binding, i.e. only 1% to 3% unbound, is needed for the desired effect. Warfarin possesses a tremendous potential to become harmful to the patient with an increase in only a few fractions of a percent of free drug.

Such an increase may occur when another drug such as aspirin competes with the binding site normally occupied by warfarin. If this occurs, we will be presented with a haematological risk to the patient as the INR rapidly rises and uncontrollable bleeding results. The most serious of these being an intracranial bleed following the concurrent administration of warfarin and aspirin[35].

Therapeutic index and therapeutic margins

If we pause for a moment to consider another safety parameter and that is the Therapeutic Index (TI) of a drug. The therapeutic index is the ratio of median toxic dose (TD_{50}) divided by the median effective dose (ED_{50}), or the dose that will cause a toxic effect in ½ of the patients taking the drug, divided by the dose that results in a beneficial effect in ½ of the patients taking the drug:

$$\text{Therapeutic Index} = \frac{TD_{50}}{ED_{50}}$$

The higher the TI, the safer the drug will be, as the dose range from effective to toxic is wider. The TI might also be termed the Protective Index (PI) but the extent of toxicity in the patient must be clearly defined. Alternatively rather than a subjective toxicity with TD_{50} an objective: LD_{50} could be used instead.

The advantage of an LD_{50} in our pharmacological estimations is that it provides a defined end-point, i.e. the established dose that is lethal in ½ of the experimental subjects.

The disadvantage of such extreme calculations is obvious and rather than having lots of dead rabbits and lab rats to account for, we now mercifully and thankfully can model our drug calculations *in-silico* and not *in-vivo*, down to a defined toxic but not a lethal level.

Notwithstanding the many animal sacrifices in the name of medical science, the TI or PI does give a clear safety index or risk versus benefit with which we can work. The problem with warfarin and many highly bound drugs is that the TI is incredibly low.

For comparison:

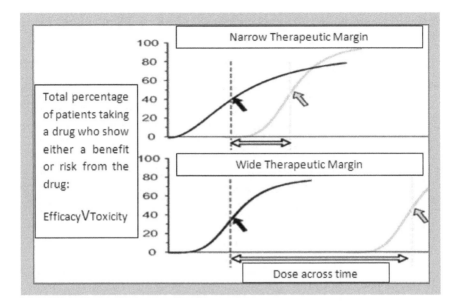

All drugs will exhibit a dose and efficacy relationship or <u>Benefit</u> (Black plot) together with a dose and toxicity relationship or <u>Risk</u> (Grey plot). The arrows on the diagram are the ED_{50} and TD_{50} points. Measuring between these points across the curves can provide an indication of the TI or PI of a drug[37]. Warfarin has a very narrow TI, factors such as genetic and metabolic variation in enzyme action can transform the relationship between efficacy and toxicity and thus risk versus benefit for any individual.

Returning to warfarin, the biggest problem with dentistry and warfarin is bleeding. A recent study (not confined to dentistry) revealed major and fatal bleeding arose every 7.2 and 1.3 per 100 patient-years respectively[38]. Following from the findings of that study, because of such adverse effects, warfarin is now the third most common reason patients end up in hospital needing a corrective medical intervention.[39]

Moving on, warfarin's narrow TI makes it extremely awkward to maintain patients within their prescribed anticoagulation range. A recent analysis of nearly 6,500 patients prescribed warfarin for atrial fibrillation revealed half the time, their INR was outside the target range of 2–3![40.] Just to put this in some perspective: An INR greater than 3 will increase the risk of bleeding, while an INR less than 2 increases the risk of a thrombotic event[41]. This problem is only made worse because every patient will have different warfarin doses due to the diversity of factors such as pharmacogenetics and other issues such medication the patient will be taking concurrently[42]. Many drugs will interfere with another drug's plasma protein binding.

Of relevance to dentistry and warfarin, those drugs we need to be vigilant about can be arranged into five groups as follows:

Drug Group	Common Example	Interaction and Result
I. Analgesic	NSAIDS such as Aspirin	Compete with protein binding sites: INR increases.
II. Antibacterial	Broad spectrum bactericidal drugs	GI tract Vit K bacteria eliminated: INR increases.
III. Antifungal	Azole derivatives	Hepatic metabolim reduced: INR increases.
IV. Antiviral	HAART and HIV Protease Inhibitor.	Hepatic enzyme pathways occupied: INR increases.
V. Antidepressant	SSRIs	Hepatic enzyme pathway interrupted: INR increases.

We are fortunate, that in clinical dentistry we would only routinely prescribe drugs from the first three of these groups. In the last two groups; the Highly Active Anti Retro-viral (HAART) drugs, the Protease Inhibitor anti-HIV drugs and the Serotonin Specific Re-Uptake Inhibitors (SSRIs) are the sole preserve of the prescribing medical specialists, whose tasks are to preserve the quantity and quality of life for those with HIV and those living with clinical depression.

With respect to the first three groups, we can rationalise our drug-safety approach as follows:

I.   We would, for sure avoid using and most certainly discourage our patient on warfarin from using Aspirin. This is due to its interference with platelet function with the risk of gastric and intracranial bleeding. Instead we would advocate their short term use of a non-NSAID e.g. paracetomol at a dose of 500mgs four times daily for up to 5 days as an antipyretic analgesic. Use of other analgesics for longer than a few days will interfere with the hepatic enzymes and once more, their INR would increase; as would the use of paracetomol or any other acetaminophen containing preparation in doses and/or durations above/beyond those recommended levels.

II.   Antibacterial use is more problematic; however, our strict adherence to the principles of antibiotic stewardship should reduce, if not entirely remove the risk that comes from the blind-prescribing of broad-spectrum bactericidals. These drugs influence the warfarin metabolism either directly by interfering with hepatic enzymes or indirectly by removing much of the Vitamin K producing GI tract flora. Rather, we should consult with medical microbiologists and then use appropriate narrow spectrum bacteriostatic drugs. In particular, we should avoid using Metronidazole and macrolide antibiotics such as Erythromycin, both of which can increase a patient's INR.

III. Topical Antifungal prescribing is well within our dental remit and a good selection is available in the BNF DPF. However, we might do better to first address the underlying cause of a fungal infection in the patient rather than treat the clinical signs with an antifungal drug. If an antifungal is needed, then topical non-azole drugs such as nystatin and amphotericin are preferable to the systemic and topical azole antifungals, which will inhibit the hepatic metabolism of warfarin, leading to a rise in INR.

Please see below for more information on this interaction.

In addition to drugs, diet can influence warfarin metabolism too. In our patients who (really) like their greens, INR values can markedly drop when a rich intake of Vitamin K from spinach and the like is eaten. Just so you know: ½ cup of spinach contains 1,284% of your daily recommended intake of vitamin K and apparently you can't ever have too much or overdose on the stuff!

Just before leaving the pharmacodynamics of warfarin, when revising the safety issues of this subject we should bear in mind the following factors; while they go beyond drug interaction, your firm grasp and understanding of pharmacology still serves to underpin your safe clinical practice:

I.   Our patients are; each and everyone: overall: individuals and require bespoke treatment plans not only medically but dentally too.

II. Of fundamental significance and of paramount importance for safe prescribing, we must review all of our patient's medical histories, renewing their medicine histories at every dental visit. As previously stated, 1% of our patients will be taking warfarin, in many cases in addition to other drugs their medical practitioners will have given them for preventing or controlling disease. Our medical colleagues will be doing this with an increasing sense of defensive prudence in the litigious times within which both they and we now practise.

III. We must be especially vigilant that our dental prescribing does not impact on their established medical treatment.

IV. Moving from the dental prescription to the dental procedure for our patients on warfarin, we should adopt a conservative approach i.e. *endodontia* rather than *exodontia*.

V.   For those patients on warfarin undergoing dental surgical procedures, such as simple forceps extraction of 1-3 teeth, their INR must be less than 4. This has to be verified ideally at 24 hours but no greater than 72 hours prior to their dental procedure.

Management of the anticoagulated patient

The following algorithm is based on the UK NHS National Patient Safety Agency National Reporting and Learning Service (2004) guideline and this is available online from:

http://www.nrls.npsa.nhs.uk/EasySiteWeb/get resource. axd?AssetID = 60028&

Such flow charts are indispensable in our assessment and management of our anti-coagulated patients:

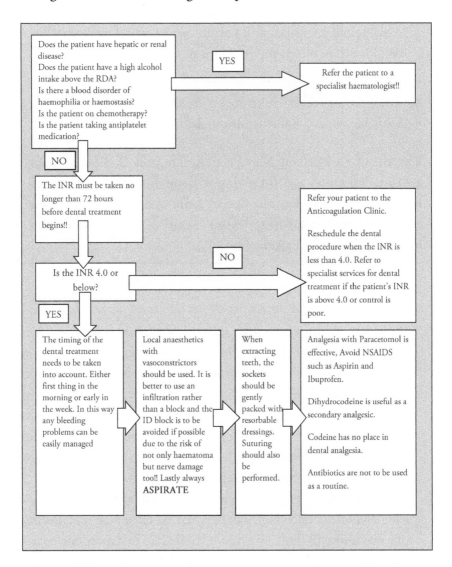

Does the patient have hepatic or renal disease?
Does the patient have a high alcohol intake above the RDA?
Is there a blood disorder of haemophilia or haemostasis?
Is the patient on chemotherapy?
Is the patient taking antiplatelet medication?

YES

Refer the patient to a specialist haematologist!!

NO

The INR must be taken no longer than 72 hours before dental treatment begins!!

Refer your patient to the Anticoagulation Clinic.

Reschedule the dental procedure when the INR is less than 4.0. Refer to specialist services for dental treatment if the patient's INR is above 4.0 or control is poor.

NO

Is the INR 4.0 or below?

YES

The timing of the dental treatment needs to be taken into account. Either first thing in the morning or early in the week. In this way any bleeding problems can be easily managed

Local anaesthetics with vasoconstrictors should be used. It is better to use an infiltration rather than a block and the ID block is to be avoided if possible due to the risk of not only haematoma but nerve damage too!! Lastly always **ASPIRATE**

When extracting teeth, the sockets should be gently packed with resorbable dressings. Suturing should also be performed.

Analgesia with Paracetomol is effective, Avoid NSAIDS such as Aspirin and Ibuprofen.

Dihydrocodeine is useful as a secondary analgesic.

Codeine has no place in dental analgesia.

Antibiotics are not to be used as a routine.

Of note: This algorithm begins with a reminder to assess and update the relevant aspects of the patient's medical history (top left) and ends (bottom right) with essential advice to:

I. Avoid concurrent NSAIDs such as ibuprofen and diclofenac, which both interfere with hepatic enzymes, irritating the stomach lining to the point of causing bleeding ulcers[43].

II. Avoid opioid analgesia, as it has no role in dental pain relief[43].

III. Avoid routine (blind) prescriptions of antibiotics[43].

> To this we must add the note of caution when prescribing not only systemic but topical Azole Antifungals:
>
> **The death in 2016 of Mrs Patricia Thomas in Wales, from a brain haemorrhage following a drug interaction between topically applied Miconazole gel from a dental prescription and warfarin is a salutary lesson for all of us on the hidden hazards from drug interactions.**

Continuing from this:

IV. If we are to extract, then the surgical procedure begins with risk reduction in local anaesthetic administration. An infiltration, rather than a block being preferred, there being anecdotal evidence of haematoma risk in the anticoagulated patient from Inferior Alveolar Nerve Blocks[44]. Following anaesthesia, the least invasive and most atraumatic procedure involving minimal tissue disruption to the socket is chosen, (e.g. buccal approach for lower 8's) with preservation of alveolar bone and soft tissues.

V. Once the tooth is extracted, with crown from root separation and root division if necessary, (as opposed to chiselling and drilling our way through bone on an industrial scale to expose the roots): We must close the socket with resorbable (vicryl) sutures over a cellulose or gelatin haemostatic dressing.

An assortment of haematologists, armchair dentists and working-parties (you cannot get a better oxymoron) advocate the use of tranexamic acid mouthwash post extraction to minimize the risk of excessive bleeding in our patients taking warfarin. (Tranexamic acid binds to plasminogen and inhibits the subsequent lysis of fibrin to achieve clotting).

Despite there being several studies with a wealth of data to support its use [45,46,47,48,49] in the UK, tranexamic acid is not yet available for the dentist in primary care, due in part to cost considerations. Despite the consensus and wisdom of the haematologist and the findings from their clinical studies, the application of simple dental measures (detailed above) are still considered equal to the complex medical proposals of the laboratory-based haematologist.

In considering this recommendation, we should remember the risk to the patient of ceasing their warfarin (even for a few days) and the ensuing complications from a thrombo-embolic event present the risk of far greater hazards than the relative inconvenience of the post-extraction haemorrhage.

Half life and drug clearance

From the previous diagrams of drug dose and time, you will see that the level of a drug in the body is neither stable nor static; looking at them once more:

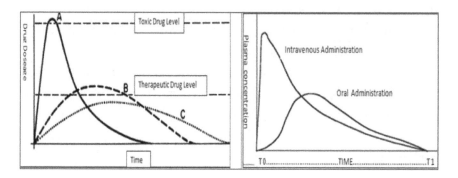

We can see from these graphs, that in a short time following the administration of any drug, not only will the plasma concentration fall; this decline heralds the onset of a decrease in the clinical effectiveness of the drug too.

Such a process can be marked and then expressed
by the half-life of a drug or **t 1/2**

The drug half-life is simply the time it takes for a drug's plasma concentration to become half of what it was from any defined start point. This time will depend on how quickly the drug can be metabolized, then eliminated from the plasma and there are several processes determining the t ½:

Any drug in plasma has been actively transported from one tissue, organ or body space to another, from the extracellular, to the intracellular and back to the extracellular again.

Once in plasma, the drug might become deactivated, or it can be removed entirely by excretion in an unchanged state.

> The removal of a drug from the plasma is the: **Drug Clearance** and the distribution of the drug in the various body tissues is the: **Drug Distribution**
>
> The Drug Clearance and Drug Distribution volume are the two pharmacokinetic factors that determine the Drug Half Life or t ½.

When we introduce any drug to our patient by those routes mentioned earlier, repeated dosing results in the plasma concentration increasing to a steady state of therapeutic or clinical effectiveness. This state will be maintained as long as repeated drug doses are being given.

Due to metabolic uptake processes, the time to achieve the steady-state will always be longer than the half-life and so larger loading drug doses might be used initially; to get the patient on their way to a state of effective medication.

A good example of this aspect of pharmacokinetics can be seen if we return (for a moment) to warfarin, which takes several days to reach the therapeutic steady state.

Heparin and the coagulation cascade

Rather than a loading dose, the introduction of another drug: Heparin (Low Molecular Weight Heparin LMWH) is used as an anticoagulation bridge until the patient achieves their steady "warfarinization" state. Heparin is a sulphated glycosaminoglycan and when injected subcutaneously, immediately blocks the conversion of fibrinogen to fibrin by binding to anti-thrombin lll and thus, coagulation cascade proteases are inhibited.

The end-point is that thrombin becomes inactive. Although the heparin half-life is expressed in minutes, three separate dose-dependent mechanisms are utilized in both heparin metabolism and heparin excretion[50]. So strictly speaking, the heparin half-life is variable. As heparin enters the blood stream, rapidly acting endothelial and macrophage receptors instantaneously begin to depolymerise heparin. Following saturation of this mechanism, a slower first order enzymatic metabolism begins to degrade the remaining heparin and finally a non-saturable renal excretory mechanism contributes to round off the heparin half-life profile[51].

Despite these complexities, heparin displays a predictably short half-life, but one that is nevertheless dose dependent:

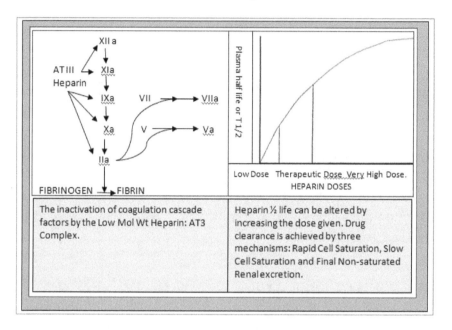

The inactivation of coagulation cascade factors by the Low Mol Wt Heparin: AT3 Complex.	Heparin ½ life can be altered by increasing the dose given. Drug clearance is achieved by three mechanisms: Rapid Cell Saturation, Slow Cell Saturation and Final Non-saturated Renal excretion.

As stated, the clinical effect of heparin is almost immediate, with one dose lasting for 6 hours[52]. While the warfarin INR is an expression of the Prothrombin Time (PT), for heparin, it is the Activated Partial Thromboplastin Time (APTT) that is used to monitor the clinical effectiveness of this drug. Large and continuous doses of heparin can increase the PT (and thus the INR) and when administered for longer than 5 days, a heparin induced thrombocytopaenia might be seen.

Whereas topical tranexamic acid might be considered as a means to control excessive dental bleeding in patients who are taking warfarin, in the heparinised patient, bleeding can be controlled with intravenous protamine. Both these measures should not be thought of as dental safety procedures, but rather as emergency medical interventions deployed by the experienced haematologist to whom defeat should be ignominiously admitted when all else fails in the dental clinic.

Knowing something in general about a drug's half-life, together with something in particular about the pharmacokinetics of warfarin and heparin, should ensure that events such as these would never happen to you or the 1% of your patients who are anticoagulated.

From this one common clinical example, we can understand that the final two pharmacokinetic processes of destruction and disposal, determine the destiny of a drug.

These processes are also referred to as: <u>Metabolism</u> and: <u>Excretion.</u> The former process occurring in the liver (and to a lesser extent, the GI tract and kidney), while the latter process occurs almost entirely in the kidneys. The degree of metabolism versus excretion varies from drug to drug and from patient to patient.

The factors governing drug metabolism

There are five factors governing drug metabolism that account for the variation we see in our patients:

I. Genetic expression
II. Age of patient
III. Physiological status
IV. Pathological state
V. Environmental influences

Considering these five factors further and in turn:

I. Expression of genetic factors are thought to account for anything from one fifth to absolutely all of the variations in a patient's drug metabolism[53]. The expression of a genetic code can control and interact with the other four factors listed above to determine the outcome of treatment with any drug. However, both the fields of pharmacogenetics (the study of an individual gene's effect on drug action) and pharmacogenomics (the study of all the genes in a patient's genome on drug action) are still in their infancy. Nevertheless, a considerable amount of data is now being revealed and at an alarmingly rapid pace, driving the move away from dogmatic assumptions on pharmacokinetics and pharmacodynamics based on a patient's race or ethnicity, towards clinical facts based on firm pharmacogenetic findings from genotyping[54]. Such a move has fuelled the drive towards personalised medicine and there is a relevance to dentistry. The US Food and Drug Administration has already advocated genetic testing of patients taking warfarin, in an attempt to lessen the impact of enzyme polymorphisms that are responsible for extreme variations in warfarin metabolism[55]. Such a measure could be used to determine the initial warfarin loading doses, with direct application to altering anticoagulation in those patients undergoing extraction.

This is especially useful for those patients who are genetically <u>slow warfarin metabolizers</u>, making them more susceptible to the risk of post extraction bleeding when compared to <u>rapid warfarin metabolizers,</u> for whom anticoagulant control is more predictable[56]. The same principles apply for our dental patients who are taking medication for asthma and cardiovascular conditions. In the next section, we will look more closely at the some of the hepatic enzymes involved in drug metabolism.

II. The age of a patient can also influence the effect of drugs. From early adulthood onward, there will be a progressive and relentless degradation in the ability of the hepatic and renal systems to metabolize then excrete drugs. Despite this being accepted wisdom, it is difficult to isolate age as a single factor in reduced pharmacokinetic activity given that throughout life, several disease processes occur in a patient, for whom medication would be beneficial. Thus, the pharmacodynamic effects of drug interactions will be present in our ever-ageing patients too!

With age, the hepatic and renal mass diminish as will the rate and volume of tissue perfusion due to a decrease in cardiovascular efficiency. Because of these processes, with the first pass metabolism, the bioavailability of certain drugs could increase with age, whereas for other drugs, it might decrease. If we also consider the changes in body composition with age, the distribution volume and half-life of lipophillic drugs increases with age, whereas the opposite occurs for the water-soluble aqueous drugs[56].

In older patients, the hepatic drug clearance of some drugs can be reduced by up to $1/3^{rd}$ with first pass hepatic enzyme activity being markedly age dependent, whereas the second phase of enzyme activity governing the processes of conjugation and detoxification seem to be age resistant, these being well preserved in the elderly[56]. Of considerable relevance to dentistry; the hepatic enzymes governing midazolam metabolism seem to be well tolerant to ageing, with no significant differences in their activity being seen between young and old patients. However, as stated previously, renal excretion is decreased by up to ½ in $2/3^{rd}$ of elderly patients. Complicating factors such as increasing blood pressure and heart disease will adversely influence renal function. Thus, age-related pharmacokinetic variations as well as multiple medications and geriatric processes will certainly complicate our use of drugs in elderly patients[56][57].

III. Changes in physiological status can also alter the effects of a drug. Once more, it is difficult to isolate the physiological status from the other four factors. Nevertheless, theoretical concepts and experimental approaches have been successfully used to account for the effects of changes in a patient's physiology on both pharmacokinetic and pharmacodynamic drug actions and interactions respectively.

Specifically there are Physiology Based Pharmacodynamic and Pharmacokinetic Drug Models (PBPD and PBPK combined to PBPKPD) to explain the relationship between drug dose and effect.

On a more precise note; such a model states that a patient's intrinsic homeostatic feedback mechanisms will affect the mechanism of a drug's action in terms of target site drug distribution, target site drug binding and target site activation, which in turn, will then affect drug transport metabolism and further feedback to alter the physiological status of the patient[58]. Most of the work on physiology and drug action has been established from the work of Levy in the 1980's and it is accepted that in common with the physiological state, a pathological state will determine drug action and clinical effect and these two processes will be linked[58].

IV. The pathological state. The state of health or otherwise of a patient will affect the way a drug behaves. This kind of... really is: stating the obvious.

Taking an alternative view, healthy patients do not need medication.

However, while the healthy patient may not harbour a pathogen, they may harbour a pathological fear of their attendance with you, your dental practice or dentistry in general just as those patients who are quite ill are also scared of the dentist.

With this in mind, we need to account for variations within the population of patients we care for and for both types of patient; be they healthy or ill, there could be a tremendous variation in the way drug metabolism influences drug effect, especially with the anxiolytic and analgesic drugs we might use.

The PBPKPD not only accounts for physiological variations in drug behaviour, it can explain those variations caused by pathological processes too. Of critical clinical importance are those conditions affecting the thyroid, the liver and the kidneys. Pathological processes in these organs will determine the metabolic rate of drug activity, the extent and effect of first pass enzymes on drug metabolism and lastly, the rate at which drugs are excreted. From a patient safety point, the updating of the medical history is essential in identifying not only the presence, but also the progress of diseases, in not only the thyroid, the liver and the kidneys, but diseases of the entire organ systems, with respect to drug administration for your patient.

V. Environmental influences. In common with the previous four internal factors altering a drug's action and effects, (by exerting an influence on a patient's metabolism), a multitude of external or environmental factors can produce similar clinical results. Perhaps the most common of these environmental factors in the UK, European and Western dental clinics, are variations in a patient's diet, in terms of the food quality and food quantity being available to the patient. Diet and specific foodstuffs are proven to significantly affect a drug's action[59]. The extent of this problem is not limited to smoking tobacco, eating meat that is burned, or cabbages that are over-cooked, all of these can induce the drug metabolism of antibiotics. In addition to these, the not-so-innocent fresh fruit juices can increase the oral bioavailability of the high clearance drugs such as benzodiazepines, eg: midazolam or calcium channel blockers eg: nifedipine, felodipine and so on and they do so by inhibiting the pre-systemic (intestinal) elimination of these drugs.

Rather, the range of this particular problem spans from the adolescent or older patients who are anorexic, through the bulimic, on to the mature adult but obese patients, all of whom we see with an alarming increase in frequency in primary dental care. To these patients, we might also include the smaller but still significant number of our patient's with alcohol and/or drug dependencies, for whom not only malnutrition presents a problem resulting in prolonged drug action, there may very well be pharmacodynamic interactions between drugs that are prescribed by the doctor and those that are acquired by the patient.

Setting physiology to one side, the pathological structural derangement of a cirrhotic liver, together with biliary obstruction and resulting jaundice, provide a clear clinical sign that our patient has both a reduction in hepatic function together with a decrease in renal excretion of drugs, two complications that are frequently seen in the dental patient who suffers from chronic alcoholism.

We must also be aware, that patients who are malnourished tend to have prolonged drug effects, whereas obese patients will have shortened drug effects due to a more rapid phase two metabolism. In the malnourished patient, a decreased rate of hepatic metabolism frequently leads to hepato-toxicity and almost certainly, further complications in their other organ systems are present.

As an aside, before we consider this problem in further detail in the following section, drug dose reductions should be considered to reduce or eliminate adverse drug effects in the patients at extremes of the body mass range. Conversely, those drugs metabolized by the extra-hepatic phase two pathways may need to be administered more frequently and in higher doses in obese patients, since the desired clinical effect may not be seen with normal drug doses due to their increased hepatic metabolism. Rather than altering the drug, altering the drug dose should be the first consideration when faced with either an increased-effect or a nil-effect in our patients for whom such environmental factors can adversely affect their drug metabolisms.

The last of the pharmacokinetic factors is drug excretion. With the exception of nitrous oxide, (which is both absorbed and excreted from the lungs) and some drugs that are excreted into bile, the most important organs for all other drugs to be excreted are the kidneys.

Drugs can leave the patient's body exactly as they entered, unaltered, or from the processes noted previously, drugs can leave in a metabolically altered form. Understanding something of how the kidneys achieve drug excretion is important.

The kidneys, their function and relevance to dentistry

In dental care, we rarely consider anything above the patient's eyelids or below their collarbones. An unfortunate complication of such inflexible dogmatic training in dentistry is that anything outside the mouth is relegated to being patient life support and transport; enabling dental problems to arrive in our clinic and with some luck, rapidly take them away again.

The kidneys are well below the clavicles and so the following diagrams might be useful to remind us what a kidney looks like and what it is they do for our patients:

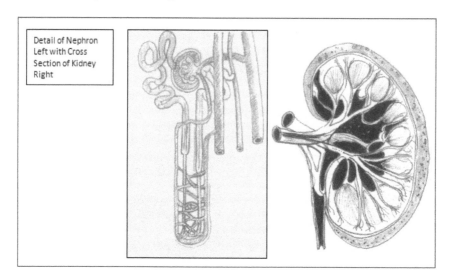

Detail of Nephron Left with Cross Section of Kidney Right

In the proximal convoluted tubules essential reabsorption and secretion of electrolytes, H_2O and drugs takes place. In the descending and ascending Loops of Henle, concentration of the excreted solution occurs with H_2O being resorbed. Finally in the distal convoluted tubules, a non-essential reabsorption and secretion occurs. Drugs are excreted from the kidney either by passive <u>glomerular filtration</u> or by active <u>tubular secretion</u>. Glomerular filtration only removes unbound drugs (the plasma free drugs). While those bound to protein and drugs present as organic acids will be actively secreted. Following filtration, passive <u>reabsorption</u> can return a drug to plasma then into circulation once more.

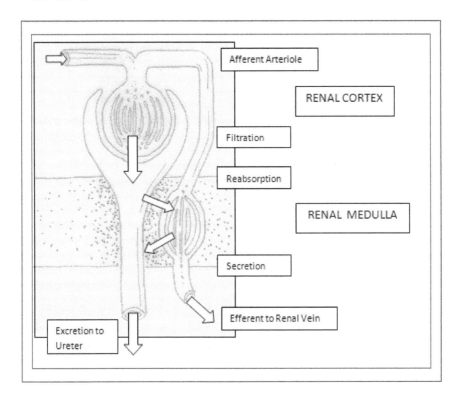

From the previous diagram:

<u>Filtration (1) – Reabsorption (2) + Secretion (3) = Excretion (4)</u>

Generally, drugs can only enter and leave cells in the uncharged or non-ionized state. By altering the pH of urine or plasma with respect to a drug's alkalinity or acidity, the rate of excretion or absorption can be altered. The passive and active reabsorption of non-ionised acids and non-ionized weak bases occurs in the renal tubules. Weak acids will be excreted passively when the tubular fluid becomes too alkaline.

The opposite occurs with weak bases. If the pH of urine can be altered we can control how much of a drug is retained or eliminated from the patient.

This is important to know for reasons of drug safety. The treatment of poisoning can utilize certain properties of the proximal and distal tubule's membranes to increase drug elimination if necessary. By alkalizing urine, <u>forced diuresis</u> can promote the excretion of drugs that are weakly acidic, such as aspirin. When an acidic drug becomes <u>ionised</u> in urine, it cannot passively re-enter the <u>renal membranes</u>. Once in the collecting tubule, it will be blocked from entering plasma and cannot return to the patient's circulation. Acidifying the urine will have the same effect for those drugs that are weakly alkaline, such as amphetamines which dental patients often acquire and use recreationally.

Variations on the above noted elimination pathways do exist. Antimicrobials such as those of the aminoglycoside class eg: streptomycin are eliminated as a glomerular filtrate with no tubular secretion or reabsorption occurring due to the high level of this drug's positive charge.

In contrast, the high excretion rate of penicillin is entirely due to active tubular secretion with little or no contribution from glomerular filtrate. Of interest, this high elimination rate can be reduced with probenicid (more commonly used to prevent nephrotoxicity associated with antiviral agents), thus enhancing the effect of penicillin by prolonging elevated drug concentrations.

Other drug elimination pathways occur, but overall these are less important than the renal processes outlined above. (The lungs also play a role in drug elimination not only for nitrous oxide but for alcohol too). Drugs can be conjugated in bile and enter the intestinal tract. Conjugated drugs, together with any unabsorbed drug fraction in the gastro-intestinal tract can either be eliminated directly from the bowels, or with further absorption, eliminated from the kidneys as noted above.

We must also consider the importance of drug elimination for mothers who are breast-feeding. Many drugs can be eliminated in breast milk. Metronidazole being a good example of a drug, it apparently taints or somehow alters the taste of breast milk[61]. (The things people do in the name of research!) The result being the baby is put off, resists and then ceases taking milk from the mother altogether.

Other effects are noted such as gastro-intestinal upset, nausea and vomiting in the mother or other adults who simultaneously take alcohol with metronidazole.

From this one example, you can see that even when a drug has been eliminated; it might exert an influence on a child. Even more so, if we consider that a neonate's liver and kidneys are anatomically and physiologically undeveloped and will not be able to deal with a drug in the same way an adult's organs would.

More recently, it has been established that despite certain concerns, there are no adverse effects or risks for the breast-feeding neonate whose mother is taking metronidazole[62]. The current advice is while it can be used, single large doses should be avoided (BNF DPF 70 January 2016).

First order and zero order drug metabolism

We have already considered the plasma concentration of a drug, with respect to its therapeutic and toxic level, the half-life and drug clearance. Having now considered the clinical and pharmacokinetic factors in turn (Introduction, Administration, Delivery, Distribution and Metabolism) ending with Elimination, it would be helpful, before we turn our attention to look at pharmacodynamic drug metabolisms to consider a variation on those graphs we have previously looked at.

First-order pharmacokinetics

The next graph is a plot of oral drug elimination annotated to show at which points the pharmacokinetic factors of absorption then elimination will affect the drug concentration. The oral route of drug administration initially results in a rapid rise in concentration, then drug redistribution and metabolism causing the concentration to fall as the drug is finally eliminated through passive or active means in the renal and other organ systems.

This is first order metabolism and elimination:

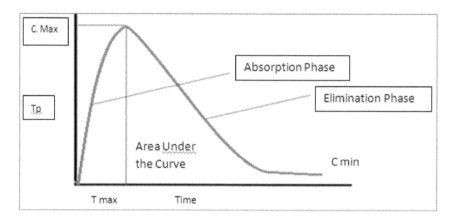

C_{max} is the maximum concentration of drug. t_{max} is the time to reach maximum concentration. AUC is the area under the curve, referring to the total drug exposure per unit of time. AUC is a definite integral.

To assess drug concentrations, approximation with the trapezoidal rule is an acceptable means for drug-dose calculations.

(Essentially using a defined grid multiplying along the X-Y axis to calculate the summed areas)

First-order (mostly oral) pharmacokinetics applies to some 95% of all drugs. Exponential elimination, proportional to drug concentration is seen. If we introduce more of the drug, the rate of elimination will increase.

With first order pharmacokinetics, the half-life is constant, being independent of drug concentration. The elimination process does not actually end, but tends towards zero with exponential reduction. With first-order elimination, a plasma concentration of the drug will be reached that is no longer pharmacologically effective. At this point, the drug ceases to exert a clinical effect.

Zero-order pharmacokinetics

Zero-order pharmacokinetics are seen in 5% of drugs with saturation of elimination enzymes and these are mostly the intravenous drugs.

In dentistry, controlled IV infusion sedation is a zero-order process. The rate of drug elimination is linear and constant, regardless of the drug concentration introduced. With zero-order pharmacokinetics, the half-life is dependent on the initial drug concentration.

The process will end when a cut off point is reached, or after the drug is no longer introduced. The action of the drug and its clinical effects will diminish as its concentration falls away.

The next two diagrams summarise the differences between these two elimination mechanisms:

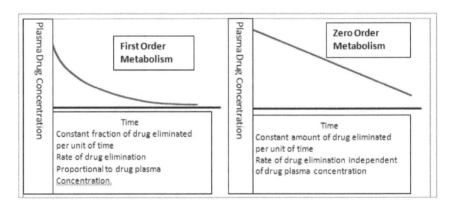

In addition to first-order and zero-order pharmacokinetic drug elimination, there is the possibility that a drug displaying first-order properties can shift to a zero-order pattern when saturation of carrier proteins or metabolizing enzymes occurs. A shift from an initial first-order to zero-order kinetic might be seen but overall the kinetic elimination is of a zero-order pattern.

In clinical dentistry, anticonvulsants, anticoagulants, anti-thrombotics, alcohol, anti-inflammatory and asthma medications are all drugs that display zero order elimination pharmacokinetics. We can remember this lot as:

P>WHEAT: Phenytoin > **W**arfarin **H**eparin
Ethanol **A**spirin **T**heophylline

Summary of pharmacokinetics

In summary, the five points of pharmacokinetic drug
actions that are important to remember are:

I.   Drugs can be administered: Topically, Orally, Intranasally,
     by Inhalation or by Injection either Transmucosally,
     Transcutaneously or Intravenously.

II. The most important mechanism of drug absorption is passive
     diffusion and non-charged lipid soluble drugs commonly
     achieve this by passing down a concentration gradient to cross
     a cell's membrane.

III. Drugs can be effective in very small concentrations by binding
     to specific cell receptors to exert their influence.

IV. Different drugs can competitively bind to one receptor, these
     antagonistic effects from one drug can block the action of
     another drug.

V.   The process of drug elimination begins with liver enzymes and
     ends with excretion through the kidneys, the lungs or other
     organ systems eg: in tears, perspiration or saliva.

References to Drug Actions

1. Cawson RA Spector RG Skelly AM. Preface to Basic Pharmacology and Clinical Drug Use in Dentistry. 6th Edition Edinburgh and London: Churchill Livingstone, 1995.

2. Seymour RA. Drug Interactions in Dentistry. Dental Update. 2009. 36 October. 458- 470.

3. Seymour RA. Dentistry and the medically compromised patient. Surgical Journal Royal College of Surgeons Edinburgh. 2003. 4: 207-214.

4. Mc Evoy GK editor in: Benzocaine. AHFS Drug Information 2007. American Society of Health-System Pharmacists; Bethesda Maryland. 2007: 2844-5

5. Dahshan A and Donovan GK. Severe methemoglobinemia complicating topical benzocaine use during endoscopy in a toddler: a case report and review of the literature. Pediatrics. 2006 Apr; 117(4).

6. Verster JC and Penning R. Treatment and prevention of alcohol hangover. Curr Drug Abuse Rev. 2010 Jun; 3 (2): 103-9.

7. Rowland M. Influence of route of administration on drug availability. Journal of Pharmaceutical Sciences 1972. 61 (1): 70–74.

8. Pond S, Tozer M, and Thomas N. First-Pass Elimination. Clinical Pharmacokinetics. 1984. 9 (1): 1–25.

9. Walsh F and Hoyt W. Clinical neuro-ophthalmology. 3rd ed. Baltimore, Williams and Wilkins; 1969: 2501-2.

10. Goldenberg A. Transient diplopia from a posterior alveolar injection. J Endod 1990; 16: 550-1. 7.

11. Goldenberg A. Diplopia resulting from a mandibular injection. J Endod 1983; 9: 261-2

12. Poland GA, Borrud A, Jacobson RM, McDermott K, Wollan PC, Brakke D, et al. Determination of deltoid fat pad thickness: Implications for needle length in adult immunization. JAMA. 1997; 277: 1709–1711.

13. Shaw FE jnr, Guess HA, Roets JM, Mohr FE, Coleman PJ and Mandel EJ, et al. Effect of anatomic site, age and smoking on

the immune response to hepatitis B vaccination. Vaccine. 1989; 7: 425–430.

14. Groswasser J, Kahn A, Bouche B, Hanquinet S, Perlmuter N and Hessel L. Needle length and injection technique for efficient intramuscular vaccine delivery in infants and children evaluated through an ultrasonographic determination of subcutaneous and muscle layer thickness. Pediatrics. 1997; 100: 400–403.

15. Zuckerman JN. The importance of injecting vaccines into muscle : Different patients need different needle sizes. BMJ : British Medical Journal. 2000; 321(7271): 1237-1238.

16. Lipinski CA, Lombardo F, Dominy BW, Feeney PJ (Experimental and computational approaches to estimate solubility and permeability in drug discovery and development settings. Adv. Drug Deliv. Rev. 46 March 2001. (1-3): 3–26

17. Emmanouil DE and Quock RM. Advances in Understanding the Actions of Nitrous Oxide. Anesthesia Progress. 2007; 54 (1): 9-18. Available online from: https://www.ncbi.nlm.nih.gov/pmc/articles/PMC1821130/ Accessed November 2015.

18. Anderson, Douglas M editor in. Dorland's illustrated medical dictionary pp859-861 (29th edition). Philadelphia 2000. Saunders p. 860

19. Mutlu EA, Keshavarzian A and Mutlu GM. Hyperalbuminemia and elevated transaminases associated with high-protein diet. Scand. J. Gastroenterol. 41 June 2006 (6): 759–60.

20. Mahmood I, Staschen C-M, Goteti K. Prediction of Drug Clearance in Children: an Evaluation of the Predictive Performance of Several Models. The AAPS Journal. 2014; 16(6): 1334-1343. Available online from: http://www.ncbi.nlm.nih.gov/pmc/articles/ PMC4389735/ Accessed November 2015.

21. Gibaldi M. Biopharmaceutics and clinical pharmacokinetics. 3. Philadelphia: Lea and Febiger; 1984. Gastrointestinal absorption: Physicochemical considerations.

22. McNammara PJ, Alcorn J. Protein binding predictions in infants. AAPS PharmaSci. 2002;4:1–8. Available online from: http://www.ncbi.nlm.nih.gov/pmc/articles/PMC2751289/ Accessed November 2015.

23. Blanco JG, Harrison PL, Evans WE, et al. Human cytochrome P450 maximal activities in pediatric versus adult liver. Drug Metab Disp. 2000; 28:379–82.

24. Cresteil T. Onset of xenobiotic metabolism in children: toxicological implications. Food Addit Contam. 1998; 15:45–51.

25. Loebstein R, Koren G. Clinical pharmacology and therapeutic drug monitoring in neonates and children.Pediatr Rev. 1998; 19:423–8

26. Klotz U. Pharmacokinetics and drug metabolism in the elderly. Drug Metab Rev. 2009; 41(2): 67-76.

27. Shi S and Klotz U Age-related changes in pharmacokinetics. Curr Drug Metab. 2011 Sep; 12(7):601-10.

28. Cusack BJ. Pharmacokinetics in older persons. Am J Geriatr Pharmacother. 2004 Dec; 2 (4): 274-302.

29. Tan JL, Eastment JG, Poudel A and Hubbard RE. Age-Related Changes in Hepatic Function: An Update on Implications for Drug Therapy. Drugs Aging. 2015 Nov 7.

30. Kamali F, Pirmohamed M. The future prospects of pharmacogenetics in oral anticoagulation therapy. Br J Clin Pharmacol. 2006; 61(6):746–51. Available online from: http://www.ncbi.nlm.nih.gov/pmc/articles/PMC443443/ Accessed November 2015.

31. Wadelius M, Pirmohamed M. Pharmacogenetics of warfarin: current status and future challenges.Pharmacogenomics J. 2007 Apr; 7(2):99-111

32. Aguilar MI, Hart R. Oral anticoagulants for preventing stroke in patients with non-valvular atrial fibrillation and no previous history of stroke or transient ischemic attacks. Cochrane Database Syst Rev.2005; 3 Jul 20;(3):CD001927

33. Freedman MD. Oral anticoagulants: pharmacodynamics, clinical indications and adverse effects. J Clin Pharmacol 32 March 1992 (3): 196–209.

34. Whitlon DS, Sadowski JA, Suttie JW Mechanism of coumarin action: significance of vitamin K epoxide reductase inhibition. Biochemistry 17 1978 (8): 1371–7.

35. Scully C. Chapter 8: Haematology in Scully, Medical Problems in Dentistry. 6th Edition Churchill Livingstone Elsevier. pp 194-196. Edinburgh 2010.

36. Muller P Y and Milton M N. The determination and interpretation of the therapeutic index in drug development. Nature Reviews Drug Discovery 2012. 11 (10): 751–761

37. Roden DM, Johnson JA, Kimmel SE, Krauss RM, Wong MW et al. Cardiovascular Pharmacogenomics. Circulation Research Review. 2011; 109: 807-820.
Available online from: http://circres.ahajournals.org/content/109/7/807.full
Accessed November 2015.

38. Linkins LA, Choi PT, Douketis JD. Clinical impact of bleeding in patients taking oral anticoagulant therapy for venous thromboembolism: a meta-analysis. Ann Intern Med. 2003; 139(11):893–900.

39. Pirmohamed M, James S, Meakin S, Green C, Scott AK, Walley TJ, Farrar K, Park BK, Breckenridge AM. Adverse drug reactions as cause of admission to hospital: prospective analysis of 18 820 patients.BMJ. 2004;329(7456):15–9.
Available online from: http://www.ncbi.nlm.nih.gov/pmc/articles/PMC443443/
Accessed November 2015.

40. Boulanger L, Kim J, Friedman M, Hauch O, Foster T, Menzin J. Patterns of use of antithrombotic therapy and quality of anticoagulation among patients with non-valvular atrial fibrillation in clinical practice. Int J Clin Pract. 2006; 60(3):258–64.

41. Jones M, McEwan P, Morgan CL, Peters JR, Goodfellow J and Currie CJ. Evaluation of the pattern of treatment, level of anticoagulation control and outcome of treatment with warfarin in patients with non-valvar atrial fibrillation: A record linkage study in a large British population. Heart. 2005; 91(4):472–7.

Available online from: http://www.ncbi.nlm.nih.gov/pmc/articles/ PMC1768813/

Accessed November 2015.

42. Pirmohamed M. Warfarin: almost 60 years old and still causing problems. British Journal of Clinical Pharmacology. 2006; 62(5): 509-511

43. Baxter K (Ed), Anticoagulants and NSAIDs miscellaneous. Stockley's Drug Interactions. 7th edition. London: Pharmaceutical Press.

Available online: www.medicinescomplete.com

Accessed November 2015.

44. Perry DJ, Nokes TJC and Heliwell PS. Guidelines for the management of patients on oral anticoagulants requiring dental surgery. British Committee for Standards in Haematology.

Available online from:

http://www.bcshguidelines.com/documents/ WarfarinandentalSurgery_bjh_264_2007.pdf

Accessed November 2015.

45. Blinder D, Manor Y, Martinowitz U, Taicher S and Hashomer T. Dental extractions in patients maintained on continued oral anticoagulant: comparison of local hemostatic modalities. Oral Surg Oral Med Oral Pathol Oral Radiol Endod 1999; 88 (2):137-40.

46. Zanon E, Martinelli F, Bacci C, Cordioli G and Girolami A. Safety of dental extraction among consecutive patients on oral anticoagulant treatment managed using a specific dental management protocol. Blood Coagul Fibrinolysis 2003; 14 (1): 27-30.

47. Sindet-Pedersen S, Ramstrom G, Bernvil S and Blomback M. Hemostatic effect of tranexamic acid mouthwash in anticoagulant-treated patients undergoing oral surgery. New England Journal of Medicine 1989; 320 (13):840-3.

48. Ramstrom G, Sindet-Pedersen S, Hall G, Blomback M and Alander U. Prevention of postsurgical bleeding in oral surgery using tranexamic acid without dose modification of oral anticoagulants. J Oral Maxillofacial Surg. 1993; 51(11): 1211-6.

49. Carter G and Goss A. Tranexamic acid mouthwash-a prospective randomized study of a 2-day regimen vs 5-day regimen to prevent postoperative bleeding in anticoagulated patients requiring dental extractions. Int J Oral Maxillofac Surg 2003; 32 (5): 504-7.

50. de Swart CA, Nijmeyer B, Roelofs JM, et al. Kinetics of intravenously administered heparin in normal humans. Blood. 1982; 60: 1251–1258.

51. Olsson P, Lagergren H and Ek S. The elimination from plasma of intravenous heparin: an experimental study on dogs and humans. Acta Med Scand. 1963; 173: 619–630.

52. Bjornsson TD, Wolfram KM and Kitchell BB. Heparin kinetics determined by three assay methods. Clin Pharmacol Ther. 1982; 31:104–113.

53. Kalow W, Tang BK and Endrenyi L. Hypothesis: comparisons of inter- and intra-individual variations can substitute for twin studies in drug research. Pharmacogenetics. 1998; 8(4): 283–289.

54. Wilson JF, Weale ME, Smith AC, et al. Population genetic structure of variable drug response. *Nat Genet.* 2001; 29 (3):265–269.

55. U.S. Food and Drug Administration. The Pharmaceutical Science Advisory Committee. November 14–15, 2005.

56. Aquilante CL, Langaee TY, Lopez LM, et al. Influence of coagulation factor, vitamin K epoxide reductase complex subunit 1, and cytochrome P450 2C9 gene polymorphisms on warfarin dose requirements. Clin Pharmacol Ther. 2006; 79 (4): 291–302.

56. Klotz U. Pharmacokinetics and Drug Metabolism in the Elderly. Drug Metab Rev. 2009; 41 (2):67-76.

57. Jancova P, Anzenbacher P, and Anzenbacherova E. Phase II drug metabolizing enzymes. Biomed Pap Med Fac Univ Palacky Olomouc Czech Repub. 2010 Jun; 154 (2): 103-16.

58. Danhof M. Kinetics of drug action in disease states: towards physiology-based pharmacodynamic (PBPD) models J Pharmacokinet Pharmacodyn. 2015 Oct; 42(5):447-62 Available online from:
http://www.ncbi.nlm.nih.gov/pmc/articles/PMC4582079/
Accessed November 2015.

59. Walter-Sack I and Klotz U. Influence of diet and nutritional status on drug metabolism. Clin Pharmacokinet. 1996 Jul; 31 (1): 47-64.

60. Tarek A. Ahmed. Pharmacokinetics of Drugs Following IV Bolus, IV Infusion, and Oral Administration, Basic Pharmacokinetic Concepts and Some Clinical Applications. 2015. Dr. Tarek A Ahmed (Ed.) InTech.
Available online from:
http://www.intechopen.com/books/basic-pharmacokinetic-concepts-and-some-clinical-applications/pharmacokinetics-of-drugs-following-iv-bolus-iv-infusion-and-oral-administration
Accessed January 2016.

61. Golightly, P. E. and Grant, E. Breast feeding and drug therapy 2: Problem areas. Pharmacy International, 1985: 6, 279-284.

62. Passmore CM, McElnay JC, Rainey EA and D'Arcy PF. Metronidazole excretion in human milk and its effect on the suckling neonate. British Journal of Clinical Pharmacology. 1988; 26(1): 45-51.

Drug action and drug interaction

In the previous section, the basics of drug metabolism were revised, with certain drugs and their importance to dentistry being discussed with respect to their metabolic activity and clinical effects. In this section, our exploration of drug metabolism continues, but will move on from the simple pharmacokinetics to focus on both pharmacokinetic and pharmacodynamic drug interactions.

To remind ourselves:

I. Pharmacokinetics are what the patient's metabolism will do to the drugs they take.
II. Pharmacodynamics are what the drugs will do to the patient's metabolism, the disease process or medical condition for which the patient is taking drugs.

By adding multiple drugs to these processes we now have to consider both the pharmacokinetic and the pharmacodynamic interactions, what one drug will do to another drug, together with the effects that such interactions will have on the patient.

Pharmaco-vigilance

As stated previously, the numbers of medicines our patients are being prescribed from their doctors and those they choose to obtain as over counter medicines (OCMs) without prescription are increasing every year. As patients live longer, the numbers of medicines they take will increase and with this, the risk of an adverse drug interaction will similarly rise. The World Health Organisation has reported that drug interactions are a leading cause of morbidity and mortality[1]. In the United States, Adverse Drug Reactions (ADR) are now the fourth greatest cause of mortality[2]. In the United Kingdom, some 16% of all hospital admissions are due to an ADR, while across Europe this figure is around 10%[3,4,5]. From such figures, the burden on any health service, whether socialized, nationalized or privatised, of any country in dealing with this issue will be severe. Indeed it has been estimated that up to one fifth of a country's hospital budget could be taken up by this problem alone[6].

The problem does not begin nor does it end with an ADR. Adding to this phenomenon, we have to consider inappropriate or irrational prescribing patterns, particularly the continued lack of antibiotic stewardship (see previous section), together with self-medication by the patient. These two problems only serve to confound the ADR issue. Lastly, into this dilemma, we must add the very recent rise, or at the least, a rise of something we have only recently began to consider in dentistry; the presence of counterfeit medicines and equipment.

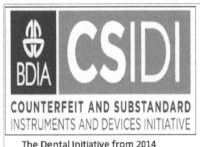 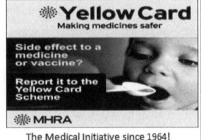

The Dental Initiative from 2014   and   The Medical Initiative since 1964!

The July 2014 initiative from the British Dental Industry Association (BDIA) is only a recent one and it follows the well established Yellow Card reporting program of the Medicines and Health Care Products Regulatory Authority (MHRA) to eliminate, or at least control the spread of counterfeit medicines and medical devices in the UK; should such entities present as an ADR.

This 1964 initiative came in the wake of the 1962 revelations of the side effects of a drug commonly prescribed as a sedative and anti-emetic. At that time, there was inadequate clinical trialling and unrestricted global release of this drug and many others too. Pregnant women were using this drug to alleviate the symptoms of morning sickness and in over 10,000 cases, the catastrophe of children being born with horrendous limb deformities or entire limb deficit both shockingly and unexpectedly began to follow in the UK and across Western Europe. At the time, the US based Richardson-Merrill company attempted to circumvent US Food and Drug Administration (FDA) regulations by distributing some 2.5 Million non-approved tablets to 1,200 doctors they had targeted to dispense the un-trialled drug to their unsuspecting patients.

Standing in the way of intense pressure and lobbying from multinational pharmaceutical companies poised to release this drug onto the US population, Dr Francis Kathleen Oldham Kelsey expressed a doubt based on just one three-paragraph observational paper written by the Scottish GP: Dr Leslie Florence, published in the BMJ, enquiring:

"Is Thalidomide to blame?"

Florence's observations of: Coldness of the extremities, neuropathy, ataxia and nocturnal cramps, were significant to merit publication in the BMJ[7]. This publication was then sufficient to temporarily block the release of Thalidomide into the US market, until Kelsey could establish the mechanism of action causing the side effect and whether such a metabolic action clearly capable of crossing the blood-brain barrier could also, as we now know: cross the placental barrier too.

Today Thalidomide is still available in the UK BNF as an immune-modulating drug for the treatment of multiple myeloma. It also has clinically beneficial effects in treating Erythema Nodosum Leprosy (ENL). Between 2005 and 2010, some 5.8 Million prescriptions for Thalidomide were issued in Brazil. Perhaps not due to poor preparation, but due to poor drug prescribing controls in a country which has the world's second greatest prevalence of leprosy behind India, over 100 cases of teratogenic birth defects resulted[8].

Thalidomide is an example of a drug with a relatively simple chemical formula: $C_{13} H_{10} N_2 O_4$. Many other drugs have similarly simple chemical formulas. Mass manufacturing, with poor preparation, combined to illicit marketing without prescription, will form a significant part of the Adverse Drug Reaction (ADR) problem. Throughout the world, medicines with dangerous side effects continue to be both inadequately prepared or inappropriately prescribed.

The presence of poorly prepared or intentionally counterfeited medicines present a global health risk as the legitimate drug supply chain becomes contaminated with substandard or ineffective products. Not only is there a risk of illicit medicines entering into the legitimate supply chain, within the counterfeit market, there is a risk of cross-contamination with compounds closely matching those of Thalidomide. The most commonly affected drug categories are the antimicrobials and the antiviral medicines, with a clear relevance and impact in dentistry from this problem. It has been reported that 10% of all drugs are counterfeit, with the proportion rising in those countries with poor pharmaceutical controls or limited regulatory mechanisms in place[9].

Other sources are now reporting globally that over one in five of all anti-infective medicines are counterfeit[10]. Furthermore, nearly two thirds of countries affected by this problem have no measures that are adequate to report on the extent of this problem[10]. In the UK, the MHRA Yellow card program into which all dental professionals have a duty to report, together with further stringent quality-control measures has kept the presence of: Substandard, Spurious, Falsely-labelled, Falsified or Counterfeit medical products (SSFFC) to the less than 1% level[11,12,13].

Although the abbreviation: **SSFFC** is now favoured in place of the term: **Counterfeit**, as it encompasses most if not all aspects of the problem, using one term to cover a multifaceted global issue has itself met with criticism. This has been due to the different causes of SSFFC, some requiring very different approaches if this problem is to be successfully tackled and eliminated[14].

It is interesting to note the UK dental profession's (only very recent) effort to deal with the SSFFC problem come 50 years after the medical profession's and that reaction followed the truly deplorable attempts of the US pharmacy industry to circumvent stringent FDA guidelines.

Of course, counterfeiting and SSFFC is nothing new, perhaps the most well known example can be found not in any clinic but from the cinema:

The Third Man was a 1949 film adaptation of Graham Green's novel. Directed by Carol Reed it is critically acclaimed as being the best British film of the Twentieth Century. The story recounts the black market in counterfeit medicines in a bombed-out, destroyed post war Vienna divided between the allied armies in four parts. Stolen penicillin was repeatedly diluted and administered to children with meningitis.

Although we don't see any children, the words spoken by Major Calloway (played by Trevor Howard) to Holly Martins (played by Joseph Cotten) as they both look down on a child dying in a hospital bed provide a picture as powerful as any screen image could...

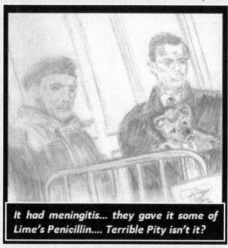

It had meningitis... they gave it some of Lime's Penicillin.... Terrible Pity isn't it?

It is truly amazing to think that in 1960, a clinical observation by a rural Scottish GP amounted to no more than a grain of sand in the well-oiled machinery of the multinational pharmaceutical industry. By 1962, with the US Kefauver Harris Amendment, then in 1965, with the European 65/65/EEC Directive, every pharmaceutical company had to prove both the efficacy and the safety of their drugs before they could be released. Such outcomes attested to the ability of Leslie Florence's grain of sand, in bringing the combined might of all chemical companies' machinery; not only to a halt, but also in affirming the important role of <u>all</u> clinicians in pharmaco-vigilance.

Human Factors and Drug Safety

Another way to look at our work in the dental clinic with respect to the drugs patients are taking and those we might prescribe, is to compare this aspect of our work with those who work in another safety critical arena: The aviation industry, specifically: Air Traffic Control.

By comparing the same way an air traffic controller (ATCO) operates with an advanced consideration of the risks that could actualise if the movement of one aircraft was to be permitted with respect to the flight plan of another; in the same way we must consider the effect on our patients if we were to permit the introduction of a drug for our patients if they are concurrently taking other medications.

> Returning to the cinema, in 1999 despite the biggest names in Hollywood: Jolie, Cusack, Blanchett and Thornton starring in "Pushing Tin" a film about the high-pressure work environment of air traffic controllers was both a critical and commercial failure.
>
> Despite this film's lack of success, there are lessons to be learned from the consequences arising from the conduct of the characters in this film. Lessons that can be applied to the safety critical arena of the dental practice:
>
> > I.   Interpersonal conflicts in the high-pressure environment of air traffic control also apply to dentistry.
> > II. We must be mindful of this, especially when considering the safety of our patients with respect to medicines and the risk of drug interactions.
> > III. Adverse personal interactions between patients and practitioners are stressful.
> > IV. Adverse professional interactions can add to the stress.
> > V.   In any safety critical environment, with an increase in stress the risk of an adverse event will also increase.
>
> The following quote from an Air Traffic Controller, (New York TRACON, Westbury Long Island) can also be applied to dentistry when we reflect on all the patients we treat without any adverse interactions:

> **You land a million planes safely;**
> **then you have one little mid-air**
> **(collision) and you never hear the end of it!!**

In these times of restrictive legislation coupled to aggressive litigation it is well worth critically thinking about the consequences that follow if two drugs with an adverse interaction should inadvertently meet in one patient

Returning to drug safety, the comparison between aviation and dentistry is both interesting and useful. The aviation terms italicised in brackets in the following paragraph can equally apply and do fit well into the clinical environment:

We have a duty to control the prescription *(Movement)* of drugs and medicines, preventing any Adverse Drug Reactions/ADR or Interactions *(Deconfliction)* and then to document and report any reactions or side effects *(Infringements)* or dangerous drug occurrences *(Near Misses (aka an AIRPROX))* that could, or do affect patient safety; from whatever source they may arise.

Just as an Air Traffic Controller will file a Mandatory Occurrence Report *(MOR)*, in the clinical environment, we have a duty to complete and submit similar reports up to and including the MHRA Yellow Card if an ADR were to occur. In aviation, if there is a concern or even a perceived risk, then both pilots and ATCOs can file reports and from this point, the analogy between dentistry and aviation becomes a dichotomy.

The following five points should be considered:

I.   Whereas for all aviation professionals, the filing of an MOR could result in a board enquiry, the investigation that follows comes from a mature no-blame culture seeking to establish reasons from which preventive lessons can be disseminated across the industry so others can learn from active CPD that: Pilots Recognize for Operational Up-skilling and Development, that is: PROUD.

II. However, in dentistry, at the time of writing, investigations are combative and litigiously driven to find fault, apportion blame and then publicly shame those the professional regulator, the GDC believes to be guilty. From such an immature approach, one can neither learn lessons, nor develop strategies to prevent clinical accidents from re-occurring. The CPD process is never considered from the beginning, to the end or at any point along this route.

III. Whereas in aviation a mature culture seeks to find the truth, learn then grow, in dentistry an immature culture seeks to find fault, blame and maintain control.

IV. By actively thinking of our dental patients in the clinic with respect to drug administration, whether: prescription, over counter medicine (OCM) or recreational in the same way an air traffic controller will work the pilots in their sector whether: commercial, military or general, we can begin to promote a drug safety culture, to learn and grow as professionals.

V. By doing so, we can further reduce the risks to patients in a climate where rapidly increasing varieties and numbers of medicines are being taken. We should adopt such an approach well before the advent of mandatory CPD in Drug Safety comes from a regulatory body. In doing so we will continue to treat patients and the risks of that one in a million mid-air or ADR will be reduced significantly.

Adverse drug reactions

We can think of Adverse Drug Reactions in five broad terms[5]:

I. An adverse drug reaction (ADR) is a noxious unintended response to a medicine or a drug used in the normal dose range. A drug is defined as a pharmaceutical product administered for the prevention, treatment, control of a physiological process, or the diagnosis of a disease and treatment for a pathological process in humans. The ADR is the response of the patient to a drug in which individual factors may play an important role in producing the noxious effect.

II. An unexpected therapeutic response, may be a side effect but this is not an adverse reaction. A side effect is any unintended effect of a pharmaceutical product occurring at doses normally used by a patient that are related to the pharmacological properties of the drug. The important parts of this definition are the adverse effect is pharmacological in nature, the phenomenon is unintended and there is no overdose.

III. In contrast, the ADR is unexpected and the nature or severity is not consistent with the drug's characteristics for which it was authorised for release or prescribed for use. An adverse event or experience is an untoward medical occurrence presenting during treatment with a medicine but which does not necessarily have a causal relationship with the treatment. The basic point here is there is a coincidence in time, without any suspicion of a causal relationship.

IV. An ADR may become a Serious Adverse Drug Reaction, in that: Serious is defined as an ADR being:
    i.   Fatal or life-threatening.
    ii. Permanently or significantly disabling.
    iii. One requiring or prolonging hospitalization or needing referral to a specialist.
    iv. Causative of a congenital abnormality or a teratogenic birth defect.
    v.   Requiring an intervention to prevent the risk of permanent impairment or damage materialising.

V. With a suspected ADR, the event should be reported with data on the possible causal relationship between an ADR and a drug, especially if the relationship was unknown or incompletely documented previously. Usually more than one report is required to generate an ADR signal, with an MHRA response, but this depends on the seriousness of the event being reported, together with the quality of the information being supplied.

The number of drugs with variations in their doses and preparations available is simply staggering. A quick internet search might reveal no definitive answer to the question:

"How many drugs are listed and available in the UK BNF?"

However, the index to BNF 70 has 42 pages with some 180 drugs (+/- 10) on each page. Therefore, some 7,500 drugs might be available for our patients. In addition to this number, there will be the OCM's, the homeopathic remedies and the recreational drugs our patient's will be taking. Please consider the following illustration:

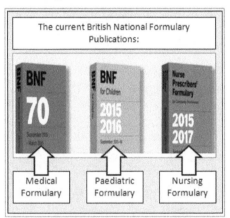

You will see that nurses and children also have their very own BNF, while dental professionals do not. Not because you cannot be trusted with drugs, in fact you can prescribe from the entire range of drugs in the BNF. However, the numbers of drugs actually necessary or beneficial in dentistry are surprisingly small. Remember, dentistry is a surgical discipline, not a medical one and certainly not a pharmaceutical one. Whenever appropriate, all attempts to cure by removing the cause with simple means, rather than treating the symptom with complicated measures must be followed, eg: incision and drainage of an abscess, rather than treating the swelling with antibiotics should be the rule rather than the exception. Such an approach provides a safe way to proceed in reducing the effects of drug interactions and side effects, which are discussed below:

Pharmacodynamic interactions

When our patient takes more than one drug, it is highly likely that an effect other than that intended from single drug use might result. We should remember that not only prescribed medicines interact, as discussed previously; certain foods eaten at the same time as the administration of a drug can increase or decrease the absorption of that drug. As noted above, we must be vigilant to those interactions between prescribed medicines and recreational drugs or prescribed medicines and alternative therapies.

Pharmacodynamic drug actions and interactions occur in five groups: Agonism, Antagonism, Synergism, Potentiation and Summation:

I. Agonism. This drug effect results from compounds binding to receptor sites. Agonists can be endogenous (produced naturally by the body, eg: hormones or neurotransmitters) or agonists can be exogenous (administered or introduced as drugs eg: morphine which binds to opioid receptors in the Central Nervous System). Super-agonists produce a greater response when bound to the receptor than an endogenous agonist, while partial-agonists can bind to and activate a receptor site but will only elicit a partial effect even at maximal or saturation concentrations. A good example of a partial-agonist is buprenorphine, which binds to opioid receptors. In addition to this agonist, there are inverse agonists and irreversible agonists. Such compounds do not elicit the response of an antagonist (see below) but express an opposite effect. An example of such a drug is rimonabant used to reverse the effect of cannabinoids such as marijuana, another drug group recently reclassified as an inverse agonist are anti-histamines; these were previously considered to be antagonists of the H_1 Histamine receptor site[16].

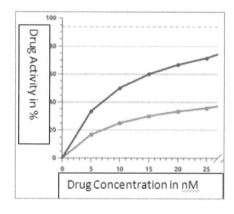

II. Antagonism. This is the blocking of a receptor site by a drug. It should be noted that an antagonist will not produce a physiological effect, but it will prevent an endogenous or exogenous agonist (a drug) from producing its action or effect. While agonists turn a cell on, an antagonist will prevent a cell from being turned on, but it will not turn a cell off. In strict pharmacological terms, antagonists have an affinity but no efficacy when bound to a receptor. Antagonists can be reversible or irreversible and exert their effect by competitively binding to receptor sites. Some examples of antagonists you will have noted your dental patients taking are Alpha and Beta Blockers and Calcium Channel Blockers. The definition of an

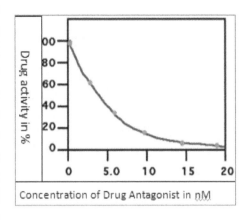

Concentration of Drug Antagonist in nM

antagonist lies with its pharmacological effects resulting from occupancy of receptors on the cell surface or within the cell itself. Such a definition can also be applied to the physiological effects of agonistic drugs that behave as antagonists. For example, histamine lowers arterial pressure through vasodilation at the histamine H_1 receptor, while adrenaline raises arterial pressure through vasoconstriction mediated by alpha-adrenergic receptor activation.

Our understanding of the mechanisms and biochemical definition of antagonists continue to evolve from those models originally proposed in the 1950's[17] [18.] From the two state agonist-antagonist model, we now have multistate models and intermediate conformational receptor models.[19.] From such an understanding, functionally selective drugs targeting receptors with highly defined messenger systems are available for those particular downstream effects we wish to inactivate[19]. Essentially, the efficacy of antagonists may depend on where receptors are located, either intracellularly or on the cell surface, altering the view that efficacy at a receptor is receptor-independent property of a drug.[20]

III. Synergism This occurs when one drug interacts with another drug in a way to enhance one or more intended clinical effects or accidental side-effects of either of the drugs. With OCMs for dental analgesia, synergism has been used in combination preparations, such as the mixing of 3-methyl morphine (codeine) with acetaminophen or ibuprofen to enhance the action of codeine as a pain reliever. The knowledge of negative synergism can be the basis of drug contraindication. The combination of CNS depressants such as alcohol when used with any of the benzodiazepines eg: Oral valium or IV midazolam will result in a greater clinical effect than the simple sum of the individual effects of each drug if these drugs were to be

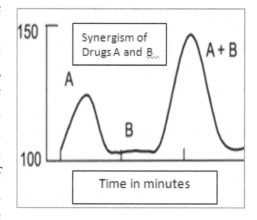

used in isolation. With relevance to IV dental sedation, if a patient were to have taken ethanol and then IV midazolam, the most serious consequence of this particular drug synergy could be an exaggerated respiratory depression, which if left untreated could prove to be fatal.

The taking of a social and medical history to identify alcohol misuse, or any form of substance abuse is an essential safety requirement for your patient requiring dental sedation.

The inadvertent mixing of drugs can produce potentially fatal reactions within the brain, such as the Serotonin Syndrome. This condition is due to synergistic reactions changing chemical and receptor activity in the CNS. We will return to consider the human impact of this syndrome later. For now, please consider the following clinical triad of abnormalities which are indicative of this syndrome:[21].

i. Cognitive effects: headache, confusion, hypomania, hallucinations and coma.
ii. Autonomic effects: shivering, sweating, vasoconstriction, tachycardia.
iii. Somatic effects: muscle twitching, hyper-reflexia and tremor.

Additionally, be aware of following drugs being implicated in the synergy of the Serotonin Syndrome:

i. Antidepressants eg: Mono-Amine Oxidase Inhibitors (MAOIs), Tri Cyclic Antidepressants (TCAs) Serotonin Specific Reuptake Inhibitors (SSRIs) and Bupropion (now in common use as an adjunct for smoking cessation).
ii. Opioids eg: Pethidine, Tramadol, Fentanyl, Oxycodon, Hydrocodon, Pentazocine and Buprenorphine.
iii. CNS Stimulants eg: Cocaine, MDMA Amphetamines
iv. Psychedelic drugs eg: Lysergide.
v. Other drugs, foods and preparations eg: St John's wort, nutmeg, olanzepine.

Drug synergy can arise from pharmacodynamics and from <u>pharmacokinetics</u> too, the commonality of metabolic enzymes that can become saturated results in drug combinations remaining in the bloodstream for much longer and in higher concentrations than if drugs were individually taken.

IV. Potentiation Is the interaction whereby one drug, induces the enhancement of another drug's effect with an overall increase in the activity of that drug so an increased clinical effect will result. While this may seem similar to Synergism as noted above, the important points and differences are as follows:

i. <u>Synergism</u> is the interaction of two or more drugs. The resulting effect is greater than the sum of the individual effects.

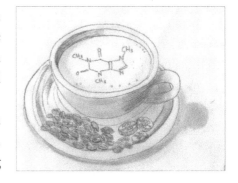

ii. <u>Potentiation</u> is the action of one drug on another, the second drug becoming more effective as long as it remains in a synergistically augmented relationship.

iii. While Synergism is the interaction of two or more drugs, Potentiation is the effect of one drug on another and the way in which a second drug acts while in synergy or under influence of the first drug.

Drug potentiation can be a useful property for medical treatments, one example being the combination of caffeine and ibuprofen to increase the nociceptive targeting properties of this and other NSAIDs[22]. However, in dentistry, potentiation can be troublesome. The most common potentiation problem we need to consider is the effect of alcohol on the post-synaptic $GABA_A$ receptor site potentiating the action of IV Midazolam. Although there is no defined receptor for alcohol, it acts as a CNS depressant through its dissolution in lipids and proteins of neural cell membranes. Alcohol will increase the permeability of post-synaptic $GABA_A$ receptors allowing Chloride ion influx and hyperpolarization of the neuronal membrane with reduced firing will then cause an increased sedative effect. In dentistry, the potential for over-sedation can move the patient out of the safe arena of prescribed conscious sedation into the dangerous domain of unintended out-patient General Anaesthesia[23].

The corollary of alcohol-midazolam potentiation is that a controlled regimen of prescribed oral benzodiazepines can be used to treat alcohol withdrawal symptoms and is useful in treating the recovering alcoholic[24].

V. Summation Is the arithmetic accumulation of similar drug effects from different drugs combining to give a simple additive effect. This is different from synergy where the effect is enhanced rather than just being additive, or from potentiation where the effect of only one

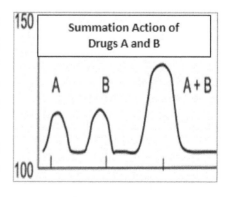

drug in the relationship is enhanced. An example of the summation effect can be found with the drug combinations used to treat cancers, specifically ovarian cancer. Cisplatin (a cycle specific but non-phase specific cytotoxic drug) has been combined with cyclophosphamide (an alkylating agent). As the two drugs differ in their mode of action, an additive anti-neoplastic effect is seen with fewer side effects than if one of the drugs was used on its own[25].

It is entirely possible that this principle and similar regimens will be applied to the oral cancers too.

There are advantages in using drug combinations when the outcome is not a synergism but only a summation. Even with an additive effect, the treatment will be enhanced, especially so if the mechanism of action of the two drugs is different. Drug combinations have been used for treating diseases for many years. The three advantages in doing so are:

i.   It is possible to increase of efficacy of the therapeutic effect, especially when drugs in sequence differ in their mechanism of action, but give similar effects.

ii. Using additive drug regimens allows reduced dosages of each component and thus toxicity risk is reduced resulting in lower adverse effects of each component.

iii. The potential for developing drug resistance is also lower when multiple drugs are used.

The last of these presents the most important challenge for ourselves in dentistry as it does for medicine, being both a critical limitation in drug use and a difficult problem to avoid, not only when dealing with cancer but for the treatment of bacterial infection too.[26.]

Drug interactions in dentistry

The drug interactions we face in clinical dentistry can be summarised in the diagram below [27]:

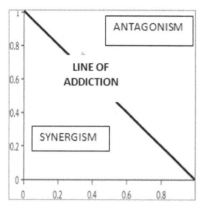

The 2 axes represent the concentrations of two drugs. Those points plotted above the line represent drug antagonism, while those below represent all forms of synergy noted above. In mathematical terms the following formula defines this isobologram:

$$\frac{a}{A} + \frac{b}{B} = \gamma$$

A and *B* are the initial drug concentrations required for the desired clinical effect. While *a* and *b* are those concentrations of the two drugs when combined that will give the same effect. If the resultant value is greater than 1 then the effect is Antagonistic, less than 1 it is Synergistic and if it is equal to 1 then it is Additive.

From the above you will see that not all drug interactions are accidental or harmful, indeed some of those noted above are intentional and beneficial. There are three broad categories of interaction we need to consider in dentistry:

1. Pharmaceutical interactions. These arise from the chemical incompatibilities of one drug when mixed with another. These reactions were principally seen with the IV route of drug administration, most commonly damage arising from emulsion forming on the endothelial lining. This reaction was a frequent outcome where Propofol was given with Diazepam, especially if the IV line was not flushed between drugs. In the advent of the 2015 Standards for Conscious Sedation in the Provision of Dental Care report (from the Royal Colleges of Surgeons and Anaesthetists), it is now extremely unlikely that you will see such pharmaceutical interactions in a dental patient as we have moved towards single drug use (Midazolam) for IV sedation which is diluted with physiological solutions.

2. Pharmacodynamic interactions can be grouped into the five categories listed above which result in adverse receptor site activity, either at the cell surface or within the cells of various tissues and organ systems throughout the body. One pharmacodynamic interaction of particular note in dentistry is that of Propofol and the benzodiazepine: Midazolam.

In the advent of the 2015 Standards for Conscious Sedation in Dentistry, Propofol doses will be restricted, but this drug will still be available for dental sedation. The pharmacodynamic interactions and misuse of this drug did little to enhance Dr Conrad Murray's credibility or career. However, it certainly worked wonders for Michael Jackson's career, which died long before he did. By (ab)using copious amounts of Propofol and Midazolam, he promptly became the highest earning dead person ...ever.

The world over, dental practitioners do have access to all manner of drugs. As previously noted in the UK BNF there are some 7,500 or so drugs to choose from.

In the USA, Dr Lester Hoffman; a dentist, was responsible for an upper central incisor which became known as the "King's Crown" however it has not been established whether he may or may not have had a hand in the unfeasibly large amount of post-mortem prescription medications found in Elvis Presley's bathroom, or his bloodstream.

For those of us who work in the UK, we would do well to remember the two salutary lessons of Jackson and Presley and not become enchanted or influenced by our patients who happen to be musicians or are world famous, as we are not immune to the risks that come from their fame and fortune. In the UK, the composer Lionel Bart was famed for carrying a briefcase so full of recreational and other drugs it became known as Bart's Hospital. More recently, the life and untimely death of George Michael on Christmas Day 2016 and the death of Tom Petty on 2nd October 2017* are poignant, but precious reminders that celebrity

---

* Petty died from an accidental overdose o of fentanyl, oxycodone, temazepam and citalopram.

status confers no immunity from, but is undoubtedly helpful in the illicit acquisition of medicinal substances.

The PIS...

Setting these lessons aside, for those of us in clinical practice, the risk to most of our patients does not come from success but from adverse drug interactions, one example we can learn from is the Propofol Infusion Syndrome.

From a point of dental safety, the Propofol Infusion Syndrome (PIS) is seen in those patients with pre-existing mitochondrial abnormalities being exacerbated by Propofol given in doses above 5mg/Kg and for periods exceeding 48 hours. Most importantly, the syndrome is expressed when Propofol is administered with corticosteroids when treating inflammatory diseases.[28,29.]

One early sign of PIS is the passing of bright green urine as a result of metabolic acidosis and rhabdomyolysis with myoglobinuria. This is an important clinical sign not to be missed, because by the time cardiac arrhythmias are seen, hepatomegaly with renal failure is well established and the patient's heart muscle will be irreversibly damaged. The ensuing cardiac and multi-organ failure is the invariably late and fatal signs of PIS.

The doses of Propofol with Midazolam used in dental sedation are unlikely to initiate PIS. Nevertheless, a patient's genetic pre-disposition to mitochondrial disease combined with established levels of stress and corticosteroid medication might theoretically precipitate PIS. Of note, is that excessive endogenous catecholamine release and exogenous corticosteroid use can only magnify the tendency for Propofol to inhibit the breakdown of fatty acids, promoting a rapid and irreversible cardiac muscle injury.[30]

Susceptible dental patients may generally remain well until they are in stressful situations ie: the dental surgery and the risk of PIS can only be aggravated by their use of corticosteroids. Adrenaline containing dental local anaesthetics accidentally injected into the vasculature (this does happen on an improbably frequent basis) can transiently reduce blood flow to the viscera thus causing a rapid increase in the relative amount of Propofol in the patient's systemic circulation. The high mortality from PIS induced cardiac arrhythmia is due to the cardio-depressant antagonism of β-adrenoreceptors and calcium channels causing reduced myocardial contractility with rapidly fatal consequences.

When all things are considered, dental patients being given Midazolam with Propofol even in the small dental doses for conscious sedation do remain at some risk from PIS and we must be vigilant to this.

Should our dental patient have been pre-medicated with corticosteroids and then be given an adrenaline containing local anaesthetic, the risk of inducing PIS can only increase.

The reasons for combining Propofol with Midazolam and then using dental local anaesthesia are:

Propofol is a rapidly acting sedative anaesthetic and it is quickly metabolized but it confers no analgesic effect whatsoever[31]. The reduction in blood pressure from Propofol is an example of a non-intentional pharmacodynamic action enhanced by its interaction with other drugs. Propofol will be discussed again in greater detail along with other sedatives used in specialist dental practice in the last section in this chapter.

Diuretics and dentistry

In contrast to this effect, diuretics exert a similar albeit intentional and non-cardiogenic lowering of blood pressure. Being among the most prescribed and studied of all drugs, at least in the UK, the EU and the USA, diuretics form part of a peculiarly effective medical response to the high prevalence of diet and lifestyle induced cardiovascular disease. (NB prevention is better than cure and diuretics are a treatment not a cure.) There are several different classes of diuretics exerting their clinical effects by distinct actions at various sites and cell receptors throughout the nephron. From a drug safety point, it is important to consider these in some detail.

Diuretics induce the loss of water from the nephron while preventing the reabsorption of Na^+ ions across tubule and collecting duct membranes. In broad terms, the five main classes of diuretic we should be concerned with are:

i. **Carbonic Anhydrase Inhibitors** enzymatically act in the Proximal Convoluted Tubules to decrease Na^+ absorption and increase bicarbonate and H^+ excretion.

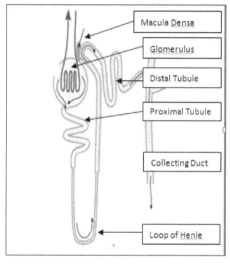

ii. **Osmotic Diuretics** exert simple pressure effects at the proximal tubule and descending limb of Henle.

iii. **Loop Diuretics** inhibit Na^+ reabsorption in the thick ascending limb of Henle.

iv. **Thiazides** are the most commonly prescribed diuretics inhibiting the Na^+ Cl^- Symporter in the distal convoluted tubule.

v. **Potassium Sparing Diuretics** although not site-specific do enhance Thiazides in Cortical collecting ducts. One notable example is the Spironalactone inhibition of Aldosterone.

In addition to these five classes of diuretic drugs, there could be up to ten drug groups and individual chemical types with distinct diuretic properties[32.] Included with these are the Xanthines (such as caffeine), various salts, ethanol and dopamine, which act on the proximal tubule to increase Na^+ secretion. Generally: Thiazides are the most frequently prescribed diuretic class with Hydrocholorothiazide being a common example, while loop diuretics are the most effective with Furosemide being the drug given to most patients with Congestive Heart Failure (CHF).

NSAIDs, COXs and ADIs

The Adverse Drug Interaction (ADI) of NSAIDs and diuretics should be borne in mind. It is entirely probable that by the time a patient attends the dental surgery, they may well have over-medicated with OCM NSAIDs for pain relief. NSAIDs taken in this way have an ability to alter renal function by their inhibition of:

i.   The Cyclo Oxygenase 1. Pathway (COX 1), that is concerned with every day physiological regulation and the control of kidney blood flow and filtration in the glomerulus.
ii. The Cyclo Oxygenase 2. Pathway (COX 2), that is involved in the reaction to injury and systemic pathology, which regulates Na+ and CL⁻ excretion in the nephron.

The following diagram shows COX 1 and COX 2 involvement in the inflammatory response. All NSAIDs inhibit either COX 1, or COX 2. These enzymes convert Arachidonic acid to a series of Prostanoids. In this way, pain sensations, inflammatory reactions and temperature regulation can be modulated. Prostaglandin H_2 (PGH_2) is converted into five primary prostaglandins, including:

i.   Thromboxane A_2: Initiates platelet aggregation and blood clotting.
ii. Prostacyclin: Vasodilates the endothelium inhibiting platelet aggregation[33].

COX 1 is constitutively expressed, being involved in protecting the stomach from excessive acid secretion (COX 1 inhibition by Aspirin is implicated in gastro-intestinal ulceration) and in the production of Thromboxane by platelets. In contrast to this, COX 2 expression follows the release of chemical mediators from tissues affected by inflammatory processes. However, COX2 can be constitutively expressed too and as noted above, it can control the function of the kidneys as well as that of the reproductive organs, osteoclasts and neurotransmission[33][34].

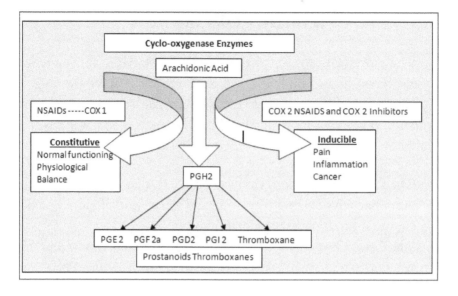

While Aspirin, Ibuprofen and Naproxen are NSAIDs, Paracetomol is not, as it has little or no discernable anti-inflammatory properties. However, Paracetomol can reduce pain by blocking COX 2 in the CNS but not in PNS. More than 5 days use of an NSAID may reduce the ability of a diuretic to lower or control hypertension.

ACE and RAAS

Although this effect was small and not clinically relevant in clinical trials on healthy volunteers [34,35], there may be serious implications for those patients who are cardiovascularly compromised or those patients taking Angiotensin Converting Enzyme (ACE) Inhibitors to lower their blood pressure, either in the advent or the wake of a cardiac event. It should be noted that ACE inhibitors are not diuretics as such, but do act to lower blood pressure by blocking the conversion of Angiotensin I to Angiotensin II in the Renin Angiotensin Aldesterone System (RAAS), Renin being released from cells in the Macula Densa in response to lower renal blood pressure and flow.

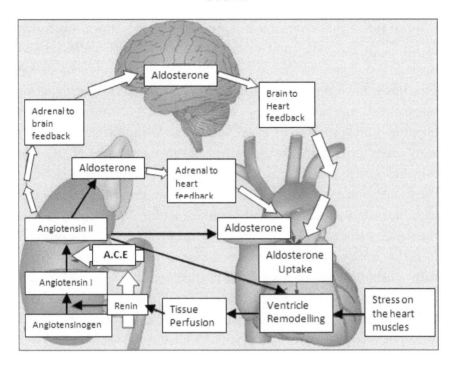

I. The importance of the kidneys and adrenal glands in homeostasis and its place in the negative feedback of the RAAS can be seen from this diagram.

II. Of note is the effect that cardiac injury or cardiac stress has on this system[36].

III. Interestingly, the RAAS has become something of a scapegoat for all the cardiovascular ills arising from hypertension and the use of Angiotensin Converting Enzyme (ACE) inhibitors, Angiotensin Receptor Blockers (ARBs) and Direct Renin Blockers (DRB)s stems from this belief.

IV. Although this hypothesis is now being challenged with new evidence:

V. It is important that the use of drugs in dentistry do not impact on the medical use of ACE Inhibitors, ARBs or DRBs

Our approach to dental prescribing must be safety critical, observant of the latest guidelines and cautious to the medical conditions and medicines our patients are taking. With such an attitude, our dental prescribing must not adversely impact on the medical prescribing for our patients; especially when we consider the RAAS and what could potentially be at stake from an ADI or Direct Drug Interaction (DDI) with either those NSAIDs the patient has taken or those NAIDs we might choose to give them.

In addition to such pharmaco-vigilance, we must keep up to date with the latest findings from evidence based studies. With regard to this, the newer selective COX 2 inhibitors when used in combination with NSAIDs available as OCMs, presents further hazards for our patient, with a demonstrable increased risk of myocardial infarct and stroke. This effect is especially noticeable with combinations of COX 1 and COX 2 inhibitors. Such combined drug regimens are not recommended due to the increased risk of myocardial infarct as follows:

i. **In patients with no previous heart disease, this risk might be doubled [38].**

ii. **For patients with a pre-existing history of heart disease, there could be a tenfold increase [39].**

The risk of raised blood pressure, peripheral oedema, sodium retention and possibly an accelerated descent into CHF with COX 1 or 2 inhibitors will be increased in those patients who are older, diabetic, overweight, medicated and with an existing heart condition. This problem is so serious that in the USA the FDA has now made public its warning about the risk from NSAID use[40].

Lastly we must be aware that the kidney as an organ of pharmacokinetic action (drug elimination) is itself at risk from damage and ultimately organ failure from the pharmacodynamic interactions of NSAIDs, ACE inhibitors and Diuretics which are in essence nephrotoxic when taken in combination.

3. Pharmacokinetic Drug Interactions. The third category of drug interaction we are interested in arises when one drug interferes with the ability of another drug to reach its target tissue or cell receptor. We have already considered pharmacokinetics in the previous section, just to remind us, the five pharmacokinetic factors are:

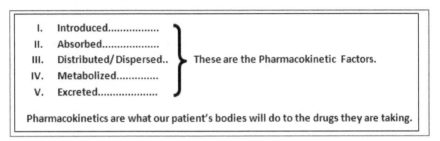

In the previous section, the principles of pharmacokinetics were described as they apply to a patient taking one drug. When two or more drugs are involved, the pharmacokinetic processes become even more interesting! When a drug is introduced orally, absorption begins in the mucosa of the mouth eg: GTN spray and in the stomach eg: alcohol and certain antibiotics. After eating or due to drug action, the stomach will become transiently less acidic. With a rise in the stomach pH, the absorption of some drugs will be reduced.

$$\uparrow \text{Stomach pH} = \downarrow \text{Drug Absorption}$$

A clinically relevant example of this absorption-interaction is that affecting the antibiotics:

i.   Ciprafloxacin (A Quinolone useful against Aerobic Gram Negative species eg: Shigella and Salmonella)

ii. Tetracycline (A broad-spectrum antibiotic previously very useful but now in decline due to resistance, but highly effective for Lyme Disease and MRSA cases)

While we may never need to prescribe the former, the latter is still effective against the anaerobic species causing destructive periodontal disease. The gastric absorption of these two drugs is significantly reduced if the patient is taking Antacids, Calcium supplements or on a diet with a high mineral content. In addition to Calcium, these minerals can include: Iron, Magnesium and Zinc. The absorption of minerals and antibiotics will be reduced by their affinity and binding.

Medications reducing gastric acid secretion, such as Proton Pump Inhibitors (PPIs) eg: Omeprazole and H_2 Blockers (antihistamine antagonists) eg: Cimetidine and Ranitidine, while increasing the stomach pH, might not diminish the absorption of the above noted antibiotics, but they will reduce the absorption of antifungals such as Ketoconazole that relies on a low pH for dissolution and absorption. (This is now something of an academic point as oral Ketoconazole, being extremely hepato-toxic was suspended by the UK CHMP from July 2013)

Drugs such as PPIs can and do significantly reduce the uptake of Folate, Vitamin B12 and Iron. Interestingly PPI use has resulted in an alteration of GI tract flora with an increase in pathogenic species. A 1.5 X risk increase of clinical cases of Clostridium *difficile* has been documented[41].

Tetracycline will compete with B12 receptors, so a reduction in Vitamin B12 levels will mean relatively more antibiotics will be absorbed, but this does not mean a reduction in pathogenic species will be seen for two reasons:

i. Tetracyclines are useful for Oral, Bronchial and Genito-Urinary Infections but not GI tract pathogens.
ii. Even if more antibiotics are absorbed, the distribution metabolism and excretion rate is unaltered.
iii. An increase in antibiotic use and patient exposure is associated with ablation of commensals and proliferation of pathogens being resistant to the antibiotic prescribed.

From the above, once more you will see the importance of Antibiotic Stewardship and Pharmaco-vigilance in drug prescribing. Every one of our incorrect prescriptions in the dental clinic might lead to the necessity for a corrective intervention in the Gastro-Intestinal Clinic.

In this respect, the treatment of C. *difficile* in the first instance will be with Metronidazole (due to cost). This is followed by Vancomycin or Fidaxomycin. If this regimen does not work then Faecal Bacteriotherapy has been reported to be more successful[42]. It doesn't matter how much you hate working in a dental clinic, or how bad a day you're having, but would you really perform faecal bacteriotherapy for a living?

Despite the offensive nature of this procedure, for the patient suffering from C. difficile, the alternative could be a surgical resection of their Colon and permanent colostomy. Remember, please: One cause of this outcome is the inappropriate prescription of antibiotics. Therefore, from a position of safety, we must seek the effective promotion of alternatives to the routine and invariably blind prescribing of antibiotics for our patients.

Most drugs are absorbed in the upper GI tract, more frequent and perhaps more significant than drug absorption-interactions are the diet absorption-interactions. The rate and extent of stomach emptying, the level of acidity and the presence of food, surely must affect drug absorption more than if another drug was being taken simultaneously.

Although NSAIDs do cause gastric irritation and there is a risk of ulceration, especially with Aspirin, paradoxically if the drug is taken on a (relatively) empty stomach, then more of the drug will be absorbed and distributed faster than if taken with food as recommended by the friendly local dispensing pharmacist. The required analgesic effect can thus be attained faster and with lower doses. As dental professionals, we must have a say in this and we do have a responsibility when prescribing, to advise our patients accordingly and not just refer them to the instructions on the back of the packet of pills we told them to use.

In addition to minerals binding to antibiotics, nutrients can bind to other drugs preventing their absorption. Notably a diet rich in fibre can reduce the absorption of Tricyclic Antidepressants such as Amitriptyline.

Of the two fibre types, insoluble fibre binds to and reduces uptake of Digoxin (a cardiac glycoside), whereas soluble fibre binds to and reduces the uptake of a variety of drugs such as Penicillin, Paracetamol, Statins, Lithium and Carbamazapine. The last two of these you will recall are of clinical importance in the treatment of depressive mental illness and neuropathic pain, both of these symptoms being associated with Trigeminal Neuralgia. Another way to look at the absorption-interactions is to consider that drugs also affect the absorption of foods due to the duality of enzymes involved in both nutrient and drug metabolism, we shall return to consider drug metabolism in detail after this short paragraph on drug distribution:

Following from drug absorption, drug distribution plays an important role in pharmacokinetic drug interactions. Drugs distributed in plasma are bound to proteins and are pharmacologically inactive. Only when a drug is free or unbound, will it become active and then: its clinical effects will be seen. In the previous section, we considered in some detail; the effect of one free drug on a bound drug, if the latter had a low Therapeutic Index or Ti. Specifically, due to the high prevalence of its use and the safety-critical relevance to dentistry: Warfarin is a good example of a drug with 99% binding and such a narrow Ti, that should Aspirin be taken concurrently; there is a risk of an unmanageable rise in INR with serious and clinically uncontrolled bleeding resulting.

However, that is from a dental point of view. From a medical point of view; the haematologist faced with the patient who has artificial heart valves may take an entirely different stance and the evidence strongly suggests the benefit of co-medicating with Aspirin and Warfarin to prevent a thrombo-embolic event far outweighs the risks of serious bleeding specifically associated with these patients[43].

The chore of biotransformation

The most common and perhaps the most complex of all pharmacokinetic drug interactions are those involving the metabolizing enzymes responsible for drug biotransformation in the liver. The acronym: **CHORE** describes those busy processes hard at work and these are:

> **Conjugation**
> **Hydrolysis**
> **Oxidation** } These are all the phases of Biotransformation
> **Reduction**
> **Excretion.**

When a drug is administered, the pharmacokinetics of metabolism can either activate an inactive Parent Pro-Drug or deactivate an active Parent Drug. These processes of biotransformation principally occur in the liver and the kidneys in the following order:

> **Phase 1:** **O**xidation, **R**eduction and **H**ydrolysis, before.
> **Phase 2:** **C**onjugation becoming H20 soluble prior to **E**xcretion

The enzymes associated with Phase 1 Metabolism are those principally involved in drug interactions while those associated with Phase 2 Metabolism are concerned with drug processing for renal excretion. The Phase 1 enzymes are located in the Smooth Endoplasmic Reticulum (SER) of hepatocytes and the SERs of other cells in the mucosa of the GI tract, the lungs, the kidneys and exocrine glands of the skin. While the Phase 2 enzymes are located in SERs of renal tissues, principally in cells of membranes in the loop, duct and collecting tubule of the nephrons.

As stated, the Phase 1 metabolic enzymes are the most frequently implicated in drug interactions, with up to 75% of such metabolic processes being mediated by these enzymes[44].

The cytochromes, drugs and dentistry

The Phase 1 enzymes comprise the hepatic microsomal system and have been identified and catalogued as part of the Cytochrome P450 (CYP 450) super-family group containing heme cofactors or hemoproteins. These are complex biologically active and reactive molecules based on porphyrin rings containing Iron. In total, some 21,000 of these hemoproteins are present in almost all forms of life from viruses, bacteria, fungi, plants and animals, to your dental patients whose multiple drug regimens reveal the clinical effects of these enzymes at work.

While Cytochrome refers to the terminal oxidases responsible for electron transfer along the hemoprotein chain, the 450 refers to the characteristic spectrophotometric peak displayed at 450 nm identifying these molecules.

The CYP 450 group are membrane bound molecules that transfer electrons from NADPH to NADP via the Cytochrome Reductase enzyme pathway.

Most commonly this is a mono-oxygenase reaction where one O_2 molecule is inserted into the drug being metabolised and another O_2 is reduced to water [45]:

$$RH + O_2 + NADPH + H^+ \rightarrow ROH + H_2O + NADP^+$$

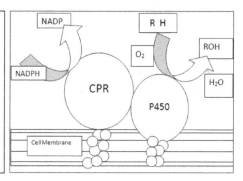

So far, some 57 genes coding for a range of drug interactions mediated by the CYP 450 system have been identified in humans. Tremendous efforts are being directed towards the identification of the mutations responsible for variations in pharmacokinetic metabolism that create the diversity of drug reactions seen in patients[46]

Polymorphisms in the CYP450 system are responsible for variations in drug handling; specifically mutations in the CYP450 reductase enzyme have been identified as a source of altered drug metabolism.....

While almost all drugs are metabolized by the CYP450 system, relatively few enzymes are responsible for the huge range of different metabolic drug responses we will see in our patients. To date only some of the locatons of the mutations have been mapped in this small number of CYP450 oxido-reductase enzymes

In CYP450, nature has provided us with a molecule that is both elegant and efficient, a creation to which we can attach any drug we've ever made, or are likely to make in the future! CYP450 quite literally, in the words of Springsteen, is:

Like a gold and diamond ring to ease the pain that living brings.

(Lyric from Beautiful Reward in the album:
Lucky Town released on Columbia records in 1992).

In contrast to the medical profession's fascination with and success from attaching various drugs to CYP450, the scientific community's attempt at producing an easily understandable classification system for this enzyme super-family have ended in a complicated disaster.

If you ever feel the need to look there is even web-site dedicated to this very subject:

The Cytochrome P450 Homepage: (http://drnelson.uthsc.edu/CytochromeP450.html)

Thankfully in clinical dentistry the only two subsets of the CYP450 family we need to consider are:

CYP 3A4 and CYP 2D6

You can see from the slices of the CYP pie of enzymes involved in dental drug metabolism that these two enzymes account for the vast majority of the drug interactions in dentistry[47]:

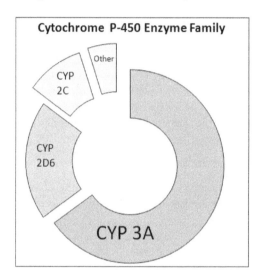

Cytochrome P-450 Enzyme Family

The administration of various drugs either alone or in combination, may increase or decrease the CYP 3A4 or CYP 2D6 activity either by <u>enzyme-induction</u> or by <u>enzyme-inhibition</u>. Such actions are the initiators of adverse <u>drug interactions</u>.

Variations in enzyme action affect both drug <u>metabolism</u> and drug <u>clearance</u>. If one drug induces the CYP metabolism of another drug, the latter may not reach a pharmacologically effective dose enabling the desired pharmaco-clinical effect to be reached. Conversely, if one drug inhibits the CYP metabolism of another drug, the latter drug may accumulate reaching rapidly toxic levels.

The OCP and the CYP

Two clinical examples of such drug interactions resulting from antimicrobial administration are:

i. The Rifampicin induction of CYP450 leading to diminished Oral Contraceptive Pill (OCP) levels and a failure in contraception.
ii. The Erythromycin inhibition of CYP3 A4 leading to elevated Statin levels resulting in myopathy.

In the previous section, the interactions of the OCP and antibiotics were considered with respect to their possible effect on GI tract flora. The antibiotics implicated in that potential interaction are commonly prescribed in dentistry: Amoxycillin and Metronidazole which are bacteriocidal and Erythromycin which is bacteriostatic. Rifampicin being an anti-tuberculosis drug is unlikely to be used in dentistry and its interaction with the OCP, is neither a result of elimination nor reduction of GI tract flora, but rather, it exerts a pharmacokinetic interaction on the enzymes responsible for OCP metabolism.

Rifampicin and related compounds are the only antimicrobials that induce CYP enzymes. With such an action they have been shown to reduce serum levels of Ethinyl-estradiol (EE2), which is the most common synthetic oestrogen component in the Combined Oral Contraceptive (COC)[48 49]. Pregnancies have allegedly been reported following simultaneous use of antimicrobials and COC.

The drugs involved in this context include Penicillin, Tetracyclines and Erythromycin, with Imidazole antifungals also being implicated. Yet none of these antimicrobials are considered to be enzyme inducers.[50 51] In fact Erythromycin is renowned for its inhibition of CYP 3A4 and thus potential increases in EE2 levels[52].

Oral contraceptives are absorbed from the small intestine undergoing extensive first pass metabolism in the mucosa of the upper GI tract and liver before being released into the circulation. While the bioavailability of Progesterone will vary, (it does not undergo entero-hepatic recycling), nearly $2/3^{rd}$ of EE2 will be metabolised and the remaining $1/3^{rd}$ will become bio-available.

As noted in the previous section, the theory behind this type of contraceptive failure comes from the reduction in colonic bacteria, which in turn may reduce the enterohepatic recycling of EE2 (conjugated EE2 is hydrolysed by commensal bacteria in the colon, causing oestrogen release, which is then resorbed suppressing ovulation).

There is however no clear evidence to support this interaction.

When prescribing antibiotics, it was generally an accepted approach and considered advisable to inform our patients that additional precautions should be used for up to three weeks until the GI tract flora returned to those levels sufficient to ensure contraceptive efficacy would no longer be compromised following the simultaneous use of antimicrobials and a COC.

From 2009/2010, the World Health Organization Medical Eligibility Criteria for Contraceptive Use (WHOMEC)[53] strongly advised that COCs are not affected by the simultaneous use of such antibiotics (as noted above) and there should be no restrictions on antibiotic use with COCs.

In short, after considering the evidence from direct studies, randomised and non-randomised, prospective and retrospective clinical trials, WHOMEC essentially stated that additional precautions are not required even for short courses of those antibiotics that are not enzyme inducers such as Metronidzole and Amoxycillin, which are frequently used in dental practice.

Clinical practise is now based on evidence

In summary, the evidence upon which the recommendations from WHOMEC were based came from all levels of the Guyatt hierarchy: --------→

As a reminder, this diagram neatly explains the strength of evidence upon which clinical decisions are made. The <u>strongest</u> evidence coming from the top of the pyramid, from Cochrane Meta-analytic reviews.

However, putting all that to one side, the most remarkable results came from cases of women who had undergone colectomy or ileostomy. In these Case Reports (from the base of the pyramid) there could be no enterohepatic EE2 circulating (due to a complete absence of bacterial hydrolysis, as there is no colon and there are no bacteria!) Yet the efficacy of COC was not reduced as evidenced by these case reports [54].

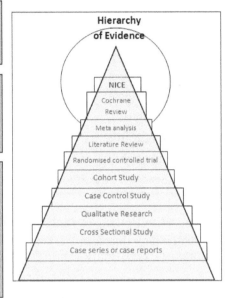

Hierarchy of Evidence

NICE
Cochrane Review
Meta analysis
Literature Review
Randomised controlled trial
Cohort Study
Case Control Study
Qualitative Research
Cross Sectional Study
Case series or case reports

Other explanations have been given to account for contraceptive failure although none can be either readily proven or easily repeatable eg: reduced absorption due to antibiotic-induced diarrhoea or vomiting, alternatively that the patient has simply forgotten to take their COC in the first place!

When considering the effect of medication on the COC, it follows that we should think about the effect of hormonal contraceptives on the metabolism of other drugs the patient may be taking too! The plasma concentrations of concurrent medications can increase or decrease with contraceptive use. The table below is an abridged version of that published from the 2012 Royal College of Obstetrics and Gynaecologist's Faculty of Sexual and Reproductive Healthcare Clinical Guidance, with the most commonly affected classes of drugs we might see in clinical practice and their effects as follows:

i. Anti-epileptics* ii. Antidiabetics iii. Antihypertensives iv. Thyroid hormones v. Diuretics**	**The clinical effect of these drugs are decreased with OCPs**
i. Antifungals ii. Anxiolytics iii. Bronchodilators iv. Immunosuppressants v. Potassium Sparing Diuretics	**The clinical effect of these drugs are increased with OCPs**

*Our patients taking the anti-epileptic: lamotrigine should be aware of the potential for reduced seizure control during the COC cycle, with the risk of increased lamotrigine toxicity during the COC-free week[55].

**Of note while diuretics are antagonised by EE2, with Potassium Sparing Diuretics the effect is reversed with a risk of hyperkalaemia and increased diuresis being seen[55].

Women taking drugs affected by contraceptive hormones may require monitoring of drug levels or their physiological effects when starting, stopping or altering a contraceptive schedule. From a dental perspective while we do not have to give advice on contraception to our patients, with regard to those drugs that could be affected by hormonal contraception, it remains our duty to monitor and to advise the patient and their medical practitioner or specialist of any relevant clinical findings in relation to interactions of contraceptives and drug.

Food and pharmacokinetics: Diet and drugs

The interactions of metabolic pharmacokinetics are not limited to drugs, both food and drink can either induce or inhibit the actions of CYP enzymes too:

i. Alcohol, tobacco and benzopyrines from cooked meat have been reported to induce CYP 1A1 and CYP 1B1 enzyme action. Although these enzymes are not primarily involved in drug action and thus drug interaction; the induction of these enzymes serves as a protective step in preventing the epoxide-diol products of the benzopyrine metabolism from corrupting the tumour suppressor genes such as p53; with the risk of cell cycle alteration and altered DNA transcription leading to neoplasia then arising[56][57].

ii. In contrast, grapefruit and pomegranate juices can inhibit the CYP 450 3A 3, 4 and 5 enzymes responsible for benzodiazepine metabolism with a doubling in plasma concentration of Midazolam being observed with these drinks. While most dental patients will not be at risk from such an interaction, those patients at the extremes of age, health or weight (especially the latter group who may be taking excessive quantities of these drinks as part of a weight control programme) might be. This food-drug pharmacokinetic interaction serves to underline the importance of updating not only the Medical History but also the Diet History of our patients in being an important consideration for clinical safety[58].

Being aware of these interactions may necessitate our reduction of drug dose or restriction in drug use, so the risk of an adverse interaction involving the CYP enzyme system can at worst be managed or at best be eliminated.

If we are to be safety critical, then we must be cognizant to the fact that all drugs will display altered plasma levels if the CYP enzymes are implicated in <u>drug metabolism</u> in any way. Such an approach is essential when prescribing drugs with a narrow therapeutic window or those drugs with demonstrably harmful side effects (such as Warfarin as previously discussed). It is important to consider the risk of adverse clinical effects arising from any alteration in CYP enzyme action.

In broad terms, for those drugs in clinical dentistry, enzyme-induction proceeds at a slower pace than enzyme-inhibition. While the drug interactions arising from enzyme-induction become clinically evident in a week to ten days, interactions arising from enzyme-inhibition usually present themselves almost immediately following administration of the drug. This clinical picture is even more evident with drugs displaying a short half-life. Many dental drugs (such as local anaesthetics) have incredibly short half-lives and a rapid onset of action, so the potential risk for CYP enzyme-inhibition is an incredibly important consideration in clinical practice.

Drug classes in dentistry

In dental practise, the classes of drugs we might use are actually quite small (when compared to those used by our medical colleagues). The classes of these drugs; briefly covered in the previous section are:

I.   **Non Opioid Analgesics: i NSAIDs and ii Paracetamol**
II. **Opioid Analgesics**
III. **Antidepressants**
IV. **Anxiolytics**
V.   **Antimicrobial: Antibiotic, Antiviral or Antifungal**

While such a classification is useful, it could also be considered overly simplistic, as certain drugs may fall into one or more of the five classes, *e.g*: Aspirin (as previously considered), Aspirin being both analgesic and anti-inflammatory. Nevertheless, working through the classes in some detail reveals information of interest and importance to clinical safety:

I. Non Opioid Analgesics:

The painkillers we might prescribe in dental practice can be either:

i.   Non Steroidal Analgesics the NSAIDs or
ii. Paracetamol

Perhaps the most frequently utilised non-opioid analgesics used in dental practice are the:

NSAIDs

i. Non Steroidal Anti-Inflammatory Drugs (NSAIDs). If not prescribed, these are frequently acquired by the patient as Over Counter Medicines (OCMs) for a relatively short period, this being anything from a few days up to one week, or longer if the patient cannot access a dentist or is frightened of doing so. Even with the low doses of OCM analgesics, there are several pharmacodynamic interactions that we must be aware of, advise our patient of and then inform the patient's medical practitioner of. From a position of patient safety, we need to do so, if we believe there is a risk these interactions could lead to undesirable clinical presentations. One problem we face as dental professionals is the widely held belief, not only with analgesics but also perhaps with most medications and this is:

If one dose, tablet or pill is good, then taking two doses, tablets or pills must be twice as good and so on. If we take this pharmaco-runcibelia one stage further, if two doses are better than one, then combining two different NSAIDs must be better by far.

---

a. Runcible and runcibelia are made up words from Edward Lear, meaning: Non-sense or Silliness, based on nothing in particular.
b. In the case of analgesia, the runcible we face, stems from the patient's fear of being in pain fuelled by drug companies advertising ie:
c. If patients use up their medication twice as fast, then sales of NSAIDs double and so on....business is business after all.

There is no evidence to support the combination of different NSAIDs for improved post-operative analgesia. However, combinations of NSAIDs may increase the risk of adverse drug interactions. NSAIDs either on their own or taken in combination are implicated in renal toxicity, fluid retention with hypertension, gastrointestinal complications, and cardiovascular events[59]. In the last two decades in the

US, every year, some 100,000 patients were hospitalised with NSAID-related GI tract complications. One in twenty of such complications proved to be non-recoverable[60][61].

NSAIDs are associated with an increased risk of adverse cardiovascular events such as myocardial infarction, heart failure, and hypertension and the increase in risk appears to be dependent on duration of exposure to NSAIDs[62]. NSAIDs in general and diclofenac in particular (one of the most widely dispensed of the NSAIDs in the UK) are also associated with drug-related hepatotoxicity, this result was seen with abnormalities in clinical trial results and case reports of fatal liver injuries among NSAID users[63].

There are a number of risk factors for the NSAID-associated morbidities as noted above, including high doses of NSAIDs being consumed with long exposures to NSAIDs often from non-prescription or self-medication. These were seen in addition to the more common factors such as older age and poor general health.

However, it was the concurrent use of OCM NSAIDs, together with low-dose aspirin, anticoagulants, or corticosteroids, which proved to be the most harmful[64][65][66]. Of note and of some concern was the concurrent use of low-dose aspirin for cardiovascular prophylaxis being is seen in ¼ of all NSAID users[67][68].

Furthermore, the presence of chronic co-morbidities in many patients, especially the elderly suffering with arthritis requiring NSAIDs, were also associated with greater risks of complications resulting from the need to conduct surgical interventions with yet even more prescriptions for NSAIDs being issued.

Such NSAID use exacerbates the following spiral of doom:

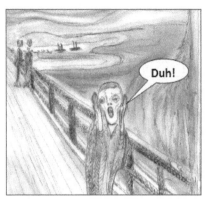

A medical intervention for a clinical sign...leads to a surgical correction for an iatrogenic complication... Meaning more medical measures attempt to improve the patient's symptoms arising from the treatments they have already received... **Which weren't working to begin with... !!**

One of the more interesting and dentally relevant pharmacodynamic interactions of different classes of NSAIDs is that of ibuprofen and aspirin. It has been noted, that if a patient has taken ibuprofen before aspirin: A 50% reduction in the anti-platelet action of aspirin has been observed (Seymour 2009)[69].

However, if aspirin is taken first and then ibuprofen, this effect is negligible. The pharmacodynamics behind this interaction are summarised as follows:

I. Aspirin irreversibly inhibits platelet functioning by acetylating the COX-1 pathway.

II. Ibuprofen blocks the active receptors on a platelet's surface by competitive binding and so aspirin cannot gain access and activate platelet receptors.

III. Although other mechanisms may be involved in this process, this explanation is sufficient for our dental clinical needs[70][71].

IV. The half-life of aspirin is some 15 to 20 minutes, if ibuprofen is given at a time longer than the half-life, possibly at 1 to 2 hours following aspirin, the anti-platelet inhibitory effect is minimised as aspirin has become bound and metabolised.

V.   Other NSAIDs such as diclofenac, selective COX2 inhibitors and the antipyretic analgesic acetaminophen (remember paracetamol is not an NSAID) do not exhibit such pharmacodynamic inhibitory effects, whereas naproxen shows a similar effect[72].

The anti-platelet effect of aspirin occurs in the drug distribution phase in the rich blood supply of the hepatic portal system, following absorption from the stomach lining and mucosa of the upper gastro-intestinal tract. The potential for interaction of ibuprofen and aspirin occurs in this location too. Although a pharmacodynamic interaction has been proven, the clinical effect and impact on patient safety may not be as critical or as important as that previously noted by Seymour.

A comprehensive study predating the observations of Seymour found thromboxane inhibition by aspirin was reduced by only 1% after 10 days of concurrent ibuprofen use![73] This result confirmed the findings of an earlier study demonstrating no increase in the incidence of myocardial infarction over not 10 days, but retrospectively: Over a period of 10 years in those patients with coronary heart disease who were taking ibuprofen together with low-dose aspirin[74].

The most common side effect of NSAID use is the risk of erosion and ulceration, not only the stomach lining but also the mucosa of the upper gastro intestinal tract. Our elderly patients with lowered dietary intake are particularly prone to such a risk becoming a reality.

Many dental patients will be taking NSAIDs and there could well be some bleeding from single drug use. However, GI tract bleeding and ulceration might become significantly greater in patients who are being co-medicated with anti-thrombotic drugs.

Once again, from a safety point, the taking and the updating of medical histories for each of our patients at every one of their dental visits is essential. In this instance, it is to identify whether anticoagulant treatment has commenced at any time, either during a course of treatment, or in the interval between regular dental check-ups in the preceding 3 to 6 month period.

Due to the increased risk of GI tract bleeding, dental prescriptions for NSAIDs must be avoided in those patients who have been prescribed anticoagulants such as warfarin or enoxaparin, or the potent anti-platelet drugs such as clopidogrel.

As noted above, although NSAIDs demonstrate an inherent ability to prevent platelet activity, the potential for this clinical effect is not as critical as the actual risk of more significant bleeding from NSAID stimulated ulceration and bleeding from the rich and finely extensive but delicate blood vessels supplying the mucosa of the GI tract[75].

The short-term use of an NSAID by a dental patient for periods of three or five days covering the post-operative pain of a procedure e.g. an extraction, is probably not a concern when combined with an existing single drug such as low-dose aspirin unless the patient is elderly. In such a case, deferring to the medical advice of the patient's general medical practitioner would be prudent.

Another interaction we must be aware of is between NSAIDs and Serotonin Specific Re-Uptake Inhibitors (SSRIs). Some examples you will have noted your patients taking are paroxetene, fluoxetene, citalopram and sertraline. Of considerable interest for your dental patient who has endured an extraction, is the role of serotonin release from platelets in response to tissue injury.

Serotonin (or 5 hydroxytryptamine 5HT) is a tryptophan derived mono-amine neurotransmitter primarily found in the gastrointestinal tract, the central nervous system and the platelets of your patients.

However when they attend for dental treatment their 5HT levels will be somewhat depleted due to a combination of dental fear and the anxiety from what you are about to do to them. All of these result in a decrease in their 5HT levels. On any other day, higher 5HT levels will contribute to a lighter mood and feelings of positivity[76].

Altering the concentration of 5HT present in synapses is the principle method and the location whereby SSRIs exert their antidepressant action. The Kulchitsky or enterochromaffin cells located throughout the GI tract mucosa release lots of 5HT into the systemic circulation (about 90% of the total amount).

Platelets then freely mop it up and store it for use when they happen upon an injury, upon other activated platelets or even upon a blood clot. 5HT is then released exerting a powerful vaso-constrictive effect, thus regulating the formation of blood clots. 5HT is also is a potent growth factor in wound healing.

In addition to the restraining effect of SSRIs on: platelet aggregation, clot formation, the inhibition of haemorrhagic control and in due course: wound healing; the parallel use of an NSAID might enhance this outcome by blocking the synthesis and release of Thromboxane.

We have previously considered the inhibitory effects of NSAIDs and Paracetomol on COX1 and COX2 in the Arachidonic Acid pathway.

In this diagram:

1. COX 1 inhibition blocks the production of Thromboxane.

2. The dysfunction of platelets ensues and no clot can form.

3. When this is combined with an irreversible

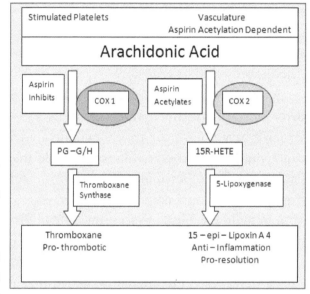

COX2 acetylation in the endothelium, anticoagulation and a bleeding event may occur.

4. If an SSRI is taken with an NSAID, haemostasis is further imbalanced.

5. The risk of a catastrophic bleeding event can increase by over 40%[77].

The evidence from the previously noted retrospective-matched and case-controlled studies; strongly suggest there is no risk of compromising aspirin's anti-platelet action, or reducing its cardio-protectant effect by the concurrent use of an NSAID. However, even stronger evidence from nearly 30,000 patients in a retrospective cohort study indicates increased bleeding in the GI tract, or a catastrophic bleed from a haemorrhagic stroke was found to be greater than 40% in those patients being co-medicated with Aspirin, Clopidogrel or other anti-platelet drug and an SSRI[77].

While such bleeding events attributable to SSRI use are rare indeed, often being subclinical or very mild, the risk to the patient will increase significantly when the patient is co-medicated with an NSAID[78]. Thus, the dental patient taking an SSRI could be placed at an increased risk in the post-operative phase of treatment if such medication is prescribed or acquired as an OCM.

An important point we must consider in the Social and Medical Histories of our patients is the presence of a current episode or the existence of a previous episode of clinical depression. With respect to this, some 1 in 5 patients with diagnosed cardiovascular illness also suffer from clinical depression and such psychopathology is a recognized risk factor for Coronary Artery and Heart Disease in healthy patients too[79]. Undeniably, depression has a proven association with higher morbidity and lower survival rates following a Myocardial Infarct (MI). This association is so strong and clear, that patients who are depressed in the week after an MI display a 3X to 4X increase in mortality in the next six months, when compared to the patient who has suffered an MI but is not depressed[80]. (In CUSPID vol. 2; chapter 5: Oral Cancer; you will read that stress and poor psychological health are also recognized risk factors for cancer!!)

The risks and benefits of SSRI use for our patient must be balanced. If the patient is prescribed an SSRI, then for sure; they will be at risk from a catastrophic haemorrhagic event, but at the same time they will, if the above evidence is considered, be at a considerably lower risk from the morbidity and mortality associated with post MI depression.

In addition to this lowered risk from using an SSRI, in the acute coronary syndrome, SSRI medication is associated with reduced rates of cardiac ischaemia and reduced levels of the enzyme markers for damage to the coronary muscles[81].

When the risks and benefits are weighed then balanced, although the pharmacodynamic interactions of SSRIs, NSAIDs and anti-platelet medication would willingly provide us with the right ingredients for an

Adverse Drug Interaction, the clinical evidence at the time of writing strongly suggests the combined use of these drugs is of considerable benefit with little risk to the patient[82].

As a dental professional, whatever side of the fence you choose to sit on, you must be aware of the interactions between SSRIs and anti-platelet medication and be alert to those risks present with the medications your patients are taking. By doing so, you will be able to discuss your clinical concerns with your patient's medical practitioner, cardiologist, psychologist or psychiatrist and do so from a position of strength borne from knowledge not weakness borne from ignorance.

Moving on to the risk of mucosal injury in the GI tract, although short-term use of NSAIDS is seldom problematic, the combination of SSRIs and NSAIDs in the longer term may give rise to some concerns. The use of SSRIs is known to produce GI tract injury and their combined use with NSAIDs heightens the risk, which may be further elevated with prolonged use in those with a prior history of mucosal injury[83].

In patients taking lithium for depression, bipolar disorder or other psychiatric conditions, or those taking methotrexate, an antimetabolite or Disease Modifying Anti Rheumatic Drug (DMARD) used to control the progression of auto immune conditions such as rheumatoid arthritis or psoriatic arthritis, the plasma concentrations of both of these drugs can be dangerously elevated by the concomitant use of NSAIDs. In such instances of combined drug use, the following clinical problems may arise:

i. Lithium can show clinical signs of toxicity including dry mouth, muscle tremor, confusion, lethargy, polyuria and seizures within a **S**yndrome of **I**rreversible **L**ithium-**E**ffected **N**euro-**T**oxicity or: **SILENT**, with cerebellar dysfunction eventually leading to an irreversible toxic encephalopathy.

ii. Methotrexate can show clinical signs of bleeding gums, bleeding and ulceration in the GI tract and mucosal tissues from lowered numbers and function of platelets. Renal insufficiency and hepatotoxicity being indicated from considerably elevated transaminase levels in serum.

In stark contrast to the NSAIDs used in dentistry to control the symptoms of which a patient complains; Lithium and Methotrexate are good examples of drugs used in medicine to control not only the symptoms of a disease, but far more importantly, the signs and progression of a disease. To prevent the toxicity issues associated with both of these indispensable drugs; your use of NSAIDs should be avoided or at least controlled in patients thus medicated, particularly for those drugs used in regimens of high concentrations and doses.

NSAIDs will interact with almost all of the anti-hypertensive medications, lowering their clinical effectiveness. However, this interaction does not seem to affect calcium channel blockers as much as other anti-hypertensives. The interaction between NSAIDs and anti-hypertensives is a pharmacodynamic one, caused by a decrease in prostaglandins that participate in the regulation of blood pressure. As previously noted, the site of this pharmacodynamic interaction is in the RAAS system located in the nephron[84]. Thankfully, there is no evidence that short-term use of NSAIDs for post procedural pain relief in dentistry presents any real risk of drug interaction. In the rare event that our patients being medicated for high blood pressure continue their postoperative NSAIDs for more than 5 days, then recall and review to measure their blood pressure might be prudent. If on such examination, the blood pressure is raised by more than 10% above their pre-procedural levels, then referral to their medical practitioner with your observations and a request to consider substitution of their NSAIDs with acetaminophen might be considered.

Of course, pre and post procedural blood pressure measurements are rarely if ever taken in the real world of general dental practice, either in the UK NHS or perhaps elsewhere. Notwithstanding the realities of general practice, the essence and theory of a safe approach to NSAID use in patients taking anti-hypertensive medication remain; if a patient is taking them for more than five days then referral to a medical practitioner for support and advice is absolutely indicated either with or without blood pressure measurements.

Paracetomol and hepatic health

ii. When the use of NSAIDs must be avoided, the use of acetaminophen (Paracetomol) provides us with a workable alternative, as few if any of the side effects and potential drug interactions noted above will be seen. On the other hand, acetaminophen is hepatotoxic and this problem is only made worse in those patients taking drugs or suffering from the disease processes that interfere with its biotransformation pathways. With regard to this and of some critical interest to clinical dentistry, are those dental patients with underlying liver disease. One unfortunate outcome of excessive alcohol use, illicit drug taking, or a result of chronic infection with HBV, HCV or possibly even a combination of some or all of these factors, is that hepatitis leads to fibrosis and then cirrhosis with hepatitis of viral origins leading to liver cancer in a significant number of cases.

While HBV and HCV have similar incubation periods (not less than 2 months and up to 5 months), HCV shows a shorter and less serious clinical illness than HBV. However, more patients with HCV rather than HBV (25% to 80%) will demonstrate persistently longer periods of atypical test results indicative of abnormal liver functioning and thus their risk of hepatoxicity from use of acetaminophen will be greater too[85][86]. Perhaps more problematic than the issue of hepatotoxicity is the risk of developing Hepatocellular Carcinoma (HCC) with up to 3% of those infected with HCV going on to develop HCC[86].

At the time of writing, data from the IARC (International Agency for Research on Cancer), confirmed liver cancer to be the second greatest cause of death from cancer globally with Hepatocellular carcinoma (HCC) accounting for 90% of these deaths[87]. While chronic infection with HBV and HCV are recognized risk factors for HCC, we must remember that HBV and HCV are different viruses. While the former is a double stranded DNA virus (of the Hepadnaviridae family), the latter is a single stranded RNA virus (of the Flaviviridae family). Thus, their oncogenic pathways in causing HCC will be entirely different. However, in addition to HBV and HCV infection, drug use, obesity and diabetes, which are all commonly associated with Non-Alcoholic

Steato-Hepatitis (NASH), also increase the risk of HCC developing[88][89]. The synergism between HBV, HCV and metabolic liver disease seems to worsen the course of the disease[90][91].

Exposure to hepatotoxic chemicals, drugs and medicines will contribute to the progression towards HCC. The oncogenicity of chronic infection with HBV, HCV and HDV leading to hepatocarcinogenesis is not in doubt as can be seen from the diagram below[91]:

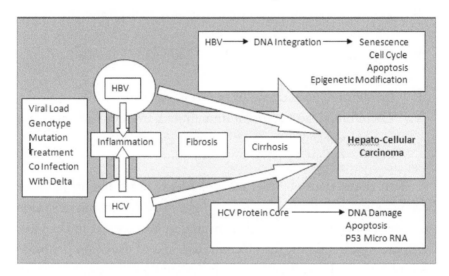

Nevertheless, we can neither ignore nor lessen the role of certain toxins and chemicals eg: acetaminophen in promoting or accelerating the onset of HCC in those with HBV or HCV. It could also be entirely possible that hepatotoxins might initiate the development of HCC in the genetically predisposed patient who has had no exposure to or infection with an oncogenic virus, but that point is *qed*.

Setting these chronic complications aside, we need to consider the acute problem associated with acetaminophen use. When the dose of paracetomol exceeds a critical limit of 200–250 mg/kg body weight, equivalent to 7 grams total ingestion within a 24-hour period, acetaminophen can no longer be conjugated to the metabolically inert N-acetyl-p-aminophenol-Glucoronide, or Sulfate or Oxide forms. Thereafter, the rapid accumulation of highly reactive N-acetyl-p-benzoquinone imine (NAPQI) within liver cells will result in hepatotoxicity[92][93.] Additional NAPQI metabolism occurs in the kidneys and GI tract too, but this is to a lesser extent than the liver.

---

4 g/day in adults and 50-75 mg/kg/day in children.

I.   This is the maximum recommended therapeutic dose of Acetaminophen.

II. The threshold for hepatotoxicity is still 75% greater than the safe limit.

III. However it is readily available and easily obtained as an unlicensed OCM

IV. In addition, paracetamol is priced in pennies.

V.   Therefore, inadvertent or intentional overdose remains a serious problem.

With doses at or slightly above 4 g/day, the sulfation pathway becomes saturated, thus an increase in glucuronidation and oxidation will commence. Paracetamol then begins to be excreted unchanged. With even greater doses, the glucuronidation and oxidation pathways become saturated and even more paracetomol will be excreted in an unchanged form. With oxidation to NAPQI now increasing, the intracellular stores of hepatic glutathione-sulfhydryl (GSH) become depleted with NAPQI binding to cysteine groups on mitochondrial proteins causing the exhaustion in cellular energy. Ion channels become blocked leading to an imbalance of Na^+ K^+ Cl^- across cell membranes. Cell death, organ failure and a descent into a fatal hepatic necrosis then follow in a matter of days.

Enzymes from the Cytochrome P450 family catalyse acetaminophen oxidation to NAPQI, whereas the involvement of CYP3A4 has not been clearly shown, the enzyme isoforms: CYP2E1, CYP1A2 and CYP2A6 are now known to be specifically involved in this process.

From the participation of these specific enzymes, one can deduce that certain drug: drug interactions involving acetaminophen will occur. In dentistry, the two interactions with acetaminophen we need to be especially aware of are:

I.   Ethanol: Acetaminophen.

II.   Phenytoin: Acetaminophen.

With both of these drugs, the CYP 450 enzymes will be induced leading to an increase in activity of oxidation pathways. Thus, GSH depletion and formation of NAPQI will be enhanced, leading to increased hepatotoxicity. The reason paracetomol poisoning in alcoholics is a well-recognized phenomenon is from the dramatic up-regulation of CYP2E1 by ethanol. Even very low to moderate doses of acetaminophen combined with a heavy consumption of alcohol lead to an abnormal liver enzyme profile, with jaundice and coagulation defects arising.

Acetaminophen demonstrates a strong inhibitory action against vitamin K. This interaction may account for some of the published data whereby prolonged use of acetaminophen has increased the anticoagulant effects of warfarin[94]. Provided daily doses of acetaminophen do not exceed 4 g per day, a healthy patient with normal liver functions will have adequate amounts of GSH to prevent the accumulation of NAPQI in the liver.

However, in those patients who are poorly nourished, suffer liver dysfunction, or are treated with other hepatotoxic drugs that are capable of inducing the hepatic enzymes responsible for creating the toxic metabolites, we must be wary of either prescribing paracetamol or even of advising patients to consider using it.

As with all the drugs we have considered so far, the use of paracetamol in the short-term for a few days only, should not concern us. However, for long-term administration, including the recently favoured IV route of acetaminophen delivery, it is safer to restrict its use and to defer to the patient's physician for specialist medical advice if we are concerned[95].

For patients taking paracetamol alone, blood pressure will increase in the short term; whereas long term, not only will blood pressure remain elevated this could be contributory to adverse cardiovascular events occurring[96]. While the incidence of dyspepsia and diarrhoea with paracetamol is not any less than for those patients taking both paracetamol and ibuprofen, with paracetamol NSAID combinations, complications such as significant blood loss (expressed as a haemoglobin drop greater than 1g/dL) are seen, possibly offsetting any observed increase in blood pressure. Such blood loss will increase with both time and the dose of paracetamol being taken and this is not related to the gastro-intestinal bleeding seen with NSAID use, but rather it was the result of COX 1 inhibition and decreased platelet aggregation solely from paracetamol use[97 98].

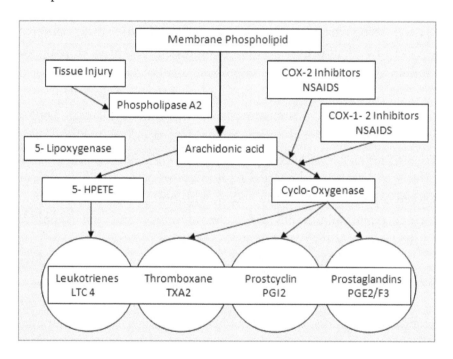

Not only are unwanted drug effects higher with combination therapies, the efficacy of using paracetamol with an NSAID is questionable. If we review the Arachidonic acid pathway, we soon realise there can be little pharmacological reason to combine paracetamol with another COX-2 inhibitor. The enzyme responsible for production of the pro-algesic: Prostagalandin E2 (Cyclo-Oxygenase) can only be blocked once. Two blockers cannot possibly achieve any more analgesia than one blocker! While any an-algesic effects from a combination of drugs will increase marginally, the risk of adverse effects can increase dramatically from combinations of COX inhibitors[99].

Based on such observations, we must question why combinations of NSAIDs and paracetamol are freely available as OCMs. As reported by Brun and Hinz, there is no scientific evidence that either a higher efficacy and/or less toxicity can be proven, but rather, the converse is true[99].

If we were to make a comparison between ibuprofen and acetaminophen, it would be of some interest. While the former is an NSAID, the latter expresses antipyeretic and analgesic properties. The former has been the focus of considerable interest and concern in part due to the risk of gastric ulceration and the potential to initiate asthma symptoms in those who are susceptible, especially in children who may have existing allergies. Whereas the latter generally, is considered to be a safe drug and therein lies the problem:

Paracetamol in moderately high doses as mentioned is hepatotoxic whereas ibuprofen is not. Paracetamol is readily available, cheap and easily accessible to the vulnerable and at-risk patients or members of the public who frequently resort to its use in either attempting suicide or successfully committing suicide.

We must never forget that suicide is a tragedy for everyone. Those who survive often make further attempts, while the personal and professional costs in terms of tissue damage, organ failure then liver transplantation with a lifetime of care are incalculable. Not only are such figures incalculable, we cannot even begin to reconcile the pennies paid for paracetamol with the ease of access to this drug against the damage caused and the complexity of corrective surgery required from an overdose[100].

> **The Facts:**
>
> I. From 1993 to 2009, deaths from paracetamol represented some 6% to 10% of all deaths from poisoning in England and Wales.
> II. In September 1998, legislation was introduced to lower the pack sizes of paracetamol and to limit the sales of this drug.
> III. The results of this legislation were striking in that 765 fewer deaths attributable to paracetamol (a drop of 43%) were recorded in the following 11 ¼ years.
> IV. Following the legislation, there was a 61% decrease in registration for liver transplantation.
> V. However, morbidity and mortality from paracetamol continue, indicating further preventive measures are needed[100].

In the reality of the dental clinic, any comparison between ibuprofen and acetaminophen is complicated by the combined use with NSAIDS or other drugs, alternating doses and the medical consequences arising from the ease with which both the vulnerable and at-risk patient's can access such medications.

No discussion on paracetamol would be complete without mentioning the work of Drs Rumack and Mathews. Over forty years ago, they developed a graph to determine whether treatment with N-Acetylcysteine (NAC) should be used to manage paracetamol poisoning and thus prevent fatal liver damage.

Today, their widely recognized Rumack-Mathews nomogram with a logarithmic plot of acetaminophen plasma concentration starting from a point four hours after ingestion is used. This point is used because acetaminophen absorption is complete and its maximum tissue concentration will be reached by four hours.

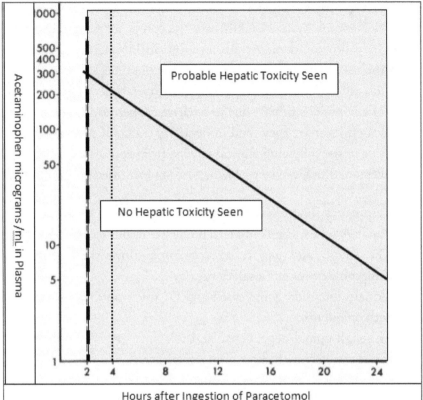

Hours after Ingestion of Paracetomol

Semi logarithmic plot of plasma acetaminophen levels –V- time

(from work of Rumack BH and Mathews H. Acetaminophen poisoning and Toxicity. Paediatrics 1975 (55) 871-876.

The plot is actually Semi-Logarithmic, with plasma concentration on the vertical and time along the horizontal axis.

If the plasma concentration of paracetamol is above 140-150 mgs/L at 4 hours post ingestion then treatment with NAC will be indicated.

Furthermore, if we take a point from paracetamol ingestion and the calculated half life is more than 4 hours, then again treatment with NAC will be needed.

II. The Opioid Analgesics. While these drugs specifically act on Central Nervous System (CNS) mu_1 receptors to exert relief from pain, they do not demonstrate any anti-inflammatory properties. Nevertheless, they are incredibly useful for the relief of both visceral and musculo-skeletal pain, especially post-operatively. The analgesic effect of an opioid is in part due to sedative properties, but opioids are neither useful nor are they used in dentistry (rarely if ever) as sedative drugs due to the following clinical effects, from activation of the CNS mu_2 receptors which can be problematic if not identified and controlled:

I.   Respiratory function is depressed.
II.   Pupillary reflexes and oro-facial protective responses are suppressed.
III. The cough and gag reflexes become diminished so airway compromise presents a safety risk.
IV.   Urinary retention is increased and GI tract motility is decreased with opioid use.
V.   Although opioid dependence and tolerance are of some concern, this is unlikely with short-term dental use.

The last of these effects is of some interest. A safety conscious dental professional may choose not to prescribe an opioid analgesic for fear of initiating an addictive effect in the patient. Given the minor nature of dental surgery and the relatively short duration of analgesia required, the chance of this risk materializing with an opioid is in reality quite small and this risk should not be a factor in choosing not to use opioid analgesia. Although in stating this, the NSAIDs and non-opioid analgesics discussed previously are in the main, perfectly adequate analgesics on their own, without the need to resort to opioids or combinations of NSAIDs and opioids to achieve the same outcome.

On balance, taking the above noted problems with the potential risks that might compromise patient safety; we would strongly encourage the safety critical dental professional to consider in the first instance using non-opioid analgesics before recourse to prescribing even the weakest of the orally administered opioids.

The most commonly prescribed opioid for postoperative pain is Codeine, together with its derivative medications. Codeine or methyl-morphine is a pro-drug. The enzyme CYP 2D6 demethylates approximately 10% of the administered parent drug to the active metabolite morphine. Of clinical importance, it is essential to note the genetic polymorphism of CYP 2D6 and the resultant variations among patients in their susceptibility to opioid analgesia.

In addition to genetic differences, drugs that inhibit CYP2D6 metabolism will also diminish the analgesic effect of codeine. Such inhibitory drugs include the widely-prescribed SSRI antidepressants such as fluoxetine and paroxetine[102.]

In contrast to drugs causing enzyme inhibition, the immunosuppressant steroid dexamethasone is a CYP2D6 inducer. Dexamethasone will enhance the conversion of the opioid parent drugs to their active metabolites. When patients are taking drugs that induce CYP 2D6, if we choose to use an opioid analgesic, then those opioids that are weakly demethylated, might be of some use. An example of such a drug might be oxycodone. The analgesic effect of this drug is almost entirely ascribed to the parent drug, with only a small fraction being demethylated to oxy-morphone.[103.] Theoretically, this could make oxycodone a better choice for patients taking those medications known to inhibit CYP2D6 activity.

In reality, there are significant problems associated with oxycodone use:

I.   With respect to the risks, oxycodone has earned the alias: "Hillbilly heroin" due to the disproportionately high addiction rates in the poor isolated rural communities of the USA. This drug problem started in 2002 in the Appalachian valley, at that time the poorest region in the US. In addition to being relatively inexpensive, it was and still is easier to misuse a legitimate drug such as oxycodone, than to obtain illicit drugs, not only in deprived rural areas of the US, but in cities and this phenomenon applies internationally too.

II.   In 2002, only 100 deaths were linked to Oxycodone abuse, however by 2008, the shocking figures released by the US CDC revealed

14,800 oxycodone associated deaths[104]. The first UK oxycodone associated death was also noted in 2002[105].

III. If we consider the previous section on NSAIDs and non-opioid analgesics, then it will come as no surprise to read that many of these deaths were from acetaminophen hepatoxicity where combination drugs containing both opioids and paracetamol were misused.

IV. Beyond these fatalities, the social effects are staggering with some towns in the US witnessing addiction rates of up to 40% with attendant increases in drug-related crime. American drugs policy experts are now claiming, this is potentially the most serious single-drug epidemic since the introduction of opium into the USA in the 19th century.

V. The major sources of Oxycodone to illicit users have been forged prescriptions, unscrupulous pharmacists and large-scale theft. There is no shortage of supply with critics noting the drug to be both widely distributed and aggressively marketed by its manufacturers[105].

If the above safety points are considered (due to the clinical potency and widespread social risks associated with this drug), it would be most unusual to prescribe oxycodone as a dental analgesic without first seeking advice and support from a pharmacist or specialist physician for alternative analgesia. If you are in the UK and considering its use, you will be aware that Oxycodone is a Class A drug, under the Misuse of Drugs Act 1971 (extant from 2010-2015). Classed as a Schedule 2 drug in accordance with the Misuse of Drugs Regulations 2001, this will provide certain exemptions from the provisions of the Misuse of Drugs Act 1971, but oxycodone is not a drug that many dental professionals would consider prescribing without firm specialist medical support for doing so.

Other opioid analgesics are available but these are also problematic due to the risks associated with drug interactions. The established medication, tramadol has gained popularity, but it does have additional effects resembling tricyclic antidepressants as it can inhibit the re-uptake of both serotonin and nor-epinephrine. Tramadol use should be avoided in patients prescribed Mono Amine Oxidase Inhibitors (MAOIs), SSRIs, or each and any of the many drugs that are substrates of CYP3A4 and CYP2D6. Any drug that induces or inhibits these Cytochrome enzymes will interact adversely with tramadol. Tramadol undergoes hepatic metabolism via the CYP 2B6, the CYP 2D6 and the CYP 3A4 enzymes, being demethylated into some five different metabolites with some having half-lives of up to 9 hours![106.] (The tramadol half-life is stated to be 6 hours, but given the genetic variation of activity in the Cytochrome enzyme family, the clinical relevance of this will not have escaped your attention).

Some 6% of the population will exhibit a reduced CYP2D6 activity, with reduced analgesic effect of opioids[107]. Tramadol use is not advised for patients deficient in CYP2D6 enzymes (being crucial to the metabolism of tramadol to O-desmethyl-tramadol.[107]). Some 6–10% of Caucasians and 1–2% of Asians are deficient in CYP 2D6 and will require a dose increase of some 30% of tramadol to reach the same level of pain relief as those with higher levels of CYP2D6 activity.[107 108.]

Tramadol, once demethylated, then enters the Phase II hepatic metabolism rendering the products water-soluble, which are then eliminated by the kidneys. The converse of increasing treatment doses (not only of tramadol but perhaps of all opioids in patients with CYP2D6 deficiency, is to decrease treatment doses and uses in patients with renal and hepatic impairment.

In this respect, the principles of acetaminophen prescribing apply equally to opioid prescribing.

In common with other opioids, tramadol use causes respiratory depression, diminished cognitive functioning and reduced GI tract motility. In contrast to other opioids, tramadol is not an immunosuppressant, but may exert an enhancing effect on the immune system[109].

In addition to the risks of decreased alertness, hepatic and renal toxicity from overdose and addiction from overuse, given the interaction with MAOIs and SSRIs, with tramadol's inhibition of serotonin re-uptake, the risk of excessive serotonin levels in the CNS and PNS should be borne in mind. Returning to consider the Serotonin toxicity syndrome or Serotonin toxi-drome; this is a predictable outcome if combinations of serotonergic drugs are being taken[110].

The clinical signs of the Serotonin toxi-drome, (this term accurately portrays the nature of the toxic-syndrome) that we might see in the dental clinic and we need to be aware of in a patient who has taken a serotonergic drug are[110,111]:

I.   Dry mouth and or excessive sweating.
II.   Spontaneous or inducible excessive or inappropriate muscle twitching.
III. Twitching of the eye muscles, with involuntary movements of the oro-facial musculature.
IV.   Muscle tremors with hyper-reflexiveness.
V.   A rapid rise in body temperature above 38 °C (100 °F)

Serotonin toxicity must be considered as a medical emergency and it is helpful to consider the causes and effects in sequence. The treatment options then appear quite logical: The cause of increased serotonin levels must be established to determine their management:

I.   Administration of any precipitating drug will have ceased by the time the patient has been admitted for specialist medical care, (this is obvious and the patient's drug history must be noted by the referring clinician)
II.   Serotonin is catabolised by monoamine oxidase in the presence of oxygen, therefore administering oxygen as an emergency measure in the first instance is incredibly helpful, whatever the cause it cannot do any harm.
III. Should the toxidrome have been caused by an MAOI, then both hydration and oxygenation are required until adequate regeneration of MAO is established.
IV.   In any event, anti-hypertensives must never be given as these can lead to hypotension and irrecoverable shock.

V. The muscle tremors and spasms causing increased body temperatures, if unchecked will lead to renal failure from the breakdown products of rhabdomyolysis. The treatment for this aspect of the serotonin toxidrome, is not to control the increased temperature with an antpyretic, as the driver is not from hypothalamic homeostatic control, but to decrease the muscle activity by using a benzodiazepine. Thus, the body temperature will return to normal levels in a matter of some 24 hours although delirium and after effects may persist for several days[110 111].

It is important from a point of safety to consider the causes, the effects and the treatment of the serotonin syndrome. Although we will most likely never see a case of serotonin syndrome, the principles in its treatment and management apply to all our prescribing for all our dental patients.

From a human and historical point, what we now understand to be the serotonin syndrome presented as an inexplicable problem to the overworked, exhausted and inexperienced junior doctors on weekend duty on the night of Sunday 4th March 1984 when Libby Zion was brought to hospital. Within hours, her condition deteriorated and she died from a cardiac arrest.

Libby Zion was just eighteen years old.

Her father Sydney Zion then took legal action to identify the issues and uncover the human factors responsible for the death of his daughter. By 2002 his relentless campaigning, resulted in the Libby Zion ruling being passed; restricting the hours that junior doctors could work in New York. By 2003, all medical training establishments in the USA had adopted this ruling as law.

More than three decades after Libby Zion's death, in the 2016 dispute over weekend working hours and conditions, in the UK NHS junior doctors backed by the BMA, took industrial action against the Department of Health's proposals that compromised patient safety. It is a sad reflection at the time of writing; both the name and legacy of Libby Zion have still gone unnoticed by those on both sides of this dispute.

At every dental visit we need to update our patient's medical and drug histories. This will allow us to take into account those drugs that may seem harmless but actually require greater vigilance. With our dental patients taking SSRIs or MAOIs, we must be especially cautious, so no prescription we might consider giving could lend itself to initiating the serotonin syndrome. As noted above, although the opioids are useful, there are many clinical and social problems associated with their use and misuse.

An increasing number of deaths from the use of opioids such as tramadol are now being reported in the UK in Northern Ireland[112]. The problem with opioid use is that it frequently leads to abuse and over-use leads to over-dose. The majority of such fatalities are associated with alcohol and illicit drug taking[112]. The recognized precipitating common risk factors include depression and a personality that is susceptible to addiction. In those patients who are at risk from opioid overdose, the opioid antagonist naloxone is the drug of choice to reverse the acute effects such as respiratory depression and mental confusion.

In almost all UK dental practices, naloxone will not be present as an emergency drug. However, naloxone must be available if you provide IV sedation using: Fentanyl, Ketamine or Propofol, (naloxone only acts as a competitive non selective opioid receptor antagonist), the properties of Fentanyl Ketamine and Propofol are outlined below: (In those dental practices limiting sedation to using midazolam, the antagonist flumazenil must be present.)

i. Fentanyl is a powerful synthetic opioid, noted to be some 100 x more potent than morphine. It acts on the CNS mu opioid receptors, giving both a rapid onset and a short half-life, albeit with a greater risk of respiratory depression, than other opioids. Fentanyl is administered intravenously, often in combination with midazolam, ketamine and propofol to give short but effective periods of sedation for paediatric patients.

ii. Ketamine is a dissociative anaesthetic drug with amnesic properties. It shows binding affinity to both CNS kappa opioid receptors, with which it is an agonist and CNS NMDA glutamate receptors, with which it is an antagonist. Ketamine does not bind to the

CNS mu opioid receptors[113]. The use of ketamine in paediatric dental sedation is supported by the demonstrated maintenance of respiration and blood pressure, together with a decreased risk of laryngospasm during its use[114].

iii. <u>Propofol</u> is an anaesthetic drug with amnesic properties, but it is not an analgesic. Acting on both $GABA_A$ receptors and Sodium channels, propofol gives both a rapid induction and recovery from sedation. The use of propofol is associated with a marked drop in blood pressure due to sympathetic inhibition causing vasodilation. Cardiac irregularities and a powerful respiratory depressant effect with apnoea are also seen. These effects are potentiated if propofol is given together with an opioid sedative. Propofol has a steep dose response curve and when used in conjunction with a benzodiazepine or ketamine its anaesthetic properties will be increased, as are the unwelcome side effects of increased respiratory depression.

Although it has been established that both propofol and ketamine have no antagonists to control or limit the clinical effects of their pharmacological actions, there has been a recent resurgence in work to investigate the effect of naloxone on patients given ketamine.

Both the mode of action and the means of delivering naloxone should be familiar to all attending staff when sedation sessions using the drugs noted above are in progress. Naloxone is a competitive antagonist for the CNS kappa opioid receptors and the mu receptors, with which it shows both high affinity and rapid binding. Naloxone is administered by IV infusion and will be rapidly distributed throughout the body.

In the intravenous drug (ab) user (IVDA), we will frequently see collapsed veins while the remaining workable veins are concealed under superficial scar tissue making access to them difficult. Therefore, in an emergency, naloxone should be delivered by intramuscular injection. Again, rapid drug distribution with a prompt clinical effect will result from this route of administration.

After two to three minutes, an improvement in respiratory function and mental state will be seen together with the clinical signs indicating that naloxone's competitive blocking of mu and kappa opioid receptors is reaching a saturation point. The resulting clinical signs of naloxone's action are essentially those of opioid withdrawal and these are:

I.   Restlessness.
II. Agitation.
III. Nausea.
IV. Sweating and possibly vomiting.
V.   Increase in heart rate.

As some of these effects are undesirable and potentially harmful, naloxone is titrated in doses of 0.5mgs/ml to 1 mg/ml every 2 to 3 minutes until a maximum dose of 10mgs has been given. Should there be no improvement in the clinical signs, an initial diagnosis of opioid overdose must be questioned. In any event, the emergency services will have been contacted and an initial definitive diagnosis of opioid overdose will have been relegated to a differential diagnosis as the patient is admitted to hospital for further testing and specialist medical care.

The median half-life of naloxone is 45 minutes and this is often considerably less than that of many opioids. By way of comparison, the half-life of tramadol is some 6 hours. Thus, the medical emergency responders will need to give repeated doses of naloxone throughout the recovery period. Should we need to use naloxone we need to be aware that with a tramadol overdose, naloxone will only partially reverse the toxic effects and its use has paradoxically resulted in an increased risk of seizures[115].

It is important to note the admitted use of illicit opioids might not be limited to one drug. Even the simple solitary admission on one medical history form may unintentionally cover many different forms of one opioid. An IVDA will frequently have no actual choice in the drugs they either acquire or are given and thus we must be alert when taking all medical histories from every one of our patients, cautious when prescribing and vigilant when medicating our patients known to have a history of illicit drug use, whether smoked, inhaled or injected.

The use of opioids either illicit or legitimate, does carry the risk of drug dependence, although (as mentioned) with the short duration of dental prescribing this is unlikely. Nevertheless, there are both physical and psychiatric problems associated with the use of opioids; there could be numbness, tingling, paraesthesia and tinnitus. These symptoms are frequently accompanied by hallucinations, paranoia, anxiety, panic attacks and confusion. With the morbidity of these physical and psychological disturbances comes the risk of mortality.

As noted in the USA, the rise of hillbilly heroin led to some 14,800 deaths in 2008 and the total number of opioid related deaths in that year was 36,450. Harm reduction programmes using naloxone in the US have now resulted in an estimated 10,000 fewer deaths from opioid overdose[116]. In the UK, the figures for opioid associated deaths released from Office for National Statistics are just as striking. From 2011 to 2014, the death rate has been steadily increasing, for all illicit drugs in general and opioids in particular. By 2014 these numbers were:

Deaths from all drugs: 3,346. Deaths from opioids: 1,786[117].

These were the highest figures since data recording began in 1993 and are likely to be an underestimate. In addition in the UK, there is sharp divide between Scotland and England as the 2013 figures for drug related deaths reveal[118,119 120]:

i.   9.6 deaths per 100,000 people in Scotland.
ii. 2.1 deaths per 100,000 people in England/Wales and
iii. 3.6 deaths per 100,000 people in Northern Ireland.

The information from Scotland's National Drug Related Death Database reveal most of these deaths were related to opioids, there is no reason to suggest there is any difference for England and Wales. Most deaths were noted to be accidental overdoses (not recorded as suicides) and most deaths occurred when others were present. Over two-thirds of those fatalities had been in drug treatment, in prison or police custody or discharged from hospital in the six months preceding their deaths[121]. Lastly, there was a stark gender difference in drug related deaths:

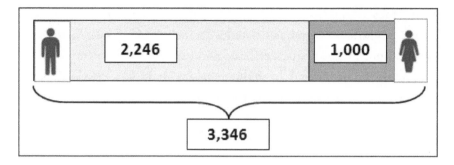

From a safety point, it is interesting to note the GDC have stressed the value of training in CPR and the importance of every dental practice having an AED. Given the numbers of premature deaths from cardiac disease; there were 42,000 in 2012[122], the GDC measures do seem appropriate. Nevertheless, if we look at the numbers of deaths noted above, although they are an order of magnitude less than cardiac disease, the numbers are still significant. Conspicuous by its absence is an approach by the GDC to reduce the risk of harm for our patients in this area.

Education and training in drug use and abuse are essential, as might be training of the dental team in not only the use of naloxone, but recognizing the problems associated with integrating dental prescribing with that of medical prescribing.

Overall, if we consider the problems associated with opioids and that satisfactory pain management can be achieved with a combination of NSAIDs and paracetamol, it is not surprising that most dental practitioners do not prescribe opioids for pain relief.

III. Antidepressants. Some of the problems associated with SSRIs and dental prescribing have already been noted in the preceding section, including increased bleeding when used with aspirin and the Serotonin toxidrome, when combinations of SSRIs, tramadol and other medications are used. In addition, we must consider the risks presented when a patient taking an SSRI is given an adrenaline containing local anaesthetic (LA). It has been suggested that blood pressure can become dangerously elevated with such combinations and therefore either non-adrenaline containing anaesthetics are used or the total number of cartridges of adrenaline containing LA are reduced in those patients taking SSRIs[123]. Conversely, it has also been suggested that in those patients chronically medicated with SSRIs, desensitization from the down-regulation of adrenaline uptake in the post-synaptic neurones takes place[69]. Of course, there are other antidepressants in addition to the SSRIs, but as stated, the range of dental prescribing is far less than that facing the medical practitioner and so we need not be too troubled by this class of drugs, other than to note the following important points on pharmacology and physiology:

Antidepressants are not available from the UK BNF DPF and their use in dentistry is the sole preserve of the oral medicine specialist when treating a patient with atypical facial pain; for which an antidepressant such as amitryptyline, a tricyclic antidepressant (TCA) may confer some analgesic effect. Adding to what has been noted above, if the dose of LA can be reduced or an anaesthetic that does not contain adrenaline is used, there should be no practical contraindications for the patient taking an antidepressant and your administration of a dental local anaesthetic.

However, the theoretical considerations must be taken into account, as the risk of a drug interaction no matter how small is still present. TCAs inhibit the neuronal uptake of nor-adrenaline. An adrenaline containing local anaesthetic will rely on vasoconstriction to achieve the depth and duration of anaesthesia that is required in dentistry. While this effect can be prolonged by the action of a TCA, there could also be desensitization in response to exogenous adrenaline as a result of down-regulation of post synaptic receptor activity.

Mono Amine Oxidase Inhibitors (MAOIs) are another class of antidepressant. They exert their effect by increasing the availability of mono-amine neurotransmitters. MAOIs are useful in the treatment of a wide range of psycho-social disorders such as agrophobia, anxiety and depression; they are also useful in the treatment of obsessive compulsive disorders and post traumatic stress disorder. Although useful for a wide range of conditions, the widespread use of MAOIs has been limited due to the risk of interaction with both diet and drugs. Together with TCAs, MAOIs can induce cardiac excitability but this effect should not be exacerbated with adrenaline containing local anaesthetics.

Whereas exogenous adrenergic drugs are terminated by hepatic enzyme transformation, neuronal uptake is the primary method whereby an endogenous adrenergic neurotransmitter is eliminated. Hepatic Mono Amine Oxidase (HMAO) will only metabolize those drugs that are not catecholamines. Thus, adrenaline (a catecholamine), will be inactivated not by MAO but by catechol-o-methyltransferase (COMT). From this, it should be clear that MAOIs do not delay the elimination of adrenaline and they should be safe to use with those dental local anaesthetics containing adrenaline. However, combinations of TCA and MAOIs will have a marked cardiotonic potential, the use of any sympathomimetic drug with these two antidepressants carries the further risk of additional cardiac excitation and thus consideration for reducing the total number of those cartridges of local anaesthetics containing adrenaline, or using a local anaesthetic that does not contain adrenaline must be given.

With patients taking MAOIS and TCAs, the total number of adrenaline containing local anaesthetics should be limited to not more than two cartridges of 2.2ml lidocaine with a concentration of 1/80,000 adrenaline[124]. This would be a sensible and safe approach to avoid both a rapid and a dangerous rise in blood pressure associated with a sympathomimetic: MAOI TCA interaction.

The last problem we really need to consider with MAOIs is the cheese reaction. Most cheeses and foods do not contain adequate amounts of tyramine to initiate this effect. The pounding headache that results from eating a well-aged slab of Stilton and/or drinking a glass of red wine, might give an idea of what patients taking an SSRI, TCA or MAOI might be faced with, if they were to develop a tyramine reaction.

Tyramine is a naturally occurring monoamine compound derived from the amino acid tyrosine that acts as a catecholamine releasing agent. As tyramine cannot cross the blood brain barrier, only systemic and not psychoactive symptoms are experienced. Many MAOIs irreversibly alter monoamine oxidase, with the clinical effects lasting until the enzyme is replenished, which can be up to four weeks.

The combination of an exogenous tyramine, together with an MAOI and a dental local anaesthetic containing adrenaline could precipitate a hypertensive crisis, which only adds to the misery that susceptible patients will experience. These effects were frequently reported with the first generation of non-selective MAOIs. With further drug development, MAOIs which target either MAO_A or MAO_B were developed. The former are the target for drugs such as moclobemide useful in the treatment of psychological problems such as social anxiety and depression and is of considerable value due to its reversible nature. The latter are the target for drugs useful in the treatment of Parkinson's disease and once more, they are reversible and of considerable clinical benefit.

Use of such selective reversible MAOIs are not associated with either drug and diet interactions, or the risks of a hypertensive crisis associated with the earlier first generation non selective MAOIs. Even with such drug development, we must maintain a high degree of pharmacovigilance. Not perhaps because of the risk of an interaction with the newer generation of MAOIs, but our patient with either depression or Parkinson's disease will have a brain chemistry that is altered. We must be mindful (no pun intended) of the potential for unforeseen interactions within such an altered pharmacological environment.

Slightly off subject but of importance and of interest are the dopaminergic COMT inhibitors used in the treatment of Parkinson's disease. Any drug that inhibits COMT metabolism will also have an effect on the metabolism of adrenaline, ultimately prolonging its duration, making the normally transient cardiogenic effects last significantly longer. With our patients who may already be anxious and have Parkinson's disease, the undesirable symptoms in addition to those of an increase in heart rate may also extend to atrial fibrillation. The discomfort in experiencing these could well lead to a temporary reduction, or a loss of the controlling effect of a COMT inhibitor in limiting the signs of Parkinson's disease.

IV. Anxiolytics. As noted, other drugs are available, however the most commonly used anxiolytic group for dental intravenous sedation are the benzodiazepines; almost exclusively midazolam. This drug together with others will be discussed in greater detail in the section on conscious sedation.

Beta Blockers and dental practise.

One drug group associated with an adverse interaction resulting in a paradoxical rise in blood pressure are the beta-blockers, specifically the non-selective beta-blockers. Their use as an anxiolytic came some time after their value in treating angina, heart failure and high blood pressure was recognized.

The clinical evidence has proven that beta-blockers are an incredibly useful cardio-protectant to control dangerous <u>arrhythmias</u> and thus prevent secondary <u>myocardial infarction</u> that follow from the primary event. The first generation non-selective beta-blocker propranolol has proven to be an indispensable treatment for <u>hypertension</u> and the management of angina pectoris, although newer generations of selective vasodilating beta-blockers have now superseded this drug.

Beta-blockers are <u>competitive antagonists</u> for the endogenous adrenaline receptor sites located throughout the sympathetic nervous system. When these receptors are stimulated, the response to stress will be seen. One such response is anxiety; this will be expanded upon below. First the basics:

Beta-blockers interfere with receptor binding of adrenaline reducing the effect of stress hormones.

The beta-receptors may be designated β_1, β_2 and β_3, their tissue locations are:

---

i. β_1-<u>adrenergic receptors</u> are situated in cardiac and renal tissue.

ii. β_2-<u>adrenergic receptors</u> are located throughout the lungs, GI tract, liver, uterus, vascular smooth and skeletal striated muscle.

iii. β_3-<u>adrenergic receptors</u> are limited to adipose tissues.

While the first generation beta-blockers such as propranolol non-selectively block activation of all types of β-<u>adrenergic receptors</u>, further development has led to cardio-selective drugs such as atenolol that only acts on the β_1 receptor. The effects of receptor stimulation are:

i. β_1-adrenergic receptors increase both heart rate and output. Additionally, in the kidneys, renin will be released, causing arterial vasoconstriction and an increase in perfusion pressure. Na+ and H20 will be resorbed from the renal tubules to maintain or raise systemic blood pressure.

ii. β_2-adrenergic receptors cause <u>smooth muscle</u> relaxation but <u>skeletal muscle</u> tremors. <u>Glycogenolysis</u> from both the <u>liver</u> and <u>skeletal muscles</u> will result in increased blood glucose levels in a preparatory advent of the flight or fight reflex.

iii. β_3-adrenergic receptor activation results in fat and lipid breakdown.

From the above, the physiological effects of receptor antagonism with beta-blockers will be evident:

I.   The release of renin is down regulated, reducing the volume of extracellular fluid and blood pressure.

II.   As the demand on the heart drops, the proportion of circulating blood being adequately oxygenated rises.

III. As adrenaline release is moderated, the risk of cardiac failure from the previously elevated adrenaline levels exerting stress on compromised cardiac tissues will be lowered.

IV.   There will be a reduction or elimination of the factors contributing to cardiac failure; increased oxygen demand, increased release of inflammatory mediators and pathological compensatory remodelling of cardiac muscle, all of which contribute to the diminishing efficiency that is seen in a failing heart, will be controlled by the action of beta-blockers.

V.   Beta-blockers counter an inappropriately high sympathetic activity, resulting in improved cardiac output, not only in the compromised heart but in the ostensibly healthy heart too.

The last of these points is of interest. While the value of beta-blockers in maintaining cardiovascular health has been established, we must recognize that our dental patients with heart conditions or hypertension will also be medicated with diuretics, calcium channel blockers and those drugs such as ACE inhibitors that act on the RAAS, (as previously discussed).

All of these have proven to be just as effective, if not more so than beta-blockers in controlling hypertension[125] and all of these will carry the risk of an adverse drug interaction as do beta-blockers.

The most significant <u>adverse drug reactions</u> associated with the use of non-selective beta blockers and β_2-adrenergic receptor antagonists include <u>bronchospasm</u> leading to breathlessness, bradycardia leading to hypotension and a reduction in distal systemic circulation (this is of critical importance for our patients who have Raynaud's phenomenon and lastly, an alteration of both <u>glucose</u> and <u>lipid</u> <u>metabolisms</u> is seen. Such effects are less common with the β_1-cardio-selective drugs. It must be stressed that receptor selectivity will tail off with higher doses of even the selective beta-blockers.

Lipophillic beta-blockers such as propranolol easily cross the <u>blood–brain barrier</u> and are perhaps more likely than the more recent range of less lipophillic beta blockers to cause psychological disturbances, such as aberrant or inappropriate dream states, or indeed a complete loss of sleep.

Should a complete block of the renal β_1 receptors located in the <u>macula densa</u> occur, then renin release will be lowered, with a reduction in aldosterone secretion following. The end-point is that a state of hyponatremia and hyperkalemia will quickly result.

Similarly, blockade of the hepatic β2-receptors which stimulate glycogenolysis and secretion of glucagon from the pancreas, will ultimately lower plasma glucose and hypoglycaemia may be seen and the relevance to the diabetic dental patient is clear. While the action of selective β1-blockers will have few if any side effects in the diabetic dental patient, there could be a masking effect of tachycardia, an important sign not be missed and often seen in the advent of an insulin-induced hypoglycaemic collapse.

The combination of diuretics and beta-blockers to treat hypertensive patients could potentially increase the risk of developing diabetes, whereas treatment with ACE inhibitors and angiotensin receptor blockers has been noted to decrease this risk. As a result of this, the use of beta-blockers should be avoided as the primary treatment for hypertension[126].

If we consider the disadvantages and set the possible benefits against the probable risks, the use of beta-blockers solely as an anxiolytic, must be carefully considered, not only for diabetics but for every one of our patients.

Additionally, beta-blockers must never be used to limit the overdose effects from cocaine, amphetamine or any other illicit alpha-adrenergic stimulant. By blocking the cardiac β_1-receptors a reduction in coronary blood flow, left ventricular function and cardiac output with reduced tissue perfusion will be seen. By leaving the stimulation of the alpha-adrenergic system unopposed, a beta-blocked hypertensive crisis could be initiated. The appropriate antihypertensive drugs given by an emergency medical specialist are vasodilators such as nitroglycerin and diuretics such as furosemide, together with alpha blockers such as phentolamine. But long before then, you will have recognized the clinical signs and summoned an ambulance....won't you?

It would seem intuitive that beta-blockers should be contraindicated in patients with asthma; remember the salbutamol in the emergency drugs box? It acts as a short acting β2-agonists or SABA, (there are long acting beta agonists (LABAs) too), so anything that blocks the receptor for salbutamol might cause broncho-constriction and in an asthmatic this might prove to be something of a problem. The most recent data seems to suggest that a dose-escalating model of cardio-selective β-blocker therapy for patients with asthma is well tolerated, does not induce acute broncho-constriction and may actually have an ameliorating impact on the airway inflammatory hyper-responsiveness.

Although these findings are clinically based, they are from a relatively small sample of patients. Before we lower our vigilance, it would be prudent to exercise caution and maintain the status quo with respect to beta-blockers and our asthmatic patients[127].

Following from this brief discourse on the principle uses of beta-blockers, we must be aware of their use as an anxiolytic and the interactions with drugs we might administer in the dental clinic. Although the precise mode of action is not known, beta-blockers do effectively reduce the signs and the symptoms of anxiety. Having treated many anxious dental patients you will recognize these clinical signs as:

> I.   **Increased heart rate and rhythm.**
> II. **Increased rate of perspiration.**
> III. **Vasoconstriction in the peripheral circulation.**
> IV. **Increased respiration,**
> V.   **Muscle tremors.**

When treating patients taking non cardio-selective beta-blockers we must exercise caution when using adrenaline containing local anaesthetics on account of an interesting interaction:

The effects of adrenaline on the myocardium will already be recognized:

I.   Adrenaline activates β-1 receptors in the Sino Atrial Node (SAN) to increase the heart rate.

II. β-1 receptors on myocardial cells will also be stimulated increasing their force of contraction.

III. This results in an increase the systemic systolic blood pressure.

IV. Adrenaline stimulates the α1 receptors in blood vessel walls closing them down.

V.   Adrenaline also stimulates the β-2 receptors in blood vessel walls opening them up.

We view adrenaline as a vasoconstrictor precisely because we need this effect to happen when we inject into the oral mucosa. The capillaries in the oral mucosa contain only α1 receptors and adrenaline will constrict them. In contrast, the walls of the larger systemic arteries contain both α1 and β-2 receptors, the latter being more numerous and stimulation of these will determine vascular resistance and changes in our patient's diastolic blood pressure will result.

If we inject a dental local anaesthetic containing adrenaline and some of the solution inadvertently enters a blood vessel, dilation of the arteries occurs with a drop in diastolic blood pressure. This effect occurs even with the extremely low doses of adrenaline used dentally; in the range of 20–100 μg. Adrenaline that is injected into an artery will preferentially stimulate the β 2 receptors.

If our patient is taking a non cardio-selective beta-blocker, the effect of adrenaline on the vasculature will be different from the patient who has not been medicated with beta-blockers. In the medicated patient: β-2 receptors on systemic arteries will be <u>non-functional</u> and so adrenaline will now activate the <u>remaining α-1 receptors</u> leading to vasoconstriction and an increase in diastolic blood pressure.

To counter this increase in resistance, the myocardium responds with a greater contraction force and the systolic blood pressure also rises! This will have the effect of increasing the mean arterial pressure. The sudden spike in arterial pressure will be picked up by the carotid sinuses baro receptors and a paradoxical cardiac reflex will then initiate a sudden and striking bradycardic response, which is then increased further because the SAN β -1 receptors have already been blocked.

The sequence of events outlined above could take place in anything up to five minutes and all being well; it will diminish in some fifteen to twenty minutes due to hepatic COMT methylation of adrenaline, thus inactivating it. It should be emphasized (again), that although cardio-selective beta-blockers might not exhibit such an interaction, with higher doses their receptor selectivity will be lost. The upshot of this is whether we treat patients on beta-blockers or not, with adrenaline in our local anaesthetics or not, as always: We need to be especially careful where we place a local anaesthetic. To achieve this, our regular revision of head and neck regional anatomy is fundamental and this matter will be considered with our revision of local anaesthetics in the next section.

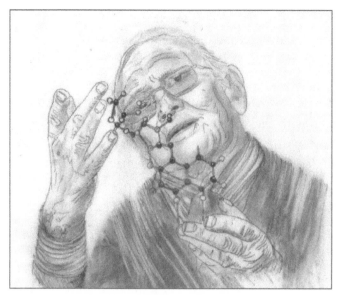

Sir James W Black, 1924 – 2010
Professor of medicine, pharmacologist and Nobel Prize winner.
An iconic Scottish academic who first discovered then
developed the beta-blocker.
His pioneering work continues to shape our
clinical practise into the 21st century

V. Antimicrobials. From reading the previous section, you will be aware of the difficulties we might encounter if we wish to prescribe certain antimicrobials when our patient is already taking another drug. The potentially adverse drug interactions and clinical reactions that follow will have been anticipated and disaster will have been averted.

As the principles of antibiotic stewardship filters downwards and outwards from academia and hospitals, becoming more accepted, then acceptable to general dental practitioners, the prescribing profiles that are viewed by some of your colleagues today as being restrictive, will on the evidence that is being established and published, become more acceptable. **Therefore:**

> ## Reduced Requesting Results in Risk Reduction

As a profession, dentistry must rightly accept this as a change and not a challenge. The risk and rate of adverse drug interactions should, if not eliminated: At least be controlled.

Against this rationale as mentioned, today more patients are being treated with more drugs and so the risk might not be as low or as controllable as we hope. Nevertheless and somewhat fortunately for the dentist, in reality; periodontal and odontogenic infections can be effectively managed with very few antibiotics.

If the periodonto-pharmaceutical approach does not work, then considering the risk to systemic health from a dental problem, as drastic as it seems, extraction must be viewed as a perfectly reasonable and a practical option from the outset and not necessarily as the last resort.

In the advent of the latest Montgomery (2015), principles of consent, when a patient blindly asks for a blind prescription; all the risks and benefits must be given to them, before you ever so politely and with the utmost professionalism, decline their offer to relegate you from being a dental surgeon to being a dental pharmacist.

Please remember that dentistry is a surgical and not a medical discipline and sometimes the surgical approach rather than the medical one is the more appropriate one.

Despite all of this, a few interactions from antimicrobials are significant, and in this section, we will first address issues regarding antibiotics in general, followed by a few more considerations in particular.

As this is the last part of this section and you have been through a lot of detail already, hold on and I'll try to make this as interesting as possible!

We have already considered the potential for reduced efficacy of the OCP when prescribing antibiotics and the dental and medical literature contains a number of publications supporting this notion[69.] Indeed, it has been suggested and it has been accepted that if not all antibiotics, then at least the majority are involved in this rapid route for your insurance provider to pay for your patient's child support.

The mechanism of GI tract commensal ablation and bioavailability reduction has been discussed, so there is no need for repetition, unless my writing has failed to sufficiently grip you and you were sleep-reading through the previous sections. Briefly (once more): OCPs deliver either oestrogen, progesterone or both. Hepatic circulation results in these being conjugated, secreted in bile and released into the duodenum where GI tract commensals hydrolyse them to release the pharmacologically active drug. However a literature search reveals no firm evidence to support the notion that antibiotics cause OCP failure!

Unless we are prescribing Rifampicin for the oral manifestations of tuberculosis, we need not worry about the interaction of an OCP and antibiotics. In any event, we will not be prescribing for patients with tuberculous lesions (unless we are working under the guidance of a medical specialist) and if we were, then the patient is extremely unlikely to be pregnant (unlikely but not impossible)

The accepted rate for unwanted pregnancies for those taking the OCP is in the range of 0.5%–1%, but your teenage dental patient taking the OCP, will be in a league of their own at a rate of 8% for unwanted pregnancies[128]. Not surprisingly, the most common reason for their OCP failure is forgetting to take the pill.

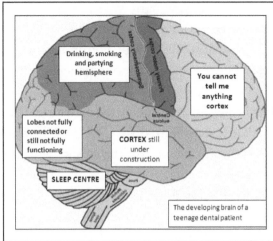

The developing brain of a teenage dental patient

This carefully researched and highly accurate anatomical view of the teenage dental patient's developing brain, highlights some of the problem areas your medical colleagues are forced to deal with, when trying to stop a teenager from turning their mum and dad into instant grandparents.

At the time of writing, there is no clinical evidence suggesting that any antibiotic other than rifampicin is affected by either the OCP or the COCP.[129] The suggestion that they are, merely adds fuel to the fires being stoked by the solicitors feeding on the weakest and lowest members of the dental profession; the professionally isolated dentist in general practice.

You will recall that warfarin inhibits the synthesis of Vitamin K, which is an essential component of the following coagulation factors: prothrombin (factor II), factors VII, IX and X, together with: proteins, C, S, and Z. As Vitamin K is derived from the activity of GI tract commensals, their ablation following the action of antibiotics will adversely affect the warfarin-medicated patient's INR. While short term dental antibiotic prescribing for five to seven days will have little impact, it would be prudent to defer to the patient's haematologist for advice and support when considering prescribing macrolides, cephalosporins or tetracyclines.

Another antibiotic interaction, not related to GI tract flora but involving the Cytochrome P450 microsomal enzymes is that of erythromycin and metronidazole for our patients taking warfarin.

This interaction has been noted in the previous section. To elaborate on what has already been mentioned, both of these antibiotics will inhibit CYP 2C9, the enzyme responsible for metabolizing warfarin.

Because of such inhibition, given the very narrow Ti of warfarin, the rise in INR that may result will be both rapid and extreme.

From a safety point in dentistry, the use of erythromycin and metronidazole must be absolutely avoided for our patients taking warfarin.

Erythromycin and clarithromycin also inhibit the activity of CYP 3A4. Therefore, any drug that is metabolized by CYP 3A4, if taken concurrently with either erythromycin or clarithromycin will also demonstrate elevated plasma levels.

Of considerable importance in this respect is the interaction between erythromycin, clarithromycin and statins.

A recently published large-scale study clearly demonstrated the increased risk of skeletal muscle breakdown, kidney damage and an increase in mortality in those patients co-medicated with erythromycin, clarithromycin and statins[130].

At the time of writing, worldwide, some 1 billion people will have been recommended to use statins with 1/3 of those reporting some form of adverse effects[131-132]. Given the sheer numbers of patients taking these drugs and the adverse clinical effects being reported, the results of the above noted study are given below:

I. Patients co-prescribed clarithromycin and a statin not metabolized by CYP3A4 were at **increased risk of hospital admission**.

II. Acute kidney injury (adjusted relative risk [RR] **1.65**, 95% confidence interval [CI] 1.31 to 2.09), Admission with hyperkalemia (adjusted RR 2.17, 95% CI 1.22 to 3.86)

III. All-cause mortality (adjusted RR **1.43**, 95% CI 1.15 to 1.76).

IV. The adjusted RR for admission with rhabdomyolysis was **2.27** (95% CI 0.86 to 5.96).

V. Among older adults taking a statin not metabolized by CYP3A4, co-prescription of clarithromycin versus azithromycin was associated with a modest but statistically significant increase in the 30-day absolute risk of adverse outcomes.

With short course dental prescribing for five to seven days, the risk should be lower than for medical prescribing, where longer durations of treatment using larger doses are the norm. Nevertheless, the same safety prescribing principles apply for dentistry as they do for medicine. Of particular interest are that the results reported in this study applied only to older patients (mean age 74 years).

In the published data, it was not made clear for what condition(s) the erythromycin and clarithromycin were being prescribed. Although chest infections of varying severity up to and including life threatening pneumonia would be a common reason. With such cases, a medical specialist will clearly make an informed decision of what drug to prescribe and when to prescribe it, balancing the benefit needed versus the risk perceived. The use of alternative antibiotics such as azithromycin did not demonstrate the morbidity or mortality associated with erythromycin and clarithromycin. Of note, the statins under investigation did not inhibit CYP 3A4. It has long been accepted that CYP 3A4 enzyme inhibition by antibiotics provided the mechanism for statin toxicity. In this study another more plausible explanation was given:

The liver-specific organic anion–transporting polypeptide (OATP) 1B1 was associated with increased blood concentrations of two non–CYP3A4 metabolized statins (rosuvastatin and pravastatin). In vitro, clarithromycin has been shown to inhibit both OATP 1B1 and OATP 1B3 and thus cause the increased levels of clinical statin toxicity. The use of azithromycin which does not inhibit either the OATP or the CYP metabolism provided the means to prove the importance of the OATP pathway in statin toxicity.

One common sense approach that has been advocated, should the need for antibiotics be indicated; is to cease statins for five to seven days. After the dental infection is brought under control, the statin treatment can then resume.

In dentistry as always, it is prudent to defer to a medical specialist for prescribing advice and clinical support. When considering a macrolide antibiotic or indeed any other treatment, sometimes the benefit versus the risk simply cannot be rationalized, reconciled or balanced.

Before considering any drug treatment, there are always pharmaceutical experts from whom we can ask for advice and guidance if we cannot find the answers in the BNF. After treatment has started and an adverse reaction begins, the choice of those we can turn to for help is invariably limited to the medical specialist in accident and emergency departments and the dento-legal advisers in the indemnity organisations.

While the risks are present, they are still vanishingly small enough to make every day dental practise a relatively safe occupation. By studying the drugs you use and the drug interactions they are capable of; you will be practising from a position of safety, while deriving professional satisfaction in developing an interest in this sometimes complicated, often dynamic, but always exciting area of your clinical working life!

References to: Drug action and drug interaction.

1. Lepakhin VK. Safety of medicines: a guide to detecting and reporting adverse drug reactions. Why health professionals need to take action. World Health Organization 2002.

2. Lazarou J. et al. Incidence of Adverse Drug Reactions in hospitalized patients: a meta-analysis of prospective studies. JAMA, 1998, 279 (15) 1000-5.

3. Moore N et al. Frequency and cost of serious adverse drug reactions in a department of general medicine. Br J Clin Pharmacol 1998, 45(3), 301-308.

4. Imbs JL et al. Latrogenic medication: estimation of its prevalence in French public hospitals. Thèrapie, 1999, 54(1) 21-27.

5. Griffin GP. The evaluation of human medicines control from a national to an international perspective. Ad Drug React Toxico Rev., 1998, 17(1), 19-50
   Available online from: http://whqlibdoc.who.int/hq/2002/WHO_EDM_QSM_2002.2.pdf
   Accessed January 2016.

6. White T et al. Counting the cost of drug-related adverse events. Pharmacoeconomics, 1999, 15(5). 445-458.

7. Florence AL. Is Thalidomide to Blame? BMJ 1960; 1954

8. Crawford A. Brazil's new generation of Thalidomide babies. BBC News. 2013 July 23rd.
   Available online from: http://www.bbc.co.uk/news/magazine-23418102
   Accessed January 2016.

9. World Health Organization. Medicines: spurious falsely-labelled falsified counterfeit (SFFC) medicines 2012.
   Available online from: http://www.who.int/mediacentre/factsheets/fs275/en/
   Accessed January 2016

10. Mackey TK, Liang BA, York P and Kubic T. Counterfeit Drug Penetration into Global Legitimate Medicine Supply Chains: A

Global Assessment. The American Journal of Tropical Medicine and Hygiene. 2015; 92 (Suppl 6): 59-67.

Available online from: http://www.ncbi.nlm.nih.gov/pmc/articles/PMC4455087/.

Accessed January 2016

11. El-Jardali F, Akl EA, Fadlallah R, et al. Interventions to combat or prevent drug counterfeiting: a systematic review. BMJ Open. 2015; 5(3)

Available online from:

http://www.ncbi.nlm.nih.gov/pmc/articles/PMC4368988/#R4

Accessed January 2016.

12. Putze E, Conway E, Reilly M et al. The Deadly World of Fake Drugs.

Available online from:

http://www.aei.org/files/2012/02/27/-appendix-a-master-2_170026856632.pdf

Accessed January 2016.

13. Faucon B. No cure for fake drugs. The Wall Street Journal 15 February 2010. Available online from:

http://online.wsj.com/news/articles/SB10001424052748704533204575047282075703998

Accessed January 2016.

14. Attaran A, Barry D and Basheer S et al. How to achieve international action on falsified and substandard medicines. BMJ 2012; 345

15. Peltzman S. An Evaluation of Consumer Protection Legislation: The 1962 Drug Amendments. The Journal of Political Economy, Vol. 81, No. 5. Sep. - Oct, 1973, pp. 1051

16. Leurs R, Church MK and Taglialatela M in Church and Taglialatela (2002). H_1-antihistamines: inverse agonism, anti-inflammatory actions and cardiac effects. Clin Exp Allergy 2002 32 (4): 489–98.

17. Ariëns EJ. Affinity and intrinsic activity in the theory of competitive inhibition. I. Problems and theory. Archives internationales de pharmacodynamie et de thérapie 1954 99 (1): 32–49.

18. Stephenson RP. A modification of receptor theory. 1956. Br. J. Pharmacol. 1997. 120 (4 Suppl): 106–20; discussion 103–5.

19. Vauquelin G, Van Liefde I; Van Liefd. G protein-coupled receptors: a count of 1001 conformations. Fundamental & clinical pharmacology. 2005. 19 (1): 45–56.

20. Urban J. D, Clarke W. P, von Zastrow M, et al. Functional selectivity and classical concepts of quantitative pharmacology. Jnl. Pharmacol. Exp. Ther. 2007. 320 (1): 1–13.

21. Boyer EW and Shannon M. The serotonin syndrome. New Engl Jnl Med 2005. 352 (11): 1112–20.

22. Granados-Soto V and Castaneda-Hernandez G. A review of the pharmacokinetic and pharmacodynamic factors in the potentiation of the antinociceptive effect of nonsteroidal anti-inflammatory drugs by caffeine. J Pharmacol Toxicol Methods. 1999 Oct; 42 (2): 67-72.

23. Varelas P and Webb Z. Chapter 12 Alcohol related seizures in intensive care unit pp 291-292. In Varelas P. Ed. Seizures in Critical Care, A Guide to Diagnosis and Therapeutics 2nd Edition. Humana Press. Springer Scientific and Business Media London 2009.

24. Stewart R, Perez R, Musial B, Lukens C, Adjepong YA and Manthous C. Outcomes of Patients with Alcohol Withdrawal Syndrome Treated with High-Dose Sedatives and Deferred Intubation. Ann Am. Thorac. Soc. 2016 Jan 22.

25. McGuire WP. Current status of taxane and platinum-based chemotherapy in ovarian cancer. J Clin Oncol.2003; 21:133–5.

26. Chou TC. Theoretical basis, experimental design, and computerized simulation of synergism and antagonism in drug combination studies. Pharmacol Rev. 2006; 58: 621–81

27. Bukowska B, Gajek A and Marczak A. Two drugs are better than one. A short history of combined therapy of ovarian cancer. Contemporary Oncology. 2015; 19 (5):350-353.
Available online from:
http://www.ncbi.nlm.nih.gov/pmc/articles/PMC4709392/
Accessed January 2016.

28. Valente JF, Anderson GL, Branson RD et al. Disadvantages of prolonged propofol sedation in the critical care unit. *Crit Care Med.* 1994; 22:710–2.

29. Vasile B, Rasulo F, Candiani A et al. The pathophysiology of propofol infusion syndrome: a simple name for a complex syndrome. Intensive Care Med. 2003; 29:1417–25.

30. Culp KE, Augoustides JG, Ochroch AE et al. Clinical management of cardiogenic shock associated with prolonged propofol infusion. Anesth. Analg. 2004; 99:221–6.

31. Vasile B, Rasulo F, Candiani A and Latronico N. The pathophysiology of propofol infusion syndrome: a simple name for a complex syndrome. Intensive Care Medicine. 2003. 29 (9): 1417–25.

32. Ali SS, Sharma PK, Garg VK, Singh AK, Mondal SC. The target-specific transporter and current status of diuretics as antihypertensive. Fundam Clin Pharmacol. 2012 April 26 (2): 175–9.

33. Rao P, Knaus EE. Evolution of nonsteroidal anti-inflammatory drugs (NSAIDs): Cyclooxygenase (COX) inhibition and beyond. J Pharm Pharm Sci. 2008; 11(2): 81s–110.

34. Moore N, Pollack C, and Butkerait P. "Adverse Drug Reactions and Drug–drug Interactions with over-the-Counter NSAIDs. Therapeutics and Clinical Risk Management 11 (2015): 1061–1075.
Available online from: http://www.ncbi.nlm.nih.gov/pmc/articles/PMC4508078/
Accessed February 2016.

35. Paterson CA, Jacobs D, Rasmussen S, Youngberg SP, McGuinness N. Randomized, open-label, 5-way crossover study to evaluate the pharmacokinetic/pharmacodynamic interaction between furosemide and the non-steroidal anti-inflammatory drugs diclofenac and ibuprofen in healthy volunteers. Int J Clin Pharmacol Ther. 2011; 49(8): 477–490

36. Dorn GW. Novel pharmacotherapies to abrogate post infarction ventricular remodelling Nature Reviews Cardiology 6, 283-291 (April 2009)

37. Cohn JN. Is activation of the renin–angiotensin system hazardous to your health? European Heart Journal 3rd August 2011. 2096-2097
   Available online from:
   http://eurheartj.oxfordjournals.org/content/32/17/2096
   Accessed February 2016.

38. Bhala N, Emberson J, Merhi A, Abramson S, Arber N, et al. Vascular and upper gastrointestinal effects of non-steroidal anti-inflammatory drugs: meta-analyses of individual participant data from randomised trials. August 31st 2013. Lancet 382 (9894): 769–79.

39. Page J, Henry D. Consumption of NSAIDs and the development of congestive heart failure in elderly patients: an under recognized public health problem March 2000. Archives of Internal Medicine 160 (6): 777–84.

40. FDA Strengthens Warning of Heart Attack and Stroke Risk for Non-Steroidal Anti-Inflammatory Drugs July 2015.
   Available online from:
   http://www.fda.gov/ForConsumers/ConsumerUpdates/ucm453610.htm
   Accessed February 2016.

41. Deshpande A, Pant C, Pasupuleti V, Rolston DD and Jain A. et al. Association between proton pump inhibitor therapy and Clostridium difficile infection in a meta-analysis. 2012 March. Clinical Gastroenterology and Hepatology : The Official Clinical Practice Journal of the American Gastroenterological Association 10 (3): 225–33.

42. Drekonja D, Reich J, Gezahegn S, Greer N and Shaukat A. et al. Faecal Microbiota Transplantation for Clostridium difficile Infection: A Systematic Review. Annals of internal medicine 2015 May 5. 162 (9): 630–8

43. Larson R J, and Fisher ES. Should Aspirin Be Continued in Patients Started on Warfarin?: A Systematic Review and Meta-Analysis. Journal of General Internal Medicine 19.8 (2004): 879–886. PMC. Web. 7 Feb. 2016.
Available online from: http://www.ncbi.nlm.nih.gov/pmc/articles/PMC1492499/
Accessed February 2016.

44. Guengerich FP. Cytochrome p450 and chemical toxicology. Chem Res Toxicol. 2008 Jan; 21(1):70-83.

45. Inui H, Itoh T, Yamamoto K, Ikushiro S-I and Sakaki T. Mammalian Cytochrome P450-Dependent Metabolism of Polychlorinated Dibenzo-p-dioxins and Coplanar Polychlorinated Biphenyls. Int. J. Mol. Sci. 2014, 15, 14044-14057.

46. Horn JR. Important drug interactions and their mechanisms. Katzung BG, Masters SB and Trevor AJ, eds. Basic and Clinical Pharmacology. 11th edition. City, State McGraw-Hill Companies Inc 2009.

47. Becker DE. Adverse Drug Interactions. Anesthesia Progress 58.1 (2011): 31–41.
Available online from http://www.ncbi.nlm.nih.gov/pmc/articles/PMC3265267/
Accessed February 2016.

48. LeBel M, Masson E, Guilbert E, Colborn D, Paquet F, Allard S, et al. Effects of rifabutin and rifampicin on pharmacokinetics of ethinylestradiol and norethindrone. J Clin Pharmacol 1998; 38: 1042–1050.

49. Barditch-Crovo P, Trapnell CB, Ette E, Zacur HA, Coresh J, Rocco LE, et al. The effects of rifampin and rifabutin on the pharmacokinetics and pharmacodynamics of a combination oral contraceptive. Clin Pharmacol Ther 1999; 65: 428–438

50. Young LK, Farquhar CM, McCowan LME, Roberts HE, Taylor J. The contraceptive practices of women seeking termination of pregnancy in an Auckland clinic. N Z Med J 1994; 107: 189–191. 47

51. Bollen M. Use of antibiotics when taking the oral contraceptive pill. Aust Fam Physician 1995; 24: 928–929.

52. Silber TJ. Apparent oral contraceptive failure associated with antibiotic administration. J Adolesc Health Care 1983; 4: 287–289.

53. World Health Organization. Medical Eligibility Criteria for Contraceptive Use (3rd edn). 2010. Available online from: http://www.who.int/reproductivehealth/publications/family_planning/9789241563888/en/index.html
Accessed February 2016.

54. Grimmer Sf M, Back DJ, Orme MLE, Cowie A, Gilmore I and Tjia J. The bioavailability of ethinyloestradiol and levonorgestrel in patients with an ileostomy. Contraception 1986; 33: 51–59.

55. Clinical Effectiveness Unit: Drug Interactions with Hormonal Contraception, Clinical Guidance, Faculty of Sexual and Reproductive Health Care, The Royal College of Obstetrics and Gynaecologists 2012.
Available online from: http://www.fsrh.org/pdfs/CEUguidancedruginteractionshormonal.pdf
Accessed February 2016

56. Pfeifer GP, Denissenko MF, Olivier M, Tretyakova N, Hecht SS and Hainaut P. Tobacco smoke carcinogens, DNA damage and p53 mutations in smoking-associated cancers. Oncogene. 2002 October 21; 21(48):7435-51.

57. Jiang H, Gelhaus SL, Mangal D, Harvey RG, Blair IA and Penning TM: Metabolism of Benzo[a]pyrene in Human Bronchoalveolar H358 Cells Using Liquid Chromatography-Mass Spectrometry, Chem. Res. Toxicol., 2007, 20 (9), pp 1331–1341.

58. Wandel C, Böcker R, Böhrer H, Browne A, Rügheimer E, and Martin E. Midazolam is metabolized by at least three different cytochrome P450 enzymes. Br J Anaesth. 1994 Nov; 73(5):658-61.

59. Jones R. Nonsteroidal anti-inflammatory drug prescribing: past, present, and future. Am J Med.2001; 110:4S–7S

60. Singh G. Recent considerations in nonsteroidal anti-inflammatory drug gastropathy. Am J Med.1998; 105:31S–38

61. Lanas A, Perez-Aisa MA, Feu F, Ponce J, Saperas E, et al. A nationwide study of mortality associated with hospital admission due to severe gastrointestinal events and those associated with

nonsteroidal antiinflammatory drug use. Am J Gastroenterol. 2005; 100:1685–1693.

62. Antman EM, Bennett JS, Daugherty A, Furberg C, Roberts H and Taubert KA. Use of nonsteroidal anti inflammatory drugs: an update for clinicians: a scientific statement from the American Heart Association. Circulation. 2007; 115:1634–1642

63. Teoh NC, Farrell GC. Hepatotoxicity associated with non-steroidal anti-inflammatory drugs. Clin Liver Dis. 2003;7:401–413

64. Laine L, White WB, Rostom A and Hochberg M. COX-2 selective inhibitors in the treatment of osteoarthritis. Semin Arthritis Rheum. 2008; 38:165–187.

65. Gutthann SP, Garcia Rodriguez LA, Raiford DS. Individual nonsteroidal antiinflammatory drugs and other risk factors for upper gastrointestinal bleeding and perforation. Epidemiology. 1997;8:18–24.

66. Huang JQ, Sridhar S, Hunt RH. Role of Helicobacter pylori infection and non-steroidal anti-inflammatory drugs in peptic-ulcer disease: a meta-analysis. Lancet. 2002;359:14–22.

67. Schnitzer TJ, Burmester GR, Mysler E, Hochberg MC, Doherty M et al. Comparison of lumiracoxib with naproxen and ibuprofen in the Therapeutic Arthritis Research and Gastrointestinal Event Trial (TARGET), reduction in ulcer complications: randomised controlled trial. Lancet. 2004; 364:665–674.

68. Silverstein FE, Faich G, Goldstein JL, Simon LS, Pincus T, et al. Gastrointestinal toxicity with celecoxib vs nonsteroidal anti-inflammatory drugs for osteoarthritis and rheumatoid arthritis: the CLASS study: a randomized controlled trial. Celecoxib Long-term Arthritis Safety Study. JAMA.2000; 284: 1247–1255

69. Seymour RA. Drug interactions in dentistry. Dent Update. 2009 Oct; 36 (8): 458-60, 463-6, 469-70.

70. Hohlfeld T et al. High on treatment platelet reactivity against aspirin by non-steroidal anti-inflammatory drugs—pharmacological mechanisms and clinical relevance. Thromb Haemost. 2013; 109.

71. Catella-Lawson F, et al. Cyclooxygenase inhibitors and the antiplatelet effects of aspirin. N Engl J Med. 2001; 345: 1809-1817.

72. Anzellotti P. et al. Low-dose naproxen interferes with the antiplatelet effects of aspirin in healthy subjects: recommendations to minimize the functional consequences. Arthritis Thrum. 2011; 63:850-859.

73. Cryer B, Berlin RG, Cooper SA, Hsu C and Wason S. Double-blind, randomized, parallel, placebo-controlled study of ibuprofen effects on thromboxane B2 concentrations in aspirin-treated healthy adult volunteers. Clin Ther. 2005; 27: 185–191.

74. Patel TN and Goldberg KC. Use of aspirin and ibuprofen compared with aspirin alone and the risk of myocardial infarction. Arch Intern Med. 2004; 164:852–856.

75. Delaney JA, Opatrny L, Brophy JM and Suissa S. Drug-drug interactions between antithrombotic medications and the risk of gastrointestinal bleeding. CMAJ. 2007; 177:347–35
Available online from: http://www.ncbi.nlm.nih.gov/pmc/articles/PMC1942107/
Accessed February 2016.

76. Young S N. How to Increase Serotonin in the Human Brain without Drugs. Journal of Psychiatry & Neuroscience : JPN 32.6 (2007): 394–399.
Available from https://www.ncbi.nlm.nih.gov/pmc/articles/PMC2077351/
Accessed February 2016.

77. Labos C, Dasgupta K, Nedjar H, Turecki G and Rahme E. Risk of bleeding associated with combined use of selective serotonin reuptake inhibitors and antiplatelet therapy following acute myocardial infarction. CMAJ September 26, 2011. Available online from:
http://www.cmaj.ca/content/early/2011/09/26/cmaj.100912
Accessed February 2016.

78. Serebruany VL. Selective serotonin reuptake inhibitors and increasing bleeding risk: Are we missing something.? American Journal of Medicine; 119 (2): 113-116.

79. Pozuelo L, Tesar G, Zhang J, et al. Depression and heart disease: What do we know and where are we headed? Cleveland Clinical Journal of Medicine. 2009; 76 (1): 59-70.

80. Pratt LA, Ford DE, Crum RM, et al. Depression, psychotropic medication and risk of myocardial infarction. Prospective data from the Baltimore ECA Follow-up. Circulation 1996; 94 (12): 3123-3139.

81. Frasure-Smith N, Lesperance F and Talajic M. Depression and the 18 month prognosis after myocardial infarction. Circulation 1995; 91 (4): 999- 1005.

82. Ziegelstein RC, Meuchel J, Kim TJ et al. Selective Serotonin Reuptake Inhibitor use by patients with acute coronary syndromes. American Journal of Medicine. 2007; 120(6): 525-530.

83. Pinto A, Farrar JT and Hersh EV. Prescribing NSAIDs to patients on SSRIs: possible adverse drug interaction of importance to dental practitioners. Compendium of Continuing Education in Dentistry. 2009; 30: 142–151.

84. Burke A, Smyth E and FitzGerald GA. Analgesic-antipyretic agents; pharmacotherapy of gout. In: Brunton LL, Lazo JS and Parker KL. Editors. Goodman and Gilman's: The Pharmacological Basis of Therapeutics. 11th ed. New York, NY: McGraw-Hill; 2006

85. Scully C and Chaudhry S. Aspects of human disease 15. Chronic liver disease. Dental Update 2007; 43: 525.

86. Modi AA and Liang TJ. Hepatitis C, A clinical review. Oral Diseases 2008; 14: 10-14.

87. El-Serag HB. Hepatocellular carcinoma. N Engl Jnl Med. 2011; 365: 1118–1127.

88. Bray F, Ren JS, Masuyer E and Ferlay J. Global estimates of cancer prevalence for 27 sites in the adult population in 2008. Int Jnl Cancer. 2013; 132: 1133–1145.

89. Ferlay J, Soerjomataram I, Dikshit R, Eser S and Mathers C, et al. Cancer incidence and mortality worldwide: sources, methods and major patterns in GLOBOCAN 2012. Int J Cancer. 2015; 136

90. Stewart BW and Wild CP, editors. World Cancer Report 2014. Lyon, France: International Agency for Research on Cancer; 2014.

91. Sukowati CH, El-Khobar KE, Ie SI, Anfuso B, Muljono DH and Tiribelli C. Significance of hepatitis virus infection in the oncogenic initiation of hepatocellular carcinoma. World Journal of Gastroenterology. 2016; 22(4): 1497-1512. Available online from: http://www.ncbi.nlm.nih.gov/pmc/articles/PMC4721983/ Accessed February 2016.

92. Whitcomb DC, Block GD. Association of acetaminophen hepatotoxicity with fasting and ethanol. JAMA. 1994;272:1845–1850.

93. Abramowicz M, editor. Acetaminophen safety—deja vu. Med Lett Drugs Ther. 2009;51:53–54. editor.

94. Abramowicz M, editor. Warfarin-acetaminophen interaction. Med Lett Drugs Ther. 2008; 50: 45. editor.

95. dela Cruz Ubaldo C, Hall NS and Le B. Post marketing review of intravenous acetaminophen dosing based on Food and Drug Administration prescribing guidelines. Pharmacotherapy. 2014 Dec; 34 Suppl 1:34S-39S.

96. Chan AT, Manson JE, Albert CM, *et al* Nonsteroidal anti-inflammatory drugs, acetaminophen, and the risk of cardiovascular events. Circulation 2006; 113:1578–87

97. Rahme E, Barkun A, Nedjar H, et al Hospitalizations for upper and lower GI events associated with traditional NSAIDs and acetaminophen among the elderly in Quebec, Canada. *Am J Gastroenterol* 2008; 103: 872–82.

98. Munsterhjelm E, Niemi TT, Ylikorkala O, et al Characterization of inhibition of platelet function by paracetamol and its interaction with diclofenac in vitro. *Acta Anaesthesiol Scand 2005; 49: 840–6.*

99. Brune K and Hinz B. Paracetamol, ibuprofen, or a combination of both drugs against knee pain: an excellent new randomised clinical trial answers old questions and suggests new therapeutic recommendations. *Ann Rheum Dis* 2011; 70:1521-1522.

100. Hawton K, Bergen H Simkin S Dodd S and Pocock P et al. Long term effect of reduced pack sizes of paracetamol on poisoning deaths and liver transplant activity in England and Wales: interrupted time series analyses. BMJ 2013; 346: f403.
Available online from:
http://www.bmj.com/content/346/bmj.f403
Accessed February 2016.

101. Rumack BH and Matthew H. Acetaminophen poisoning and toxicity. Pediatrics 1975. 55 (6): 871–6.

102. Abramowicz M, editor. Drug interactions. Med Lett Drugs Ther. 1999; 41:61–62.

103. Smith HS. Opioid metabolism. Mayo Clin Proc. 2009; 84:613–624.

104. Policy Impact: Prescription Pain Killer Overdoses Centers for Disease Control and Prevention.

105. Skrebowski L. Oxycodone explained. The Observer UK News. Sunday 24th March 2002.

106. Leppert W. CYP2D6 in the metabolism of opioids for mild to moderate pain. Pharmacology 2011 87 (5–6): 274–85

107. Rossi, S, ed. Australian Medicines Handbook (2013 ed.). Adelaide: The Australian Medicines Handbook Unit Trust

108. Samer, C. F. et al. Applications of CYP450 Testing in the Clinical Setting. Molecular Diagnosis & Therapy 17.3 2013: 165–184.
Available online from:
https://www.ncbi.nlm.nih.gov/pmc/articles/PMC3663206/
Accessed March 2016.

109. Liu Z, Gao F, Tian Y. Effects of morphine, fentanyl and tramadol on human immune response. Jnl Huazhong Univ. Sci. Technol. Med. Sci. 2006 26 (4): 478–81

110. Dunkley EJ, Isbister GK, Sibbritt D, Dawson AH and Whyte IM. The Hunter Serotonin Toxicity Criteria: simple and accurate diagnostic decision rules for serotonin toxicity. September 2003. QJM 96 (9): 635–42

111. Boyer EW, Shannon M The serotonin syndrome. N Engl J Med. 2005 Mar 17; 352 (11):1112-20.

112. Randall C and Crane J. Tramadol deaths in Northern Ireland: a review of cases from 1996 to 2012. Journal of Forensic and Legal Medicine 2014 23: 32–6

113. Mikkelsen S, Ilkjaer S, Brennum J, Borgbjerg FM and Dahl JB The effect of naloxone on ketamine-induced effects on hyperalgesia and ketamine-induced side effects in humans. Anesthesiology. 1999 Jun; 90(6):1539-45.

114. Kohrs, R; Durieux, ME Ketamin. Teaching an old drug new tricks. Anesthesia & Analgesia. November 1998. 87 (5): 1186–93

115. Rossi S, ed. Australian Medicines Handbook. 2013 ed. Adelaide: The Australian Medicines Handbook Unit Trust.

116. Wheeler E, Davidson PJ, Jones TS, Irwin KS. Community-Based Opioid Overdose Prevention Programs Providing Naloxone — United States, 2010. MMWR Morbidity and mortality weekly report. 2012; 61(6):101-105.
Available online from:
https://www.ncbi.nlm.nih.gov/pmc/articles/PMC4378715/
Accessed March 2016.

117. Office for National Statistics. Deaths related to Drug Poisoning in England and Wales: 2014 Registrations.
Available online from:
http://www.ons.gov.uk/peoplepopulationandcommunity/
birthsdeathsandmarriages/deaths/bulletins/deathsrelatedtodrug
poisoninginenglandandwales/2015-09-03#opiates
Accessed March 2016.

118. Graham, L., et al. (2012) The National Drug-related Deaths Database (Scotland) Report 2010 Available online from:
http://www.isdscotland.org/Health-Topics/Drugs-and-
alcoholmisuse/Publications/2012-02-28/2012-02-28-NationalD
rugRelatedDeathsDatabase2010-Report.pdf
Accessed March 2016.

119. Hecht, G. et al (2014) The National Drug-related Deaths Database (Scotland) Report 2012 Available online from:

https://isdscotland.scot.nhs.uk/Health-Topics/Drugs-and-AlcoholMisuse/Publications/2014-03-25/2014-03-25-NDRDD-Report.pdf?54671877623
Accessed March 2016

120. Hoolachan, J. et al. (2013) The National Drug-related Deaths Database (Scotland) Report 2011 [online]. Available online from: http://www.isdscotland.org/Health-Topics/Drugs-and-AlcoholMisuse/Publications/2013-04-30/2013-04-30-NDRDD-Report.pdf?81992739440
Accessed March 2016.

121. National Health Service Scotland Publication Report. National Naloxone Programme Scotland. Monitoring Report 2014/2015. October 2015.
Available online from:
http://www.isdscotland.org/Health-Topics/Drugs-and-Alcohol-Misuse/Publications/2015-10-27/2015-10-27-Naloxone-Report.pdf
Accessed March 2016.

122. Scarborough P, Bhatnagar P, Wickramasinghe K, Smolina K, Mitchell C, Rayner M (2010). Coronary heart disease statistics 2010 edition. British Heart Foundation.

123. Dawoud BES, Roberts A and Yates JM. Drug interactions in general dental practice – considerations for the dental practitioner. BDJ 2014 216 15 – 23. 2014.

124. Haas DA. An update on local anaesthetics in dentistry. J Can Dent Assoc 2002; 68: 546-51.

125. Xue H, Lu Z, Tang WL, Pang LW, Wang GM et al. First-line drugs inhibiting the renin angiotensin system versus other first-line antihypertensive drug classes for hypertension. Cochrane Database of Systematic Reviews 2015, Issue 1. Art. No.: CD00817.

126. Elliott WJ, Meyer PM. Incident diabetes in clinical trials of antihypertensive drugs: a network meta-analysis. *Lancet* 2007. 369 (9557): 201–7.

127. Arboe B, Ulrik CS. Beta-blockers: friend or foe in asthma? International Journal of General Medicine. 2013; 6: 549-555. Available online from: http://www.ncbi.nlm.nih.gov/pmc/articles/PMC3709648/ Accessed March 2016.

128. Sondheimer SJ. Update on oral contraceptive pills and postcoital contraception. Curr Opin Obstet Gynecol. 1992;4:502–505.

129. Back DJ and Orme ML. Pharmacokinetic drug interactions with oral contraceptives. Clin Pharmacokinet. 1990; 18:472–484.

130. Li D Q, Kim R, McArthur E, Fleet J L, Bailey D G, Juurlink D and Garg A X et al. Risk of adverse events among older adults following co-prescription of clarithromycin and statins not metabolized by cytochrome P450 3A4. CMAJ : Canadian Medical Association Journal. 2015 187 (3), 174–180. Available online from: http://www.ncbi.nlm.nih.gov/pmc/articles/PMC4330139/ Accessed March 2016.

131. Ioannidis JP. More than a billion people taking statins? Potential implications of the new cardiovascular guidelines. JAMA 2014; 311:463–4.

132. Cohen JD, Brinton E, Ito M and Jacobson TA. Understanding Statin Use in America and Gaps in Patient Education (USAGE): an Internet-based survey of 10 138 current and former statin users. J Clin Lipidol 2012; 6:20.

Local Anaesthetic Safety

Needle Phobia and Anaesthetic Failure

If we look across the entire spectrum of clinical practise, as mentioned earlier (and I am sure you will agree), almost all medicines are administered orally. However in dentistry, you will be in a unique position but perhaps a difficult one. While both the numbers and the types of medicines you might choose to give your patient are considerably lower than those from your medical colleagues, the ones you will have to give in the clinic are almost invariably: Local Anaesthetics (LA) and these are applied topically or injected, either as an infiltration or as a block.

The paradox you are faced with is that most patients avoid attending the dentist because of fear; either their fear of pain or their fear of an injection. Isn't it bizarre, that the very means with which you might remove one cause of fear is the very cause of another?

The blessing that comes from the means to relieve dental pain is the curse that now afflicts the profession of dentistry.... ...

The dreaded needle!

Adding to the feelings of despair you have when things don't go according to plan, will be the patients' feelings, usually feelings of misery that accompany their pain, while you go about trying to numb them. It was reported over three decades ago, that some 90% of dentists will have at some point in their careers experienced difficulties in achieving adequate anaesthesia for their patients[1]. In the following years up to the present day, there has been considerable development in the field of dental anaesthetics, yet the most recent figures do not differ that markedly from those published earlier:

When working on lower teeth the often used block to the inferior alveolar nerve (IAN) is reported to have a failure rate of around one in seven (15%) for those patients where there are no infective or inflammatory processes occurring[2]. As for those patients where the

440

tissue to be anaesthetized is either infected or inflamed, failure rates to block the IAN rise considerably; failures from nearly one in two, to over four out of five have been reported (44-81%)[3]

Similarly, when working on upper teeth, the failure rate of a maxillary infiltration could be as high as one in three where the tooth to be anaesthetised has an irreversible pulpitis[2].

Of interest, the patients in these studies, reported complete numbness of their lips and peri-oral areas, yet when their teeth were tested with either an electric pulp tester or ethyl chloride all reported that sensations were still present!

Several reasons for such anaesthetic failure have been proposed and some of them you will already be familiar with. One suggestion is that the inflammatory processes affecting both pulpal and periapical tissues can significantly lower the tissue pH, thus limiting the ability of the local anesthetic to provide pain control. A second possibility is that inflammatory mediators enhance the conduction potential along nerves[4.] While a third hypothesis is that the blood vessels in significantly vasodilated tissues may facilitate the systemic uptake of local anaesthetic away from the area of anaesthetic administration, thus its effectiveness locally will be simply reduced due to inadequate levels of anaesthetic being maintained in the tissues[4].

Whichever of these is correct, possibly all, possibly a combination of some, or possibly none, the fact remains that patients have a fear, a very real fear of pain and of injections. For over twenty years needle phobia has been recognized as a specific phobia of blood, an injection or an injury. The inclusion of this condition in the Diagnostic and Statistical Manual of 1994 (DSM IV) is due to the clinically significant distress and impairment in social, occupational or other functioning that this condition causes in patients. Of interest, it has been noted that some 10% of patients in the USA suffer from this condition, but if we pause for a moment to think about this, such a figure might be something of an underestimate as the needle phobic person tends to avoid not only the dental clinic, but many or any form of medical or clinical intervention, so we might not really know the true prevalence of this condition after all[5].

Fainting and fatality

Needle phobia may have both a genetic and a behavioural or a learned element to it. Of particular interest is the problem of a parent or another relative who faints upon witnessing a clinical procedure being performed on a close family member. This occurrence is not the sole preserve of the soon-to-be-father who faints in the delivery room as his child is being born, then on recovering, demands the nitrous oxide, seemingly needing it more than the mother does. There are numerous reports of dentists and doctors who cannot bear to be present when their nearest and dearest are having even the most minor of procedures and will feel quite ill at the thought or the sight of this. A professional appreciation and recognition of the early symptoms of a vaso-vagal syncope (the operating room lights getting a little bit brighter and their beginning to swirl around the ceiling) are sufficient for them to make their excuses and embark on a hasty exit for some fresh air.

From the chapter on medical emergencies, we know that vaso-vagal syncope is the most common of the medical emergencies we will see in a dental practice. With this in mind, we should consider the following: Half of those with a needle phobia will experience a faint and some 80% of those who do, will have a first degree relative doing the same. Upon questioning those with needle phobia, the clinical picture becomes a little more confusing; needle phobic patients state their fear of fainting in the (dental) clinic is greater than their fear of the needle[6]. Such a finding is both important and of concern to us in dental practice. While the simple faint may seem an innocuous event in itself and one that can be easily remedied (laying the patient out flat, loosening their collar and raising their legs...couldn't be any easier), a further investigation of fainting in connection with, or as a result of needle phobia, revealed that the catastrophic drop in blood pressure from profound vaso-vagal shock was: <u>the cause of death in 23 patients</u>[7].

Given the serious nature of this condition, when exhibited by the needle phobic dental patient, there are a number of safety strategies we might usefully deploy to diminish the distress experienced by our needle phobic patients:

Safety strategies for phobic patients

1. Treating symptoms of the needle phobic behaviour exhibited through therapy. Overall this is an effective strategy, but the outcome depends on both the severity of the presenting symptoms and the patient's behaviour type. Their acceptance of therapy combined with a willingness to continue in a treatment programme which might continue for a many months, should not be overlooked. Given the complexity of problems a needle phobic patient presents with, that might extend across the social, medical and dental domains, together with the involvement of dental, medical and nursing professionals all eager to assist the needle phobic patient first hand, there is bound to be some debate as to the effectiveness of behavioural treatment.

The results from studies where gradual exposure to the fear evoking factor together with differential re-enforcement has yielded encouraging results, not only for dental patients, but diabetic patients and even those children struggling with maths at school[8,9.] The use of relaxation techniques might be a good way to begin our support for the needle phobic patient, but in thinking about this approach, it could be contraindicated as the end point of this therapy is to encourage relaxation and that means a drop in blood pressure and that would only enhance the vaso-vagal response even further with an increased risk of syncope occurring.

2. Thinking about this problem in a different way, a better outcome might be achieved by encouraging the patient to tense up their muscles; clenching their jaws, fists (and anything else) as they sit in the dental chair, then after a few seconds, relax, then tense and to continue doing so repeatedly for several minutes. This technique of Applied Muscular Tension or AMT, where the phobic patient is encouraged to tense then relax their skeletal muscles, encourages blood flow, with greater venous return and in doing so, a high degree of cerebral perfusion can be ensured. Thus blood pressure is maintained as is their level of consciousness. While the phobic patient is concentrating on doing all of that, you can be getting on with their treatment.

As almost all men can't multi-task, or think about more than one thing at a time (an observation based on experience) the results from using AMT might work better in men rather than women although to date, a gender bias has not been investigated with this technique. AMT has been proven to be effective in reducing anxiety, needle phobia and avoidance behaviours among blood donors, and given the size of needles used in that particular clinical environment, applying this technique to a dental practice should prove to be useful. Even if smaller needles are used in dentistry, they are still being introduced into one of the most sensitive and intimate areas of our patients and so AMT should find its place and value in the dental clinic[10].

3. Topical anaesthetics or other agents can be used to minimise the discomfort experienced as an injection is given.

    a. <u>Ethyl Chloride</u> is easily administered, but provides superficial pain control only and might cause more discomfort for the patient if it ends up getting to places where it ought not to be applied eg: the gum margins of dentin sensitive patients.

    b. <u>EMLA</u> is a topical anaesthetic cream that is a: <u>Eutectic</u> Mix of <u>Local Anaesthetics usually lidocaine</u> and <u>prilocaine</u>. It is available as an OCM in the UK and the EU, but only on prescription in North America. Although EMLA does not penetrate deep into the cutaneous or intra oral tissues, the penetration is deeper than topical anaesthetics, and it works adequately for many individuals.

    c. Ametop is a gel preparation; it appears to be more effective than EMLA for eliminating pain for patients undergoing intravenous sedation[11].

The self heating <u>lidocaine</u>/<u>tetracaine</u> patch also contains a <u>eutectic</u> mix of <u>lidocaine</u> and <u>tetracaine</u> and was available up to 2010 in the UK for use in reducing the pain or discomfort experienced with needle procedures. On exposure to air and applying to the patient's skin, the patch begins to heat up while releasing both anaesthetic and heat to an area of skin that in response, soon becomes vasodilated thus increasing the absorption of the anaesthetic, quite simple and really clever, exactly the type of clinical development we all wish we had thought of first!

A study from 2009, clearly demonstrated the lidocaine/tetracaine patch provided effective anaesthesia with an application time as short as 10 minutes and was better than lidocaine/prilocaine cream at all application times shorter than 60 minutes. The results demonstrated a substantial improvement in time to onset of anaesthesia. The lidocaine/tetracaine patch gave an important alternative to lidocaine/prilocaine cream for topical local anaesthesia. However there were problems with localized irritation and the patch was contra indicated for use in patients with liver disease. By December 2010 the lidocaine/tetracaine patch was no longer marketed in the UK and had been withdrawn from MIMS and the BNF[12].

4. If the needle phobic patient is resistant to behavioural modification through therapy or topical agents, then the use of pharmacological agents systemically applied might prove to be of some benefit. Nitrous Oxide inhaled intranasally provides both a sedative and an anxiolytic effect for the patient, together with some analgesic relief too. The oral route of administration of benzodiazepines such as midazolam may be considered, but to do so will require a prescription from a medical practitioner as relatively large doses are needed. Before embarking on this route one would need to demonstrate that techniques higher up this list, but lower down the ladder of anxiety management were either inappropriate or had met with failure.

5. If oral benzodiazepines do not work, then the extreme but last resort of referring the dental patient to a hospital for an inhalation general anaesthetic may, but only in very rare cases be considered. The use of a general anaesthetic will eliminate all pain and also all memory of any exposure to a needle. However, when the ratio of benefit to risk is calculated, due to the morbidity and mortality of using a general anaesthetic for a procedure that can be managed in the outpatient

clinic using local anaesthesia, this is regarded by many if not all dental professionals as an extreme solution.

The most recent figures from the Royal College of Anaesthetists are informative[13] [14] :

I. 1/10,000 allergic reactions per general anaesthetic for all patients.
II. 1/100,000 deaths per general anaesthetic for healthy children and adults[15] [16].
III. 1/40,000 deaths per general anaesthetic for healthy children[17].
IV. 17/100,000 deaths from all causes when the procedure is a Caesarian Section[18].
V. 1/185,000 deaths annually in the UK for all general anaesthetic procedures.

However these figures are increased wherever there is:

I. Poor health
II. Extremes of age
III. Where trauma or major vascular surgery is needed.
IV. Where the patient has a complex medical or medication history.
V. Where the surgery occurs at a time (weekend) or location (certain units where the figures are higher than the National Average (eg: obstetrics and gynaecology for caesarean section as noted above)[19]

As low as these figures are, they are still high enough to persuade any reasonable person be they a patient or a practitioner against referral for a general anaesthetic. If the patient is still insistent on having (*i.e:* not needing) a general anaesthetic, then it might be the case that the patient is being unreasonable or the dentist or the dental team have not done everything practicably possible to dissuade the patient from taking this course of action.

There are only three elements involved in dental anaesthesia:

I.   The dentist or hygienist or therapist
II. The local anaesthetics.
III. The patients.

Quite simple really and everything should go according to plan as it generally does on a daily basis. Dentistry is quite straightforward, essentially undemanding; until we do anything that involves the last of these three elements: The patients and after this, things start to get interesting. The dental professional must have a good rapport with their patients, without an encouraging, helpful and empathic approach to dental care, it doesn't matter how much anaesthetic is used and how accurately it is placed, the patient who has an adverse interaction with the dental professional is the one who will be most likely to complain of an adverse reaction to the local anaesthetic too.

The following reactions are frequently complained about:

The fabled but lamentable allergy to adrenaline, or there was simply no anaesthesia; either to begin with, or the entire procedure was completed while the patient endured excruciating pain. Between these two extremes lies the patient who quite willingly tolerated the injection and the dental procedure who then complains: It was only on their way home that the numbness set in. There is no doubt you will be familiar with these sorts of complaints, having had them directed at you or your colleagues.

Critically thinking about them in turn; there is no known allergy to adrenaline, as it is a naturally produced catecholamine being released in all of us in response to; physical, physiological and psychological stresses. The very small amount of adrenaline introduced from a dental local anaesthetic will not elicit an allergic reaction. It is more probable that there may be an allergy to either the preservative or the rubber stopper in the anaesthetic cartridges, which may contain latex; but such occurrences are incredibly rare.

A literature review revealed some evidence that latex allergens can be released into solution from the stoppers in local anaesthetic cartridges; however there were no cases of a demonstrable allergy to the cartridge, the stopper or the contents of the cartridge[20]. Despite such conclusively negative findings, manufacturers of local anaesthetic cartridges have moved towards using latex-free stoppers. If such an allergy existed, it is most unusual that its first presentation would be in the dental clinic, rather than at any time in the patient's past, for example when they received injections for childhood inoculations (for MMR and tetanus) or immunizations during adolescence (BCG for TB).

We can ensure anaesthesia has been achieved by using an electric pulp tester on the teeth to be worked on and if the patient's lip is not numb, then most certainly their teeth won't be either. However if the lip is numb this doesn't always indicate the mandibular molar teeth will be numb. In some 23% of cases where lip anaesthesia has been achieved, pulpal anaesthesia was not reached[21,22.]

One way to determine if anaesthesia has reached the pulp is to probe the mucosa around the tooth to detect sensations in the nerve territories supplying the tooth, to use the refrigerants: ethyl chloride or tetrafluoroethylene on the tooth, or as stated above, to use an electric pulp tester. All of these will soon reveal if the level of anaesthesia is adequate, or if our injection has missed its intended nerve.

Lastly in dentistry, like most things in life, timing is essentially everything and perhaps nowhere is this more important than with the administration of local anaesthesia (LA). Timing is essential with the delivery of this drug (as it is for all drugs) and once delivered, timing is essential as we wait and we must observe the patient.

Observing the patient for the clinical signs telling us that anaesthesia has been reached in the intended nerve territories is only half of our duty. We will return in a moment to consider timing in more detail. For now, we need to consider the other half of our duties; our responsibilities with respect to patient safety. The following information should be helpful in maintaining our safety critical focus:

The patient, having received an LA, then needs to be observed for several minutes, as we monitor them for any untoward clinical signs, or any undesirable symptoms the patient may tell us about, which could indicate an accidental intravascular injection has occurred.

Consider the following:

The strict limit on the total number of LA cartridges for use in children, adults and those on various drug regimens is made absolutely clear to us from the Drug Patient Information Leaflet. Every box of Local Anaesthetic has such a leaflet and they are essential reading. We will return to consider these in greater detail. The data contained in these leaflets ensures us when administering dental local anaesthesia, we will never even come close to the patient or whole body toxic levels of:

I.   Lignocaine
II. Articaine
III. Mepivicane
IV. Prilocaine
V.   Or the vasoconstrictors: Adrenaline and Octapressin.

These are the most common dental local anaesthetic
agents in the UK, EU and USA/Canada.

The intravascular injection accident

Notwithstanding such data guiding the safe doses of LA, the accidental intravascular injection especially during an Inferior Alveolar Nerve Block (IANB) may mean that a sizeable proportion of the contents of the LA cartridge ends up going around the systemic circulation of the patient's head and neck, but actually nowhere near the intended intra oral target tissue; the tooth or its pulp we intended to anaesthetise.

The results of an accidental intravascular injection are that tissues supplied by the vessel into which the contents of a dental anaesthetic cartridge were emptied will be rapidly perfused with a drug concentration far in excess of the toxic dose, albeit only transiently.

While the liver will readily conjugate and the kidney will eventually excrete all of the metabolized products of the inadvertent intravascular injection, we must not forget the rich vasculature of the head and neck, especially those vessels in close proximity to the IAN in the Pterygomandibular space will mean the risk of accidental intravascular injection and its rapid after-effects will always be present.

An accidental intravascular injection with an IANB is a common occurrence. One noted study reported the incidence at 11.7%[24] while a more recent study limited to oral and maxillofacial surgeons reported the incidence of their intravascular injections to be 15.3%[25].

Which, considering their excellent working knowledge of head and neck anatomy is a disturbing and an uncomfortably high rate.

The general dental practitioner's working knowledge of the neurovasculature of the Infratemporal fossa might be far less than their specialist colleagues and thus, they may have a far greater incidence of IANB associated intravascular injection. The proof of this hypothesis may come from an observation that only 3 out 5 dentists used an aspirating technique when administering an IANB, while all of the oral and maxillofacial surgeons (in the above noted study) did so[24 25].

Hence the figures given for the general dental practitioner's rate of IANB associated intravascular injection may actually be something of an underestimate.

Accidental injection into the vasculature may occur with all intra-oral injection techniques and not only the IANB. However any highly vascularised area, such as the pterygomandibular space presents an increased risk of the intravascular injection occurring with vascular damage, haemorrhage and haematoma formation.[26] Using an aspirating syringe, with a slow injection technique during the procedure, then aspirating in two different locations, while not eliminating the risk of an intravascular injection may certainly reduce it.

If a vein is involved, then bleeding will be minimal, post procedural discomfort and stiffness might be the only clinical signs being reported back to us. However, if an artery is involved or the needle transects one of the major arterial branches of those vessels in the Infratemporal fossa, the Pterygoid Spaces, the Pterygomaxillary Space, or if any of the branches of the Maxillary Artery (the larger of the two terminal branches of the External Carotid Artery) are involved, the complications can be all together more serious.

When administering an IAN-Block, we must remember, both the Maxillary Artery and several of its branches, including the Inferior Alveolar Artery pass perilously close to the Mandibular Foramen and the path of the IAN. Particularly, the proximal portion of the Maxillary Artery actually crosses mesial to the posterior border of the mandibular ramus before giving off an inferiorly directed arterial loop which forms the Inferior Alveolar Artery just above our intended target area for an IANB: the Mandibular Foramen.

As noted, it is not only the IANB which is prone to the accidental intravascular injection, the LA infiltration and block techniques in the maxilla have their risks too. Generally, infiltration anaesthesia directed at the maxilla is less problematic than the above noted mandibular blocks. While this may apply for infiltration anaesthesia, the maxillary block techniques, especially those directed towards the Posterior Superior Alveolar Nerve (PSAN) and Anterior Superior Alveolar Nerve (ASAN) will involve penetration of the LA needle to a considerable depth. In doing so, the base of the skull, the orbit and associated neurovasculature are all at risk from haematoma and haemorrhage, which may result in the patient experiencing post procedural pain and discomfort. More alarming however, for both patient and practitioner are visual disturbances and the risk of temporary blindness caused by minor arterial bleeding from an intravascular injection into a terminal branch of the Maxillary Artery[23,27].

It must be remembered that the Maxillary Artery is the larger of the two end branches of the External Carotid and the diameter of these terminal branches can be over 2.5mm, thus a considerable volume of blood under relatively high pressure will be flowing through these vessels. Consequently, the potential for serious bleeding is present with the accidental needle puncture of an artery[23].

> **Should pain, swelling, blindness or any visual disturbances be noted, the patient must be monitored and reviewed within 24 hours, then at 48 hours post-procedure and your clinical notes will fully document this incident, until full recovery and function is regained.**

There is also a risk of recurrent arterial bleeding. Although this is rare, specialist assistance should be sought and the patient must be referred to hospital for appropriate management including the possibility of surgical ligation of the torn blood vessel. Unfortunately, should such an eventuality occur, the misery for the practitioner and the patient will continue as there is also a risk of infection and appropriate antibiotic therapy must be started.

After all of that, there is the clinical inquiry to contend with, plus the very real chance of litigation being initiated and encouraged from the patient, their friends and family... it goes without saying, that all of this can be quite stressful for all concerned.

Occasionally, as noted above, temporary blindness, or blurring of vision could follow the PSANB or the IANB that was placed too high in relation to the Mandibular Foramen. In such a situation, the injection either approached the Inferior Orbital Fissure (IOF) at the height of the Posterior Maxilla or a significant amount of local anaesthetic was delivered under excessive pressure ie too rapidly into the tissues.

Remember: <u>Timing is essentially everything</u> and this has resulted in the anaesthetic solution, not so much passively diffusing through the tissues, but being actively forced through the IOF and into the orbit. This horror story ultimately involves the optic nerve and results in blindness, albeit temporary blindness, but any form of blindness is nonetheless extremely distressing for the patient. In the event of such a debacle, it might be prudent not to continue with the dental procedure and to reassure the patient that this unpleasant incident is short-lived and their vision will return to normal as the effects of a badly placed local anaesthetic will wear off within an hour or two.

In addition to blindness and bleeding, the superficial or peripheral branches of the Facial Nerve (CN VII) can also be compromised by a rapidly or forcefully injected local anaesthetic. The facial paralysis the patient experiences could extend to the eye. Once more this is transient. Remember the CN VII innervates the eyelids and eyebrows and the effects of a local anaesthetic on the lower motor neurones of the CN VII will cause the upper eyelid and eyebrow on the affected side to appear raised, ie a temporary paralysis will result in an inability to close the eye, furrow the brow or frown with the forehead muscles on the affected side. Essentially the clinical picture you will see is that of an iatrogenic and transient Bell's (like) Palsy. Such facial paralysis is brief in nature and although unpleasant, lasts no longer than the duration of the local anaesthetic; perhaps no more than two to three hours.

A comparison of the intravascular injection accident and Horner's Syndrome

This clinical presentation <u>must not</u> be confused with a Horner's Syndrome (like) presentation, the Horner's syndrome results from damage to the Sympathetic nerve chain and consists of:

I.   <u>Miosis</u> (a constricted pupil),
II. <u>Ptosis</u> (a weak, droopy eyelid)
III. <u>Anhidrosis</u> (decreased sweating)

The key difference with a local anaesthetic accident, you will see Mydriasis (a dilated pupil) and not Miosis. The explanation for this will be provided.

In addition to this clinical presentation, there are several reports documenting the effects of intravascular injection on the cranial nerves responsible for eye movement. Due to the risks involved and the disconcerting signs associated with these intravascular accidents, it is worth taking some time to explore and explain this phenomenon in some detail:

The Third Cranial Nerve or CN III, the Oculomotor Nerve, is responsible for controlling the majority of the muscles responsible for eye movement.

If CN III is affected by an intravascular accident, a temporary Oculomotor nerve palsy will result in the affected eye displaying a classic down and out position.

The affected eyeball will be displaced downward within the orbit and outward from the orbital midline.

I.   The eyeball will be displaced downward, because the Superior Oblique muscle that is innervated by the Fourth Cranial Nerve CN IV or Trochlear Nerve) will be un-opposed by the now paralyzed: Superior Rectus, Inferior Rectus and Inferior Oblique muscles.

II. The eyeball will be displaced outward because the Lateral Rectus muscle that is innervated by the Sixth Cranial Nerve CN VI or Abducens Nerve maintains muscle tone in comparison to the paralyzed medial rectus and its effect is unopposed.

III. The eye will also exhibit a marked ptosis, or drooping of the eyelid, as the Levator Palpebrae Superioris muscle responsible for raising the eyelid will be affected.

IV. Mydriasis or pupillary dilatation is also present because the parasympathetic nervous supply, causing papillary constriction, or miosis, is also carried with the CNIII. When this nerve is affected by a neuro-vascular injection accident: Mydriasis results because the sympathetic supply will be unopposed and therefore pupillary dilatation will be seen,(thus explaining the difference between a Local Anaesthetic Accident and Horner's Syndrome.)

V.   In addition, the intra-ocular ciliary muscles can also be affected with a CN III intravascular accident. The temporary loss of the eye's ability to maintain focus on objects from near to far, with short-term blurring of the patient's vision being indicative of this loss of accommodation[28].

The CN III has a complex branched structure and the intravascular injection of anaesthetic could impact on the nerve at different points along its path. Furthermore, the clinical presentation could be a result of the pharmacological effects of the local anaesthetic, or from physical compression on the nerve from a haematoma or haemorrhage. Consequently different groups of extra-ocular muscles could be affected or different muscles could affected individually, so the clinical presentation could be quite variable.

If an intravascular accident occurs or local anaesthetic diffuses towards the CNIII from surrounding tissues, the parasympathetic fibres running along the periphery of the CN III will be affected before the motor fibres located in the core of the nerve begin to suffer from the compressive forces exerted by a haematoma or haemorrhage. Accordingly, the classic blown pupil or ptosis will be seen before the eyeball looks characteristically down and out.

The Medical Third and The Surgical Third

With intra-vascular injection accidents, the cause is predominantly pharmacological in nature and this is essentially a non traumatic or pupil-sparing oculomotor temporary paralysis sometimes termed a **"medical third"**. In contrast, the much rarer extra-vascular sequalae from an intra-vascular injection accident resulting in haematoma and haemorrhage that involves the pupil are termed a **"surgical third"**.

Just as the CNIII can be involved, the CN IV (the Trochlear Nerve) responsible for innervating the Superior Oblique muscle and the CN VI (the Abducens Nerve) which innervates the Lateral Rectus muscle can be caught up by the impact of events following an intravascular injection[29]. It is entirely possible that these muscles can be included with, or spared from those muscles affected by CN III palsy, or they can suffer from palsy in isolation. Investigating the cause of this clinical problem will mean a revision of the anatomy you learned as an undergraduate and then adding some more details to complete the picture. The following short section should prove to be useful in this respect:

A local anaesthetic can be transported to the orbital region by passive tissue diffusion, venous absorption or arterial intravascular injection.

By one, some, or all of the above means, a misplaced dental local anaesthetic (LA) can pass through the Inferior Orbital Fissure to cause direct anaesthesia of the CN III, IV or VI.

Alternatively the misplaced LA could reach the Inferior Ophthalmic Vein via the Pterygoid Venous Plexus or by any of its communicating branches. Of crucial importance, this vein contains no valves and has a direct connection to the extra-ocular muscles via the Infraorbital Foramen. Any LA that is intravascularly injected into any of these veins could therefore, in the absence of valves, quite easily reverse the blood flow. The distal innervation of the extra-ocular muscles will then be susceptible when exposed to the effects of the LA.

Another possibility could be deposition of the LA within the Posterior Superior Alveolar Artery results in back-flow into the connecting Maxillary artery and from there into the Middle Meningeal Artery. There exists a constant anastomosis between the Orbital branch of the Middle Meningeal and the Recurrent Meningeal division of the Lacrimal branch of the Ophthalmic Artery. This Lacrimal branch supplies the Lateral Rectus Muscle, the Lacrimal gland, and the outer half of the eyelids[30].

If you've read all of the above and followed it; then good, if not then please go over this text again until you can see how such neurovascular arrangements provide an explanation for the symptoms that are seen on an improbably frequent basis with IANBs and maxillary infiltrations that are delivered incorrectly.

Local anaesthetic and the cavernous sinus

A further explanation can be provided if the LA directly reaches the CN III, CN IV and CN VI as they lie in the Cavernous Sinus. A misplaced LA can enter the Cavernous Sinus through the Infratemporal Fossa and the Pterygoid Plexus and the connecting Emissary Veins as they pass through the Foramen Ovale and Foramen Lacerum[31]. The

The Cavernous Sinuses are dura-mater lined spaces being: 1cm x 2cms^2, lying on each side of the Sella Turcica on the Sphenoid bone. The paired Cavernous Sinuses extend from the Superior Orbital Fissure anteriorly, to the apex of the Petrous aspect of the Temporal Bone posteriorly. In this area of the sinuses there is an additional Intercavernous Communicating Sinus. Each of the Cavernous Sinuses receives a rich blood supply from the Superior and Inferior Ophthalmic Veins, Superficial Middle Cerebral Veins and blood from the Sphenoparietal Sinus too. On the lateral wall of each Cavernous Sinus are the CN III CN IV, CN V$_2$ and CN V$_3$ (The Maxillary and Mandibular Divisions of the Trigeminal Nerves). Within and inside each Cavernous Sinus are the CN VI, the Internal Carotid Arteries and their Sympathetic Supply.

Having read and followed all of the above, it will now be clear, that the degree of havoc resulting from a misplaced dental local anaesthetic ending up intracranially among the neurovasculature in just one Cavernous Sinus, could be as challenging for the practitioner as it is distressing for the patient. The variable clinical pictures that are observed from vascular accidents involving dental local anaesthetic and the Cavernous Sinus may be explained in terms of the intimacy of the parasympathetic and sympathetic supplies associated with the CN III and Internal Carotid Arteries respectively[32].

Of all the ocular nerves, the CN VI, (the Abducent) is perhaps the most vulnerable to the effect of a vascular or a diffusion LA accident from anaesthetic being delivered into the Greater Palatine Canal and then into the Pterygo Palatine Fossa with diffusion into the Inferior Orbital Fissure soon following. From here it is only a short journey up to the apex of the orbit where the CN IV lies on the deep surface of the Lateral Rectus Muscle. This route is very nearly a straight line from the insertion of a needle for a PSAN Block to the Orbital Apex. The entire distance is perhaps only a couple of inches (5cms) at the very most.

The architecture of the Maxilla, Ethmoid, Sphenoid, Frontal and Temporal bones all play an important role in the untoward spread of a dental LA. The Inferior Orbital Fissure communicates with the Pterygopalatine Fossa. In the orbital region, the Greater Palatine Canal also communicates with the inferior aspect of Pterygopalatine Fossa.

With such open tracts between the bones of the skull, from the orbit to the mouth, it is easy to visualize the ease with which an anaesthetic solution may diffuse through the tissues and along the bundles of neurovasculature in these cavities.

The natural variation in dento-facial profiles may in fact provide some individuals with either a natural susceptibility or a natural resilience to the spread of a dental LA within this skeletal architecture. Adding to this, it has been suggested that the recumbent position of the patient during administration of a dental LA may also play a role[33].

What is more likely, opening the patient's jaw, creates tension in their muscles of mastication in anticipation of the pain of an injection. This tension might result in the Lateral Pterygoids and Temporalis muscles actually protecting or shielding any hiatus that is present within the bone structures. Whichever proposition is correct, a dental anaesthetic, if badly placed or rapidly introduced will soon make its way into the orbit and intracranial sinuses with the consequences as noted above. From the above you will understand why the potential for disaster is ever present and should not be underestimated when administering your local anaesthetic. A literature search will reveal many case reports of LA accidents but overall, if we consider that many millions of dental local anaesthetic injections are given every year, the number of reported complications is actually very small. However, there is one paper that has reported a case of <u>permanent blindness</u> in one eye as a result of a fluid embolus of an amide local anaesthetic injected into the ophthalmic artery[34].

The badly placed needle and the misplaced local anaesthetic

If a local anaesthetic is rushed or badly placed, our obligatory monitoring of the patient could reveal the following clinical signs and symptoms:

I. Blanching of the skin in CN V $_1$ (Ophthalmic Division) and CN V$_2$ (Maxillary Division).
II. Ocular Complications: Loss of muscle control, Palpebral Ptosis and the Down and Out Orbit.
III. Ophthalmic Complications: Mydriasis, Presbyopia, Blurred Vision, Diplopia or Loss of Vision.
IV. Peri-Oral tingling, Circumoral Pallor.
V. Agitation, Drowsiness and possibly: Loss of Consciousness.

Should any of these clinical signs and symptoms be seen the following safety measures must begin:

I.   The symptoms of diplopia and blurred vision must be documented in the clinical notes, together with the type and dose of LA used.
II. The affected eye is examined for signs of muscular paralysis and pupillary involvement.
III. The patient must be reassured that their symptoms are temporary, with the affected eye being protected.
IV. The patient should be escorted home, not allowed to drive and recalled for review.
V.   If the ocular or ophthalmic complications last longer than six hours then referral to a hospital for a specialist assessment will then be required.

There are certain measures the safety critical clinician should observe so the risk of harm from the ocular and ophthalmic complications noted above are reduced to an acceptable level if not entirely removed:

I.   Inadvertent injections directed towards neurovascular tissues must be avoided.
II. The risk of the vascular accident can be controlled by aspirating before administering any injection of local anaesthetic.
III. When the injection begins it should be with a slow and steady rate of delivery.

IV. **Ideally it should take some 60 seconds in which to aspirate then inject the local anaesthetic.**

V. **The slow steady injection technique is undoubtedly far less painful than the firm but perhaps forceful, rapid and ultimately dangerous injection technique.**

Updating and revising your knowledge of the surgical anatomy with respect to the particular nerve territories and tracts to be anaesthetised is the best means of preventing the complications noted above. At the same time, following the conventional techniques of drug administration and adhering to those injection techniques established from principles of clinical safety is the surest way to avoid problems for the patient and trouble for yourself.

Timing and technique

As noted before, timing is essentially everything, not only for the onset and action of a drug, but in delivery of the drug too. Injecting with a slow rate and a low pressure will undoubtedly reduce the pain, the discomfort and the anxiety experienced by your patient[35].

The issue of needle phobia and its consequences has been discussed and we should not forget that many of our patients, perhaps all of them and maybe ourselves too, have been conditioned from a very early age to anticipate and to invariably expect or even experience pain when being injected. After all, our childhood immunizations might not have been placed anywhere as sensitive as the mouth, but they didn't contain much if any local anaesthetic either.

A significant reminder of this problem came from a study reporting that dentists could not adequately assess the pain and distress experienced by the patient they were injecting. The results of the dentists were compared to those assessments made by an independent observer[36]. Such a finding may be suggestive of a form of professional conditioning, or alternatively it may be an indication of compassion fatigue, which is symptomatic of emotional and professional burn-out[37].

One technique to reduce the pain of an injection is to reduce the rate at which an anaesthetic is given. The injection that is given slowly over 1 to 2 minutes is far more comfortable than the one given in a matter of 10 to 20 seconds. Not only is this common-sense and accepted wisdom, but the evidence from a double-blind randomized controlled trial indicates the slower injection is also more effective in producing a greater anaesthetic effect[38]. To reduce the pain and discomfort further, the injection can be delivered in two stages, the first might deliver 1/5th of the cartridge and after a few seconds, the remainder of the cartridge (or whatever amount is required) is given very... ...

---->>>> *S l l o o o w w w l l y y* ---->>>>

Considering all of the above there are five distinct stages to injecting a dental local anaesthetic:

I. **Place** the needle into the intra oral mucosa.
II. **Advance** the needle from penetration towards the intended target tissues.
III. **Deliver** the correct anaesthetic in the correct amount in the correct time period.
IV. **Assess** the patient for any adverse reactions to the Local Anaesthetic that has been given.
V. **Wait** until Local Anaesthesia develops to the level required <u>before</u> dental treatment.

Of the five stages the last two are safety critical, while the first three are technique sensitive.

It is the second stage, advancing the needle which has been reported to be the most painful for the patient.

This shouldn't be surprising, as the third stage releases anaesthetic and the discomfort of the first stage could be masked by the use of topical anaesthetic gel.

While we are at this point (that wasn't a pun) the notion that heating up the anaesthetic cartridges or getting your nurse to roll them around between her (gloved) hands somehow reduces the pain of injection is either a good thing or a complete waste of time, depending on who you work with/for or the research findings you wish to accept and adopt.

In the interests of evidence based and safety critical dental practice a mini-literature search on the subject was undertaken:

Three studies claimed that warming does little if anything to minimize patient discomfort:

I.   Martin S, Jones and Wynn BS. Does warming local anaesthetic reduce the pain of subcutaneous injection? Am. Jnl of Emerg. Med. 1996; 14: 10-12

II. Colaric KB, Overton DT and Moore K. Pain reduction in lidocaine administration through buffering and warming. Am. Jnl of Emerg Med. 1998; 16: 353-356.

III. Ram D, Hermida L B, Peretz B. A comparison of warmed and room-temperature anaesthetic for local anesthesia in children. Pediatr Dent 2002; 24:333-6.

(NB: none of these studies were dental).

Then three studies claiming the opposite were investigated:

I.   Fialkov JA and McDougall EP Warmed local anaesthetic reduces pain of infiltration. Ann. Plast. Surg. 1996; 36: 11-13.

II. Bell RW, Butt ZA and Gardner RF. Warming lignocaine reduces the pain of injection during local anaesthetic eyelid surgery. Eye (London) 1996; 10: 558-560.

III. Sultan J. Towards evidence based emergency medicine: Best BETs from Manchester Royal Infirmary. Effect of warming local anaesthetics on pain of infiltration. Emerg. Med. Jnl 2007; 24: 723-725.
     Sultan J. Towards evidence based emergency medicine: Best BETs from Manchester Royal Infirmary. The effect of warming local anaesthetics on pain of infiltration. Emerg Med Jnl. 2007; 24: 791-793.

(Again none of these studies were dental).

However the third pair of studies in the second group reviewed 720 papers on the subject, of which 11 offered the best clinical evidence to answer the question, concluding that: Overall the evidence suggests that warming local anaesthetics, either alone or in combination with buffering, significantly reduces pain of local infiltration[39][40].

Just in case you are ready to accept the above verdict, there are further studies available, one study was revealing, reporting patients could not detect the difference between room temperature and body temperature[41.] That difference, in case you were unsure, is some 15⁰C to 20⁰C, depending on whether you work in an NHS clinic with broken windows and no heating (yes I have too) or treated patients that are reptiles (no I haven't either).

Lastly, there is a study claiming, that by the time the contents of the cartridge is injected, remember it is done ---->>>> S l l o o o w w w l l y y ---->>>> the anaesthetic solution will be back to room temperature anyway[42].

Personally... ..., now that we are all wondering about this... ... the fewer stages involved in getting the LA out of the cupboard and into the patient, will mean the entire procedure will be both simpler and thus safer. Heating up drugs that are normally kept in cool dry storage, will mean the contraction of cooling and expansion of heating may lead to the seal between the rubber in the stopper and the glass walls of the cartridge being compromised, encouraging the further growth then spread of microbial species. If a heated cartridge is not used today, will it be warmed up and the contents served to another patient tomorrow?

Although the evidence is strongly suggestive of heating being beneficial, until there is a safety marker present to differentiate those cartridges which have been heated from those which haven't and therefore cannot be re-heated, it may be better to serve our anaesthetics cold, but that is just my view, both yourself and our patients may feel differently.

OK, so back to timing once more, after the first four stages have been completed and there are no adverse physiological, pharmacological or pathological effects from your delicately, accurately and:

---->>>> S l l o o o w w w l l y y ---->>>> placed local anaesthetic we will be waiting for anaesthesia to take effect.

How long do we need to wait?

Although there could be anatomical, physiological and some pathological factors contributing to variations in the time until sufficient pulpal anaesthesia is achieved and for how long it lasts, the following five factors are the perhaps most important:

I.   The type of anaesthetic, whether an amide or an ester.
II. The dose of anaesthetic, broadly whether 0.6ml, 0.9 ml or 1.2ml 43.
III. The distance from the site of injection to the tooth to be numbed.
IV. Whether the injection was an infiltration or a block.
V.   Whether the injection was maxillary or mandibular.

For maxillary injections, the published data suggests waiting for 2 to 5 minutes, before starting treatment (a reference infiltration of 1.8 ml of 2% lignocaine, with 1/100,000 adrenaline was used)[44][45]. Although maxillary infiltration injections are clinically more successful than those in the mandible, the problem lies with the duration of anaesthesia that can be maintained for the upper teeth.

While the shortened duration, when compared to mandibular injections, is not a failure as such, it does mean the patient undergoing a lengthy procedure may experience discomfort, then pain towards the closing stages of their appointment. If your work extends beyond the time for which anaesthesia can be maintained, for patient comfort and safety, consider giving another local anaesthetic at half time if you regularly undertake one hour appointments.

Adding to this, it is important to note the duration of pulpal anaesthesia in the anterior maxillary teeth declines at around 30 to 35 minutes, whereas the upper molars can keep going for up to 45 to 50 minutes[46].

Duration of local anaesthetic

The following table provides useful data on the duration of anaesthesia for maxillary infiltrations:

Local Anaesthetic Used	Upper Anteriors	Upper Molars
2% Lignocaine with 1/80,000 Adrenaline	30 to 35 minutes	45 to 50 minutes
3% Mepivicaine (no vasoconstrictor)	10 to 15 minutes	10 to 15 minutes
3% Prilocaine with Felypressin	30 to 35 minutes	45 to 50 minutes
4% Articaine with 1/100,000 Adrenaline	30 to 35 minutes	45 to 50 minutes

Note: i The differences in anaesthetic duration between the posterior and anterior teeth.

ii Without a vasoconstrictor the duration of pulpal anaesthesia ia ¼ to 1/3rd of that with vasoconstriction!

Having briefly considered maxillary infiltration (there are other techniques for maxillary anaesthesia which we will shortly consider), we should now turn our attention to mandibular anaesthesia.

When there is failure to achieve anaesthesia it is most often with the IANB (Inferior Alveolar Nerve Block). There are several studies that have investigated the success rate of the IANB and the results at the first attempt, range from 51% in the first molar down to 10% in the first incisor[47]. In these studies, it is of considerable interest, that in all cases, despite anaesthetic failure, the patient reported profound numbness in the lower lip, but there was a curious absence of anaesthesia for the teeth requiring treatment.

The failure to achieve anaesthesia at the first attempt will require a second or a third injection, possibly the use of an alternative local anaesthetic, or a change in technique or approach to the delivery of the

LA, perhaps the use of a different block to an alternative nerve supply could be considered.

Your safety net when faced with anaesthetic failure will rely on a text-book, or on your text-book working knowledge of the anatomy of the head and neck, knowing where and how to deliver a subsequent local anaesthetic to turn failure into success. Despite all of that, the first failure often heralds a subsequent failure and failure rates of 23% in the first molar to 58% in the incisors have been noted, even though, once more the patient reports profound numbing of the lower lip[48].

With an IANB, the onset of pulpal anaesthesia is observed from 5 to 19 minutes[49]. Numbness of the lips frequently occurs before LA begins to affect the tissues of the pulp, with the symptoms of lip tingling and deadness being reported at 4.5 to 6 minutes following injection[49,50]. With almost all patients, the anterior teeth become numb after the posterior teeth and 8% of dental patients will be slow responders to an accurately placed IANB with anaesthesia beginning to develop after 15 minutes[50].

In all cases, for maxillary and mandibular teeth, for IANBs and for infiltrations, the efficacy of anaesthesia can be determined by electric pulp testing or the use of ethyl chloride or other refrigerant on the tooth to determine whether the level of anaesthesia achieved is sufficient to begin your intended dental procedure. It would be inadvisable to begin our dentistry without doing so.

Just before we consider the duration of anaesthesia you might expect from an IANB with the most commonly used local anaesthetics, there is another clinical phenomenon you may have observed and that is discontinuous or intermittent anaesthesia. With such an event, the patient may initially demonstrate numbness of the lower lip and tooth (with ethyl chloride as noted above), then a period of anaesthetic loss is noted, before the anaesthesia resumes again and so on. One explanation for this might be as follows:

With an accurate delivery of an IANB, anaesthetic diffuses into the nerve which is a complex array of bundled neuronal fibres with varying properties. You will remember these from your undergraduate physiology days being the: β, Aδ and C-fibres with quite different conduction velocities and potentials. We know that stimulation of these nerve fibres will generally result in pulpal vasodilation, together with some pulpal vasoconstriction from the un-mylinated C fibres involved in axon-reflexes of post-ganglionic sympathetic neurones[51][52]. The blocking and unblocking of the sodium channels by a local anaesthetic acting on neural membranes will be asynchronous. If sufficient sodium channels become unblocked, anaesthesia will lapse. Then with further sodium channel blocking, local anaesthesia will resume once more and so on.

In contrast to maxillary infiltration anaesthesia, once IANB anaesthesia is achieved, the duration is quite considerable with anaesthesia persisting for some 2.5 hours[53]. (As with maxillary anaesthesia a reference infiltration of 1.8 ml of 2% lignocaine, with 1/100,000 adrenaline was used.)

The following table provides useful data on the duration of anaesthesia for the IANB:

Local Anaesthetic Used	Pulpal Anaesthesia	Soft tissue Anaesthesia
2% Lignocaine with 1/80,000 Adrenaline	Up to 2 ½ Hours	Over 3 Hours
3% Mepivicaine (no vasoconstrictor)	At least 50 minutes	Over 3 Hours
3% Prilocaine with Felypressin	At least 1 Hour	No Study Data Available
4% Articaine with 1/100,000 Adrenaline	At least 1 Hour	No Study Data Available

Note: i The differences in anaesthetic duration between the pulp and soft tissue.

ii Without a vasoconstrictor, the duration of pulpal anaesthesia is far less than when a vasoconstrictor is used.

However, given the technique being reported is a block rather than an infiltration, then soft tissue anaesthesia often remains unchanged, possibly due to a supply from accessory innervations[53][54]. Having considered what can go wrong when administering a local anaesthetic and what to expect after giving a local anaesthetic, we should now turn our attention to what local anaesthetic we might give and for which patients. In the UK and the EU the most common dental local anaesthetics are:

> I. Lignocaine
> II. Prilocaine
> III. Articaine
> IV. Bupivicaine
> V. Mepivicaine

Pharmacology and Biochemistry of Local Anaesthetics

Before we consider our dental local anaesthetics in detail, some revision of the pharmacology and biochemistry will help our understanding of the mode of action of these drugs. Before doing so, a review of physiology is needed. I am sorry if all this is getting on your nerves, but after all neuro-phsiology is a stimulating subject (or a subject that deals with stimulation)!

In the resting state, Sodium ions (Na^+) are prevented from entering into nerve cells as the ion channels are closed. When a neuron is stimulated, the ionophores or sodium channels open and there is an influx of Na^+ into the cell and depolarization results.

Immediately after this depolarization event, further Na^+ influx cannot occur as the ionophores become inactive while an active ion pumping mechanism returns the Na^+ to the extracellular environment once more. After the membrane becomes repolarized, the ionophores are open for business once more.

Local anaesthetics have an affinity for binding to receptor sites around Na^+ channels. However, this affinity becomes heightened when the receptor is either in a state of activity or a state of inactivity, *i.e:* local anaesthetic binding is greater with functioning ion channels.

From this information, we will be aware that those nerve fibres with rapid firing rates are therefore more predisposed to the effect of a dental local anaesthetic than those nerve fibres with slower firing rates.

In addition to this, the smaller nerve fibres are more susceptible to dental local anaesthetic than larger fibres. A dental local anaesthetic will more easily block the number of sodium channels required for the conduction of a nerve impulse in a smaller, rather than a larger fibre, simply due to the permeation being easier in smaller rather than larger fibres.

If we stop to consider the properties of these nerves, then the small but numerous rapidly firing autonomic fibres, innervating the dental pulp will be the most sensitive, followed by the sensory fibres and finally the larger somatic motor fibres will be the last to yield to the effects of a dental local anaesthetic.

In the Maxillary and Mandibular divisions of the Trigeminal Nerve (CN V_2 and CN V_3) the branches to be anaesthetized are made up of small, rapidly firing sensory fibres. However, these sensory fibres vary in their diameters, conduction potentials, velocities and firing rates. Pain fibres are more sensitive than pressure and proprioceptive fibres[55][56]. Therefore your dental patient will feel pressure but not pain, while you poke, prod and probe away at their pulpal and periodontal problems.

Having considered the physiology, we can now move onto consider the pharmacology. All dental local anaesthetics are made up of three parts:

I.   A terminal amine that can be Tertiary (lipid soluble) or Quaternary (water soluble).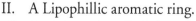
II. A Lipophillic aromatic ring.
III. An intermediate link that can be either an Amide or an Ester.

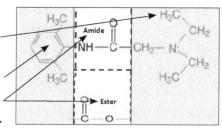

These three components contribute to the pharmacological activity of the local anaesthetic as follows: The lipophillic aromatic ring together with the tertiary amine determines the lipid solubility and therefore the ability of the LA to diffuse through the neural sheaths and membranes into the nerve cells. The more lipid soluble, the more rapid the onset and the lower the concentration of the LA needs to be for the desired effect per dose delivered, but only up to a point.

If only things were this simple, other anatomical and vascular factors might result in the LA having a greater dispersal away from the target tissue. The more lipid soluble an LA, the less likely it is to pass through tissue fluids. Actually, with a highly lipid soluble LA, a greater affinity for adipose tissue rather than neural tissue might be seen.

At this stage, this is where the terminal amine becomes useful. The tertiary form has 3 bonds and is lipid soluble, whereas the quaternary form has 4 bonds and is positively charged and water soluble.

While you have been closely inspecting your local anaesthetic cartridge batch numbers for the CQC, (we don't need to do that anymore), but we do need to make sure they are in date, not contaminated and you are giving the right drug, in the right amount, to the right patient, in the right part of their mouth... you will have read that local anaesthetics are formulated as hydrochloride salts.

This means the LA is packaged in its cartridge as a quaternary water-soluble molecule. As such, in this state, the LA can pass through the patient's mucosa into their tissues as an infiltration or a block and having read the foregoing sections, you will now, as before; be delivering your dental local anaesthetics at a slow rate with a high degree of accuracy.

However, in the quaternary terminal amine form, the LA will be unable to penetrate the neuron. Not to worry, a proportion of the terminal amine, immediately upon injection into your patient's tissues will be exposed to a tissue pH of 7.4 becoming ionized from the quaternary form to the tertiary form.

The time for the onset of local anaesthesia is directly related to the conversion rate from the quaternary to the tertiary form and there will always be a proportion of the LA doing this per unit of time. This is measured as the ionization constant or p Ka of the LA and you will clearly and vividly remember this from your undergraduate physiology lectures.

If you haven't fallen asleep by now, the Henderson-Hasselbach formula when applied by a pharmacology lecturer to the conscious brain of a dental student has the same effect as a local anaesthetic when applied by a dentist to the nerves of a patient. Both are capable of sending their intended target into a state of temporary oblivion:

$$\log (\text{cationic form/uncharged form}) = pKa - pH$$

The most important piece of this equation is the difference in pH between LA and tissue. If the LA has a pH equivalent to the tissue into which it is injected, then only ½ of the LA will penetrate the neural membranes as ½ are quaternary cationic and ½ are tertiary uncharged.

All dental LAs have a pH greater than 7.4 and so more will be water soluble rather than being lipid soluble.

When we inject into inflamed tissues (never a good idea with a patient being in a state of allodynia due to the increased sensitization to pain and the risk of spreading infective micro-organisms along the track of the needle) the acidity associated with inflammation lowers the tissue pH below 7.4, thus the quaternary, water-soluble configuration of LA will be the preferred state.

This has been suggested as a reason for the loss of anaesthetic efficacy observed when dealing with inflamed or infected tissues[55,56]. With such clinical presentations using an LA with lower pKa such as mepivicaine @ 7.6 is theoretically better than using bupivicaine @ 8.1.

The higher the pKa the lower the lipid solubility.

Once the LA enters the neuron, the tertiary amine re-ionizes to the quaternary form, which then binds to receptors and blocks the sodium channel. The following diagram explains the processes involved:

Local anaesthetics; their mechanism of action

There is a balance of the Quaternary hydrochloride salt (BH$^+$) and a lipid soluble base Tertiary amine (B).

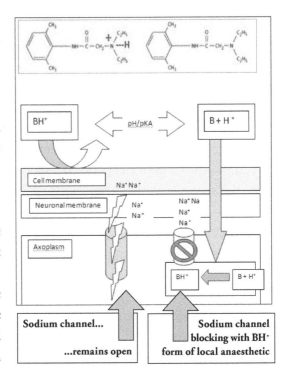

The tissue pKA determines their relative amounts. Equilibrium between (BH$^+$) and (B) is determined by the pH of the tissues and the pKa of the anaesthetic (pH/pKa).

To penetrate the nerve sheaths and nerve cell membrane, the local anaesthetic has to be in the (B) state.

Once the molecule reaches the neuron, the tertiary amine gains an H$^+$ becoming the Quaternary (BH$^+$) form that can now block the Na$^+$ channel[57].

Having looked at the two ends of the local anaesthetic, we should now apply some biochemistry to look at the bit in the middle. The intermediate link can be either an amide or an ester and gives us a useful handle with which we can classify our dental local anaesthetics as follows:

I. **Amides** are transformed and metabolised by the patient's hepatic enzymes... ... whereas

II. **Esters** are hydrolysed by plasma esterases (no real surprise there) which are present in the blood stream.

Esters are now only found in topical anaesthetics such as benzocaine. However if you look in your practice principle's lower drawer (usually beneath the old and dusty scratched-up surgical loupes) is an amide anaesthetic, that also contains an ester in a side branch that is hydrolysed. This local anaesthetic is articaine, although articaine is an amide, it begins its journey of metabolism then elimination in the same way an ester does.

Moving on from your practice principle's secret stockpile of anaesthetics, returning to biochemistry and pharmacology once more, in common with most drugs, local anaesthetics also reversibly bind to plasma proteins in the blood stream. The duration of their action can be determined by such protein binding potentials. In the previous section on drug safety we have already considered protein binding within the context of a drug's therapeutic index. Bear in mind, that property is expressed as the percentage of a circulating drug that is protein bound; it will therefore come as no surprise to you that for local anaesthetics, this figure closely correlates with a local anaesthetic's binding affinity for those receptors associated with membrane Na^+ channels too.

Highly protein bound anaesthetics will show a longer duration of action.

I.   Whereas mepivicaine has 55% protein binding and can provide some 15 to 30 minutes of anaesthesia from a maxillary infiltration and 50 minutes of pulpal anaesthesia from an IANB.

II. Lignocaine with up to 80% plasma protein binding[58], provides some 45 to 55 minutes of anaesthesia from a maxillary infiltration and up to 3 hours of pulpal anaesthesia from an IANB.

In addition to plasma and receptor protein binding, if an anaesthetic is molecularly bound both to and within adipose tissues of the nerve sheath and fascial tissues around the nerve, there could well be a delayed, continual and slow release from an anaesthetic bolus deposited in close proximity to the foramina of the IAN and Mental nerves in the mandible or the PSA or ASA nerves in the maxilla.

Adding to such anatomical factors, are pharmacological ones. Vasoconstriction of the adjacent and attendant blood vessels is an important factor we need to consider when administering local anaesthetics. Whereas a local anaesthetic such as pure lidocaine will initiate vasodilation by the blockade of nerve fibres (NB both mepivicaine and bupivicaine do not exhibit such properties), the addition of epinephrine to lidocaine or a vasopressin analog such as octapressin to prilocaine will initiate a counter vasoconstriction with the effect of prolonging the local anaesthetic effect.

Taking the issue of therapeutic index one stage further into the domain of clinical safety (the motivation for and the main reason you are reading this book), we might state that the toxicity of local anaesthetics is purely a dose related affair, simply determined by the number of cartridges of LA we should give to a patient. However, once more, things are not that simple (if only they were).

In recent years, the very essence of drug safety with dental local anaesthetics was missed, being completely overlooked, while the various UK dental regulators were mindlessly meddling and mandating the necessity to check and document the batch numbers of anaesthetics in the patient notes (a fallacy spawned from non-clinical bureaucratic imprudence).

While the systemic toxicity of most drugs is dose related, understanding the stated doses of local anaesthetics is a slightly more complex matter.

The dental cartridge contains a defined volume of a local anaesthetic, often in amounts such as 1.7ml, 1.8 ml or 2.2 ml but with variable doses expressed oftentimes in concentrations of micrograms, milligrams or sometimes as a percentage (of the total but totally variable volume). With all of that and a regulatory focus on supervising the administration of the drug in the clinic, but not supervising the delivery of the drug to the patient, a degree of recklessness with regard to doses may have slowly crept into our use of dental local anaesthetics. Adding yet more concern to the safety critical nature of local anaesthetics, the cartridges we use frequently contain two active drugs, one is a vasoconstrictor and the other is the local anaesthetic itself and both will have differing doses, concentrations and effects on our patient.

Putting all this together, we might find ourselves simply documenting in the patient notes: The total volume of the LA given; but this is only expressed in terms of cartridge numbers. Whereas the actual doses of the active drugs the patient has received are never revealed, as they were never entered in the notes to begin with. In our efforts to complete the patient records, if we do write drug doses (from the labels on the cartridges), these are often just those figures that have been committed to memory, while this practice may satisfy a cursory audit from our regulators, it is neither good practice nor is it safe practice.

From a safety perspective it is better to over-estimate the doses of local anaesthetics and their vasoconstrictors. We might begin by assuming all cartridges are 2ml (rather than the 1.8 or the 1.7 ml we frequently have to hand). Following from this, we might then use the gradations on the cartridge to note how much of a cartridge has been given. By using these measures, we will be closer to recording the volume of LA we have injected and the volumes can be more readily converted to indicate the doses of each component of the LA in milligrams or micrograms.

In the beginning of this chapter we briefly looked at drug volumes, dilutions and concentrations. Revisiting them briefly, your confidence in their use and the ease with which you can convert the following units, must form the basis of your safe working practice with all dental local anaesthetics:

I. The Concentration of Local Anaesthetic eg: Lidocaine in a Cartridge is noted:

II. Percentage concentrations can also be expressed as milligrams/millilitre

III. 1.0% is equivalent to 10mg/mL

IV. 0.5% is equivalent to 5 mg/mL and so on.

V. eg: 2.0% Lidocaine hydrochloride is equivalent to 20mgs/mL

> I.   The Concentration of Vasoconstrictor eg: Adrenaline in a Cartridge is noted:
> II. Ratio concentrations can also be expressed as milligrams/millilitre.
> III. 1/100,000 is equivalent to 10μg/mL
> IV. 1/50,000 is equivalent to 20μg/mL
> V.   The more common concentration of adrenaline is 1/80,000, being equivalent to 12.5μg/mL

By strictly limiting the total volume and thus the overall dose of local anaesthetic we give to a patient, the risk of toxicity from systemic absorption from the injection site is significantly reduced if not entirely eliminated.

The neural blockade by local anaesthetics such as lidocaine also extends to their ability to depress the CNS too. While the clinical signs of toxicity might be seen with systemic serum concentrations of c. 5μg/mL, critical toxicity only occurs with doses greater than 10μg/mL. CNS depression and respiratory collapse are seen with loss of consciousness, convulsions, coma and cardiac arrest. For these reasons when using dental local anaesthetics, we must remain vigilant to their effects on the CNS, especially in our patients who are taking drugs with inherent CNS depressant effects, such as opioids (whether prescribed or acquired by other means).

Taking such safety issues further, if we accept that a local anaesthetic has both CNS and respiratory depressant effects, then patients with compromised respiratory and cardiac functions will demand even greater vigilance as the systemic serum concentrations of LA required to elicit toxicity will be far lower than those figures given above.

If we are treating a child with compromised respiratory and cardiac capacity, their margins of physiological safety will be even lower, the risks present will be even greater and so the doses and types of local anaesthetic we are able to use will be even less.

As mentioned before, a local anaesthetic will display an affinity for receptor proteins located with those Na^+ channels which are active, in preference to those Na⁺ channels which are less active or inactive. However, bupivicaine has a broader non-selective affinity and dissociates more slowly from the inactive or resting Na⁺ channel receptor protein sites.

Thus, bupivicaine blockade lasts longer and the risk of systemic (especially cardiac) toxicity is greater. Where bupivicaine is used in far greater doses in medical procedures, cardiac arrhythmias have been noted. Thankfully in dentistry, with bupivicaine doses being several orders of magnitude less, such problems have not been observed. However the risk is present and could be raised, should a patient be cardiovascularly compromised or be at risk from an acquired or congenital cardiac conduction defect.

Dispersal of LA into the systemic circulation occurs and as noted previously, this can be from an accidental injection into a blood vessel, or by diffusion after passing through the highly vascularised soft tissues in the mouth, the head and the neck.

The safety critical factors associated with systemic spread of LA are the rate (speed) of injection, the dose or concentration (mg) of injection rather than the volume (mL) of injection.

> **When using lidocaine or any LA, regardless of their formulated concentration:**
>
> **The dosage (mg) administered and not the volume (mL or cartridges) must be considered** [59].

The use of a vasoconstrictor significantly reduces both the rate and amount of systemic spread. In any event, by adhering to the maximum recommended dosages for any local anaesthetic, the risk of an LA injection approaching toxic serum levels will be avoided.

Safety first: PPP and protective procedures

When treating children it is important to follow a **Precautionary Paediatric Protocol** (PPP), expressing the maximum dose of LA per child's body weight as the mg/Kg maximum dose of local anaesthetic to be used.

However, this calculation doesn't really apply for adults and their maximum dose of LA, in mgs, should only be used as a guideline, a limit that is rarely, if ever approached but never crossed. Given the problems with obesity and the epidemic of wobblingly oversized children being transported to dental clinics by their even wobblier and larger parents, the mg/Kg calculations may result in a permissible LA dose for children exceeding that for adults.

With such cases, a common -(safety)- sense approach dictates review, then reduction in the total permissible dose of LA to a much lower and far safer level.

The matter of parent drug metabolism and end-products accumulating to toxic levels in other tissues and organ systems, rather than through appropriate metabolism and effective excretion in the liver and kidneys, has already been considered in the previous sections.

Returning once more to this aspect of drug safety, we might look at the most commonly used dental local anaesthetic: Lidocaine hydrochloride (2%) and adrenaline in a concentration of 1/80,000 in our standardized 2ml cartridge.

We know that the neurological effect of adrenaline ends with its re-uptake into the post synaptic nerve terminals and the pharmacological effects end with metabolism in the liver by Mono-amine-oxidase A (MOA A) and Catechol-O-Methyltransferase (COMT):

Adrenaline$\rightarrow$ (MOA) $\rightarrow$ 3,4 dihydroxymandelic acid (DOMA) $\rightarrow$(COMT)$\rightarrow$ vanillyl mandelic acid (VMA)$\rightarrow$ excreted in urine.

Nearly all lidocaine is metabolically dealkylated in the liver by CYP 3A4 to mono-ethyl-glycine Xylidide (MEG- X), which has a longer half life than lidocaine but is a less effective Na^+ channel blocker, then it is metabolized to $\rightarrow$ glycine xylidide $\rightarrow$ 4-hydroxy-2,6-dimethylaniline$\rightarrow$ then excreted in urine.

While this metabolic pathway takes care of 90% of lidocaine, some 10% will be excreted unchanged in urine. The clinical effects of lidocaine are seen after 1 minute, lasting up to 30 minutes and this will be prolonged with the addition of adrenaline in the LA. Lidocaine displays a biphasic half life lasting up to 2 hours. In those who are cardiovascularly challenged, this is prolonged only slightly, whereas in those with liver pathology the half life can last over 3 hours and possibly up to 4 hours[60].

All of this is fairly straightforward simple pharmacology and so it should be, as lignocaine (lidocaine) with epinephrine really is a safe drug, as long as we stick to the maximum doses and keep it away from those patients who have:

I.   Cardiac Conduction Defects. (From partial to complete blocks and syndromes too).
II. Pacemakers.
III. Any cardiovascular condition, especially if anti-arrythmic drugs are needed.
IV. Impaired liver function.
V.   Diabetes (although, with dental doses, this is complex and theoretical only).

It is easy to see why the first four conditions would restrict the use of lidocaine, due to epinephrine increasing the force, rate and risk of arrhythmia in a healthy heart.

On the other hand, with a heart that is both physiologically and functionally compromised to begin with, or even a healthy transplanted heart either with or without a pacemaker, the effects of epinephrine would be at best unpredictable or at worst harmful[61,62].

With the last of these conditions: diabetes, while an increase in plasma glucose levels is theoretically possible, determining the physiological effects of epinephrine present in pharmacological doses in dental local anaesthetics is not so straightforward:

I.   Adrenaline may inhibit the release of insulin, with glycogenolysis and gluconeogenesis following from this[63].

II. As this effect is not insulin controlled, whether the patient is diabetic or not, should make no difference to the increase in plasma glucose that is seen after LA containing epinephrine is used.

III. If the diabetes is well controlled then the rise in blood glucose and its impact will be (if anything) a subclinical, an interesting and a theoretical consideration only.

IV. However, if the diabetes is not well controlled then we (or rather the patient and the dental team) may well have a problem.

V.   For all diabetic patients, whether well-controlled or poorly-controlled, by adopting a safety critical approach: Updating the medical history, including blood glucose tests whenever LA will be used, even for patients with previously elevated glucose levels, the additive impact of epinephrine, will be unlikely to influence either the patient or our management of the patient.

When treating our patients with any of the above problems, using an alternative local anaesthetic becomes somewhat less optional and rather more sensible.

Prilocaine hydrochloride (3% or 30mg/mL), in common with lidocaine is an amino-amide local anaesthetic, however in place of adrenaline, octapressin (felypressin 0.03IU/mL) is the non-catecholamine vasoconstrictor, which has little if any noted cardiogenic effects in low doses.

Although in greater doses than those in dental local anaesthetics, vasoconstriction in coronary blood vessels could result[64]. In addition to this potential problem, when using prilocaine, you will already be familiar with the following restrictions for patients who are or who are/ or who have:

> I.   **Impaired renal and hepatic functions**
> II. **Difficulty breathing or an allergy to:**
>   i.   **Foods**
>   ii. **Drugs or Medicines**
>   iii. **Dental Local Anaesthetics!!**
> III. **Blood Disorders.**
> IV. **Pregnancy**
> V.   **Breast Feeding**

The contra-indication and restriction of drugs with the first two conditions are straightforward matters. The next three conditions are more complex and involve the three factors of:

(i)   Drug interaction.
(ii) Drug Excretion and
(iii) Drug Metabolism

These will occur not only for the patient, but for the unborn child and infant and arise not only with prilocaine but for (m)any drugs.

Octapressin is an analog of vasopressin, being molecularly similar to oxytocin, it can induce both uterine contraction and water retention.

With breast feeding, there is a risk that the newborn may ingest octapressin, resulting in water retention. The noted risk of blood disorders not only affect the adult patient, but the neonate; whom we might not routinely treat but we must consider when choosing a dental local anaesthetic.

The last of these factors: Metabolism is of considerable clinical interest: Prilocaine is metabolized to o-toluidine and this can oxidize ferrous Fe^{2+} in haemoglobin to ferric Fe^{3+} methaemoglobin. With this adverse metabolic process, we have two problems:

Firstly: ferric (Fe3+) methaemoglobin does not readily bind oxygen.

Secondly: ferric methaemoglobin, once formed is quite stable and will affect the three adjacent haem-arms in the haemoglobin tetrameric molecule, so they in turn neither readily release, nor easily take up oxygen.

Thus, the transport efficiency of the individual red blood cell and that of the patient's blood will be significantly diminished in this process of prilocaine induced or acquired methaemoglobinaemia. Normal levels of methaemoglobin are around 1% in blood.

When the level rises and more than 15% of the total haemoglobin is affected, the patient may appear cyanotic, have shortness of breath and complain of dizzinesss or headaches. The condition becomes severe with methaemoglobin levels above 50% and rapidly becomes fatal at levels of 70% or above.

1. In the normal course of events: Methaemoglobin Fe 3^+ is reduced to Haemoglobin Fe2$^+$

2. In the main, this process occurs by the NADH methaemoglobin reductase enzyme pathway (cytochrome-b5 reductase)

3. To a lesser extent it occurs by the NADPH

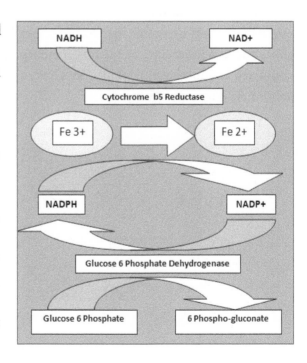

methaemoglobin reductase glucose 6 phosphate dehydrogenase hexose monophosphate shunt pathway.

4. In addition Vitamin C and glutathione enzyme systems also assist in this recycling process.

The physiological process behind the methaemoglobinaemia and tissue hypoxia can be explained by the oxygen dissociation curve being shifted to the left.

Where the use of prilocaine becomes a safety critical issue are in those patients with anaemias, cardiovascular problems and lung pathologies, or in the presence of other abnormal haemoglobinopathies such as thallasaemia, and sickle cell anaemia. With such conditions, the use of prilocaine begins to look a little more bothersome.

Even with very low levels of methaemoglobin at around 5% to 8% in these conditions, problems can result in the same clinical signs that might be seen in a healthy patient but at far higher levels of methaemoglobin[65].

Taking this one stage further, you will see from the dissociation curve in the next diagram that fetal haemoglobin has an inherent left shift, due to a lower level of NADH methaemoglobin reductase when compared to adult haemoglobin. The same shift and enzyme levels are seen in neonates up to 6 months.

Oxygen dissociation with Prilocaine, Benzocaine and Articaine

From this graph, the left shift in the oxygen dissociation curve diagrammatically shows the problems we might encounter in our very young patients.

There is a risk of inducing a met-haemoglobinaemia when using topical anaesthetic gels containing:

Prilocaine
Benzocaine
Articaine.

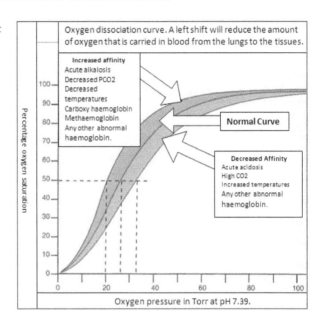

Oxygen dissociation curve. A left shift will reduce the amount of oxygen that is carried in blood from the lungs to the tissues.

Increased affinity
Acute alkalosis
Decreased PCO2
Decreased temperatures
Carboxy haemoglobin
Methaemoglobin
Any other abnormal haemoglobin.

Normal Curve

Decreased Affinity
Acute acidosis
High CO2
Increased temperatures
Any other abnormal haemoglobin.

Percentage oxygen saturation

Oxygen pressure in Torr at pH 7.39.

The last aspect of a prilocaine induced methaemoglobinaemia we need to think about is for our dentally phobic patients who require sedation. The use of pulse oximetery is mandatory when using IV sedative agents. Throughout the procedure and the immediate recovery period, it is essential to maintain both effective oxygenation and ventilation. The difficulties we might encounter with patient monitoring are that critical decreases in fractional oxygen saturation (Sa O_2) in methaemoglobinaemia will go unnoticed with simple pulse oximetry alone. With methaemoglobinaemia it has been shown and it is established that the indicated pulse oximetry (Sp O_2) levels will <u>over-estimate</u> the Sa O_2 levels by an amount proportional to the concentration of methaemoglobin present until the latter reached approximately 35%[66].

Recordings of haemoglobin saturation from pulse oximetry readings could be erroneous and we would then continue a sedation procedure with little clinical evidence of effective levels of oxygenation and ventilation[57][67]. For example, pulse oximeter readings may be greater than 90%, but the actual arterial oxygen tension (PaO_2) may be within normal range greater than 80 mm Hg[68].

Putting all this patho-physiology into a dental perspective, methaemoglobinemia attributable to prilocaine is extremely unlikely with the small doses being used. Certainly, should your patient have congenital or hereditary methaemoglobinemia, prilocaine **would not** be your local anaesthetic of choice!!

Essentially: If you choose to use Prilocaine, please do so only after taking a comprehensive and complete medical history from your patient. It is of interest that anaesthetic choices vary with both the age and the experience of dentist and between the countries in which dentistry is practiced.

In the UK, lidocaine with epinephrine is the most commonly used LA, followed by prilocaine for those patients who have cardiovascular disease or other medical conditions. After these, articaine was utilized[69]. It is of some interest that 10% of older and thus more experienced dentists used prilocaine with felypressin in their pregnant patients, whereas the recently qualified dentists absolutely desisted from doing so. Perhaps the recent graduate is cognizant of the (theoretical) risks of foetal methaemoglobinaemia inherent with prilocaine and the induction of uterine contractions with felypressin. Whether such knowledge is forgotten with time, or that experience makes the dentist more capable of independent risk assessment was not established from this survey[69].

After considering the results further, it may be the case that a process of risk normalization overrides safety critical concerns in the older but perhaps not the wiser dentist.

The experience of anaesthetic use in the UK is not the same throughout the EU. It has been reported that by far the most commonly used dental local anaesthetic in Germany is articaine/epinephrine, with lidocaine/epinephrine being used infrequently: 91% and 2% respectively[70]. Outside the EU, there are further differences, in Brazil the most commonly used dental local anaesthetic is prilocaine: 86%[71]. Such disparity may represent cultural, educational or economic factors between dentists in these countries[69]. The only factor that is common for all the dentists in the countries in these surveys is anaesthetic choice varies according to the perceived risk to the patient. The use of prilocaine/ felypressin being used in place of lignocaine/epinephrine for those patients with medical conditions such as asthma and diabetes, even if there is no clear evidence to contraindicate use of the former local anaesthetic[69].

Moving on from the pharmacology and the sociology of local anaesthesia, it is not unheard of for your patients to make claims of local anaesthetic allergy. These may be nothing more than the patient experiencing the symptoms of cardiac palpitations arising from the epinephrine in the local anaesthetic, or the immediate effects of their own adrenal glands rapidly releasing their contents into the patient's blood stream. Alternatively and more probably, the patient may have experienced the first stages of a faint or they are recounting their entire vaso-vagal episode complete with visit to the local A and E department in the back of an ambulance with everyone and the world in attendance.

Allergic reactions in relation to dental local anaesthesia are exceptionally rare and are more likely to be stimulated by the preservatives used in anaesthetic cartridges such as methylparaben (now used very rarely), or antioxidant additives such as sulphites, containing the ion: SO_3^{2-} which are only used to extend the shelf life of the vasopressin used in prilocaine. Sulphites do occur naturally and are noted to be capable of generating an adverse, but not an allergic reaction in patients who are susceptible. The clinical signs to be aware of are an asthma-like difficulty in breathing and possibly migraine-like headaches. As noted, these are physiological responses and not allergic reactions as such. Rather than generalized reactions to local anaesthetics which are extremely rare, the localized reactions are more problematic and more frequent. While injecting into the highly vascularised oral mucosa, you will have noticed the effect of the vasoconstrictor in a local anaesthetic resulting in the patient's gingival and periodontal tissues rapidly becoming pale.

Or if you have as most dentists have; initiated a vascular accident with a local anaesthetic, you will have been fairly horrified to witness an extra-oral version of this event. As blood drains out of tissues, but doesn't refill, an almost dermatome like area clearly becomes visible on the affected side of your patient's face. An ischaemic necrosis of tissues could potentially follow from the injection of a local anaesthetic. The principle reasons for this could be from a rapid increase in intercellular tissue pressure exerted by too great a volume of local anaesthetic injected at too great a rate.

Alternatively, vaso-spasticity of blood vessels with no collateral circulation will initiate a localized and irreversible ischaemia resulting in necrosis. Such a problem could arise with injections into the attached mucosa of the hard palate. Lastly, with regard to tissue necrosis, the chemical formulation may play a part too. Recently concerns have been raised with respect to the neurotoxicity of articaine in concentrations of 4% and prilocaine in concentrations of 3% to 4%.

Neurotoxicity and nerve damage from local anaesthetic use

Sometime after articaine was introduced in the 1980s in North America, there were reports of an increased incidence of paraesthesia. In 1993, there were some 14 cases reported in Canada, all related to the use of either articaine or prilocaine[72]. The US Food and Drug Administration when considering the approval of articaine did note that the paraesthesia risk was higher than that for lidocaine[57]. In a 10 year review of this problem in the USA, from 1997 to 2008, some 248 cases of dental paraesthesia attributable to articaine and prilocaine were uncovered. Some 95% of cases involved the use of a mandibular nerve block and in 89% of these cases, the lingual nerve was affected. Paraesthesia was found to be 7.3 X more likely with 4% articaine and 3.6 X more likely with 4% prilocaine[73]. The North American experience was also seen in Europe, with a Danish investigation into this problem revealing a disproportionate rate of nerve injury attributable to articaine with 292 cases reported from 1995 to 2007. The result from Denmark showed a highly significant over-representation of neuro-sensory disturbance associated with 4% articaine, especially when used to achieve mandibular blocks[74].

From this data, we could make and stand by two assumptions:

> Firstly, the greater the concentration of local anaesthetic solution, the greater the risk for toxicity and damage to nerve trunks will be.
>
> Secondly, any local anaesthetic will cause nerve damage if the intracellular concentration of anaesthetic is sufficiently high.

Certainly, if the concentration of articaine is experimentally doubled from 2% to 4%, then for up to 3 weeks after injection, concentration-dependent neurotoxic injuries will be seen.

Interestingly, from laboratory studies investigating this phenomenon, while there was no decrease in the numbers of nerve fibres, the injuries manifested as a reduction in the cross-sectional area of axons, together with a reduction in the thickness of the myelin sheath, when 4% rather than 2% articaine was injected into the sciatic nerves of rats[75]. In this experimental study, the mechanical injury from needle penetration into the nerve fibre had no significant effect on subsequent nerve histology or nerve conduction in the three weeks from injury to dissection examination of the nerve.

From these experimental findings, the safety critical practitioner will quite reasonably insist on using a local anaesthetic with the lowest possible concentrations[73]. Further safety measures might be worth implementing after considering the following:

Both the Inferior Alveolar Nerve (IAN) and the Lingual nerve are at risk from local anaesthetic injury. However, it is the IAN within its bony mandibular canal that is more at risk from both the primary toxic and the secondary ischaemic effects following an injection.

In contrast, it is the lingual nerve, located on the mesial mandibular border, within a soft tissue sheath which is more at risk from the direct physical and secondary patho-physiological damage from an IANB accident. Several suggestions have been made why this should be.

Principally, it is the structure of the lingual nerve near the lingula, which creates the increased risk of trauma from an injection. Proximal to the lingula, the lingual nerve comprises far fewer bundles or fibres than the Inferior Aleveolar Nerve. Whereas, distally the lingual nerve picks up the CNVII Chorda tympani, the following diagram illustrates the relationship of some of the more important nerves in the oral region:

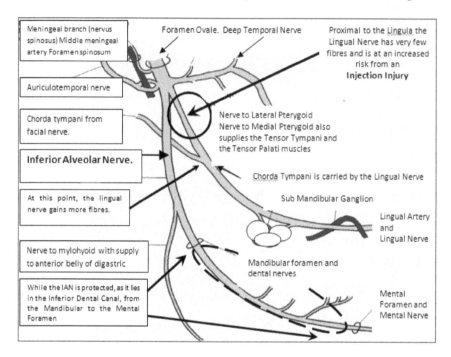

Further support for the assumptions arising from the structure of nerves comes from histological samples of the lingual nerve proximal to the mandibular foramen and lingula: In a post mortem examination: 1/3rd of all dissected lingual nerves examined under the microscope were found to be uni-fascicular, whereas more distally, beyond the mandibular foramen (the IANB target area): The lingual nerve becomes multi-fascicular, as it picks up fibres from the CN VII Chorda Tympani.[76]

In contrast to the lingual nerve, the Inferior Alveolar Nerve at the lingula is a multi-bundled complex arrangement of nerve fibres. Such a joining together with duplication of nerve fibres results in an elegant anatomical system-redundancy that provides ample reserves of safety from injury, either chemical: from the anaesthetic solution, or mechanical: from the tip of the needle used in the injection[76]. These findings could explain why 70% of permanent nerve injures from an IANB only affect the lingual nerve. The conclusion being:

> **Small nerves are more susceptible to injection injury than larger ones.**

After thinking about the risks involved with the IANB, our use of local anaesthetics in relatively high concentrations for mandibular block rather than mandibular infiltration techniques merits some further discussion.

One advantage of using articaine in preference to lidocaine is the longer duration of anaesthesia that it provides, thus making it a very useful drug for the longer dental procedures such as implant placement or the surgical removal of impacted wisdom teeth. However this longer duration of anaesthesia does come at a price:

The thiophene aromatic ring in articaine —————→

Will give greater lipid solubility than the benzene ring in Lidocaine

An Ester side chain can be rapidly hydrolysed. Giving a short half life.

From the chemical formulation of articaine, an improved ability to cross myelin sheaths will be seen. <u>However such properties do make articaine more neurotoxic.</u> One would be inclined to think these characteristics could mean that articaine should be presented in a lower concentration than the 2% that is available and used for lidocaine in dental local anaesthetics. Conversely and somewhat peculiarly, articaine is presented in a 4% concentration! Thus, for equal volumes of both local anaesthetics, articaine is 2X more potent, providing double the active anaesthetic compound than lidocaine... but the maximum recommended volumes are identical!!

Turning this problem around, looking at it another way... If we take both articaine and lidocaine in the same concentrations ie: 4%, it might be the case that lidocaine used in this level would be unacceptably neurotoxic with an even greater risk of systemic problems if accidental intravascular injection were to occur[57]. However, this is not the case as articaine has an elimination half life of 1/3 that of lidocaine, due to the above noted ester side chain of the thiophene ring being hydrolyzed by plasma esterases in 30 minutes compared to the 90 minutes it takes for liver enzymes to metabolize lidocaine. In essence, while articaine may be more neurotoxic in a 4% concentration, it is still less systemically toxic than lidocaine at a 2% concentration[73,74].

The last point to make about articaine is that it is metabolized by esterase enzymes in <u>plasma</u>, whereas lidocaine and prilocaine are metabolized by de-alkylating enzymes in the <u>liver</u>. While the former show no significant age dependent decline, by comparison, in our patients over 65 years old the levels of the latter will have fallen by some 50%[57].

Adding to this problem, many of our older patients will also have been prescribed medications that can either directly interact with the vasoconstrictors in our local anaesthetics, or which decrease renal and hepatic blood flow, further reducing the abilities of the patient's innate drug handling metabolism; that is already well established on a path of natural decline.

Certain beta blockers provide a particularly good example of a medication that both interacts with epinephrine and can significantly reduce both renal and hepatic blood flow. From a safety perspective, our use of articaine might be reduced; not only by limiting the total dose, but also in the choice of application too. It might be prudent to limit the use of 4% articaine for infiltrations only and absolutely avoid its use for IANB or other block techniques, opting instead for lidocaine or prilocaine, both being formulated in lower concentrations and both carrying a lower risk of nerve damage[73,74].

While lidocaine is the most commonly used local anaesthetic in the UK and articaine use is indicated for longer procedures, ideally we might also consider the use of bupivicaine for any dental procedure longer than the 1 ½ hours we might usefully gain from lidoccaine. Bupivicaine can provide up to 3 hours of anaesthesia, but it is noted to be irritating and more painful on injection than lidocaine.

One way around this problem is to initiate local anaesthesia with lidocaine then prolong the anaesthesia by adding bupivicaine after one hour. If such a multi-drug approach is to be used, with respect to systemic safety, then the total of all local anaesthetic doses should additive. If half of the intended or maximum anaesthetic dose is used with the first drug, this will also limit the second anaesthetic to half[77].

It was and still is widely accepted that the maximum dose of lidocaine that could be used in one dental appointment was and is 10 cartridges. This was empirically calculated from submucosal injections of lidocaine up to 400 μcg being equivalent to 10 cartridges producing no systemic or toxic effects[78]. If you consult the Oxford Handbook of Clinical Dentistry, the authors do not disagree with this figure, stating lidocaine to be extremely safe[79]. However these dose limits are given for the "ideal healthy adult": An exclusive if not elusive person; a patient few of us have had the opportunity to meet, to treat, or the privilege to apply the knowledge we have learned from dental school. As for the elderly, children and the infirm of all ages, it is difficult to see how simple dose reductions could apply either for lidocaine, or the other local anaesthetics such as prilocaine, articaine, or bupivicaine.

Rather than referring to a clinical text, perhaps the ideal source from which dose limits and drug restrictions might be taken are the Patient Information Leaflets, which under current UK legislation every manufacturer should include with every box of local anaesthetic we use.

The following information is taken from these sources for the most commonly used anaesthetics used in the UK:

Lidocaine 2% with epinephrine 1:80,000

(Septodont 94100 St Maur des Fosses France 2014)*

Adult:	A single cartridge either 2.2mL or 1.8mL is sufficient. **Do not exceed 3 cartridges.**
Adolescent: (14 to 17)	4/5th of 2.2mL or 1X 1.8mL. Do not exceed 1 3/5th of 2.2mL or 2X 1.8mL (3.6mL)
Elderly:	4/5th of 2.2mL or 1X 1.8mL. Do not exceed 1 3/5th of 2.2mL or 2X 1.8mL (3.6mL)
Children: (6 to 14)	3/5th of 2.2mL or 3/4 of 1.8mL (1.35ml). Do not exceed 1 1/5th of 2.2mL or 1 ½ of 1.8mL (2.7mL)
Children: (3 to 6)	2/5th to 4/5th of 2.2ml or 4/5th to 1 X 1.8mL. **Do not use on patients under 3 years old.**

Prilocaine 3% with Felypressin 0.03 IU/mL

(Dentsply Addlestone Surrey KT15 2SE UK 2014)*

Adult:	A single cartridge of 2mL is sufficient.	**Do not exceed 5 cartridges or 10mL** **Never exceed 8mgs/Kg body weight**
Children: (5 to 10)	½ X 2mL to 1x 2mL maximum.	**Never exceed 6.6mgs/Kg body weight** [79]
Children: (3 to 5)	¼ X 2mL to ½ X 2mL maximum.	**Never exceed 4.0mgs/Kg body weight** **Do not use on patients under 3 years old.**

Articaine 4% with epinephrine 1:100,000

(Septodont 94100 St Maur des Fosses France 2014)*

Adult:	A single cartridge either 2.2mL or 1.7mL is sufficient.	**Do not exceed 6 X 1.7mL or 5 X 2.2mL** **Never exceed 7mgs/Kg body weight.**
Child: (40kg)	3 X 2.2mL or 4 X 1.7mL	**Never exceed 7mL.**
Child: (20Kg)	1 ½ X 2.2mL or 2 X 1.7mL (3.5mL)	**Never exceed 3.5mL** **Do not use on patients under 4 years old**

1. *The manufacturers noted on the previous page supply these local anaesthetics for use in the UK.

2. If you are outside the UK or are using a different supplier, the data from the Patient Information Leaflets could differ from the information you are working with.

3. Notwithstanding such differences, the overall pattern of doses presented in the tables on the previous page should not be significantly altered from those doses you will work with.

4. With that in mind, the previous tables should provide an indication of those patterns and parameters for safe prescribing but they are not the absolute limits for the administration of these drugs!

5. When using any dental Local Anaesthetic: We should always aim to be well below the published and prescribed levels for all of our patients: Whether they are children, adults, the elderly or infirm.

From these three tables you will see the manufacturer's recommended maximum doses are actually significantly less than those doses given in the dental texts quoted and those doses we have probably been used to operating with. Why this is so, is something of an oddity. One would think the manufacturers would be keen to agree with both the clinical experts and the users of their products, the former group suggesting far greater doses are safe to use. After all business is business and if the experts believe more local anaesthetic can safely be used, then more can surely be sold.

Personally and professionally, we believe the dose limits given above are cautiously conservative, while the text book upper limit of 10 cartridges of a local anaesthetic for a healthy adult could be somewhat optimistically excessive.

After all, even with a medical history updated at every dental visit, do we really know for sure that our healthy adult patients are that healthy?

Putting patient safety first, we should not aim to use unnecessarily high doses of any drug let alone local anaesthetics, especially given the potential for a vasoconstrictor such as epinephrine to exert its cardio-tonic effects, should a vascular injection accident occur. Perhaps the best way to keep our local anaesthetic use to levels that are both safe and practical is to develop and use an injection technique that is proven from clinical evidence to be practical and safe, when correctly applied.

The techniques you choose will be both safety critical and effective, working on time, every time.

As noted previously, timing is perhaps as important as any technique you choose. You will already know from your clinical experience, that the successful dental procedure begins with the successful injection of local anaesthetic. The slow injection in the right place at the right time is the key to achieving procedural success and achieving it safely.

The heart and local anaesthetics

Just before we begin our discussion on local anaesthetic techniques, we do need to revise a few more points on the cardio-tonic effects of the vasoconstrictors in local anaesthetics. While epinephrine produces a vaso-constrictive effect on the α-1 receptors in the capillaries of the oral mucosa, (even with the small doses contained in local anaesthetic cartridges), the most commonly used vasoconstrictor: Epinephrine, increases the heart rate by activating the β-1 receptors in the Sino-Atrial Node. Epinephrine also activates β-1 receptors in heart muscle, increasing their contractility. As a result, Systemic Blood Pressure will increase. Furthermore, epinephrine activates the β-2 receptors in arterial walls, with a resulting converse vaso-dilation in the systemic circulation producing a decrease in diastolic pressure.

If the **β1** effect is balanced against the **β2** effect, very little alteration in the overall systemic arterial pressure is seen. In summary, the agonistic effects of epinephrine on cardio-vascular Beta receptors will have the following results[57]:

> I.   Heart Rate ↑
> II. Stroke Volume ↑
> III. Cardiac Output ↑
> IV. Arterial Resistance ↓
> V.   Systemic Pressure: **Unchanged.**

These effects have been observed when as little as 3 cartridges of 2% lidocaine with 1:100,000 epinephrine, (dose equivalent = 60µgm) were injected into the oral mucosa.[80] Similar clinical effects were also noted when articaine with adrenaline at 2% and 4% (60 µgm and 120 µgm epinephrine respectively) were used. A proportionately greater cardiotonic effect was seen as the dose of epinephrine was increased[81]. By way of comparison:

> In your dental clinic emergency drugs box the Adrenaline doses for anaphylaxis are:
>
> I.   **Adult (> 12 years)   500 µgm**
> II. **Child (6 to 12 years) 300 µgm**
> III. **Child (<6 years)   150µgm**

> From this table we can see the epinephrine doses in local anaesthetic are lower, but not by any order of magnitude, so they are still considerable and thus capable of exerting systemic effects too.

Certainly, the results for dental local anaesthetics are as expected and the subjects in the above noted studies were healthy adults. However, the issue of best practice will remain for those patients where the diagnosis of cardiovascular pathology has either not yet been established, or where such a history has been established and the patient is taking medication for their cardiovascular condition, the core issue of clinical safety must be addressed with respect to the types and doses of local anaesthetics we can use.

With the latter type of patient, a dose reduction in local anaesthetic dose, or switching from lidocaine with epinephrine to prilocaine with felypressin would be prudent. However this does not address the problem for the former type of patient; with occult cardiovascular pathologies, for whom epinephrine may be quite reasonably given but it may actually induce an arrhythmia or theoretically precipitate a circulatory crisis. One position that has been adopted by the manufacturers of dental local anaesthetics, as you have seen from the data in the tables presented previously, is to limit the total local anaesthetic dose that might be safely used. However, to restrict local anaesthetic doses for all patients irrespective of their cardiac health or general health does seem to be an overly simplistic if perhaps an excessively restrictive measure to take.

Possibly one safe option we might take is to ensure an updated comprehensive medical history is taken for those dental appointments where local anaesthetics are to be used and to vary the doses, setting aside the use of one anaesthetic in favour of another, or that consideration is given to deferring a dental appointment until a medical opinion is sought and only then are appropriate local anaesthetics used.

While it seems that no appropriately safe limits on dental local anaesthetics have yet been established, we do know that epinephrine will be rapidly metabolized by Catechol-O-Methyl Transferase in a matter of minutes. The maximum clinical effects of exogenous epinephrine are seen in 5 minutes, the elimination half life is 3 minutes and the total clinical effect on the cardiovascular system is barely discernible by 10 to 15 minutes after injection of a dental local anaesthetic[57,81].

With this time scale in mind, perhaps another option is to establish a baseline for our patient's heart rate, blood pressure and oxygenation, then administer local anaesthetic to that level which achieves anaesthesia but does not impact on the patient's cardiovascular system. As the level of anaesthesia declines, further doses could then be given while the patient's vital signs and physiological status are being monitored in response to supplemental or additive doses of local anaesthetic. While this may seem a little onerous, in reality patient monitoring can be achieved with equipment that is easy to use, requires little additional staff training and is relatively inexpensive to operate and maintain.

The only drawback with such additional monitoring is the burden it places on our already stretched capacity to operate safely in the clinic. The dentist already beleaguered with regulatory matters is unlikely to embrace another layer of patient monitoring, while it may be practical and elegant in principle, it will be soon become shrouded in bureaucracy if the safety conscious dental professional begins to think about attaching such devices to a patient in practice. The aphorism for new developments in the aviation industry could easily be applied here:

> *"When the weight of paperwork equals the weight of the new equipment, only then can its use be permitted."*

Lastly, the risk of drug interactions with epinephrine must be recognized. In the previous section medications such as beta blockers were considered in some detail. The risks associated with non cardio-selective β-blockers such as propranolol and epinephrine have been recognized for over thirty years. Using a dental local anaesthetic with a vaso-constrictor such as epinephrine is not absolutely contra indicated with patients medicated as such. However, both the delivery and the dose need to be, respectively; cautious and conservative[82,83]. Certainly, an IANB with its risk of a vascular injection accident needs to be very carefully considered before proceeding and in any event, the patient would need to be monitored throughout the procedure should you choose not to err on the side of caution, when using an IANB with epinephrine in a patient taking beta blockers.

Other medications our patients take and we need to be aware of are the TCAs, MAOIs, thyroid medication and certain drugs used for diet and weight control, as these drugs can exert an influence similar to the vaso-constrictors in local anaesthetics. While the use of a dental local anaesthetic with epinephrine is not absolutely contraindicated, we do need to be wary of the potential risk of interaction with drugs, be they prescribed medically or obtained recreationally.

The use of any legitimate sympathomimetic medicine or illicit stimulant drug such as cocaine will be revealed in a medical history, but only if the patient can be trusted to trust you. In other words, an empathic and non-judgmental approach to taking a medical history is more than being polite it is safety critical for the patient and for yourself.

Following both the medical and the dental assessment of your patient, the decision to use a local anaesthetic and the choice of local anaesthetic will have been made. In the preceding sections, our revision of the physiology of the patient and the pharmacology of the drugs they are taking, together with actions and potential for interactions with those you might choose to give will lead you towards the right choice of drug with the right dose. The techniques discussed in the next section will guide you towards the correct delivery of those drugs.

Maxillary local anaesthesia

Of all dental local anaesthetic techniques, the simple infiltration <u>onto</u> (and not into) the maxillary bones is the most predictable, having the highest success rate and being the easiest to perform; but actually it is quite difficult to perform well. Success in the upper arch is in part due to the unique physical properties of the maxillary alveolar and maxillary basal bones, which are different from mandibular bones and the IANB techniques which will also be discussed.

Overall, the maxilla is tremendously porous and the bone is frequently quite thin around the bucco-facial aspects of the roots of teeth. Maxillary bone demonstrates a higher degree of plasticity much more so than mandibular bone. Such differences are quite striking especially if the maxillary dentition is compared with the directly opposing mandibular dentition. Adding to this the maxilla is well supplied with nerves, arteries and veins. The rich palatal neuro-vascular bed can be seen from this illustration:

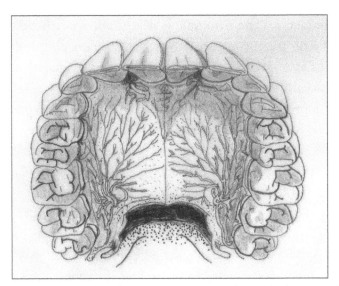

The extent of the distribution of the Greater Palatine and Naso Palatine Nerves can be seen from the above drawing of the maxillary dentition.

The cancellous alveolar and basal bone of the maxillary dental arch, possess a rich supply of blood vessels and along these lie the alveolar nerve plexuses and branches of the Maxillary Division of the Trigeminal Nerve (CN V$_2$) providing the upper dentition with its generous innervation.

As a result of these anatomical factors, with your patience, some fortitude and forbearance from the patient, the maxillary infiltration is almost guaranteed to be successful. However as always, in clinical dentistry, things are never quite so simple. For maxillary anaesthesia, one objective and repeatable definition of success is:

> The absence of a patient's perception to the
> maximum output of an electronic pulp tester.

It should be noted the duration attached to this definition for infiltration anaesthesia (the most commonly used technique for the maxillary dentition), is that the patient should be oblivious to two maximum pulp-test readings set at an interval of 15 minutes.

Whereas the definition for block techniques, (the most commonly used technique for the mandibular dentition), anaesthetic success is defined by no patient response to two maximum pulp test readings again at an interval of 15 minutes, but this level of anaesthesia should be maintained for at least 60 minutes[89].

This reproducible clinical standard has been accepted as the benchmark for pulpal anaesthesia[88]. From the literature, maxillary infiltration with lidocaine and epinephrine has been quoted to be successful between 50% and 100% of the time[84,85,86]. Such a range with a highly variable lack of success has been attributed to differences in the smoothness, the density, the porosity, and the thickness of the bone surrounding the maxillary teeth[87]. In addition to hard tissue barriers, it is possible that an intervening plane of fascial tissue, through which an anaesthetic cannot pass, or a mass of connective tissues along which an anaesthetic needle has been deflected away from the bone and the intended underlying nerves, together with individual variations in patient responses to the local anaesthetic being delivered; could all contribute to the less than 100% success rate for maxillary infiltration anaesthesia.

The three factors contributing to failure or detracting from success of maxillary anaesthesia are:

i Anatomy. The location of the teeth both in and within the arch: The incisors show a greater rate of success (in terms of rapid onset and lengthy duration) of anaesthesia than the molars. Teeth with their apices and innervations held deep within bone will possibly take longer to anaesthetize than those with roots and apices more superficially sited and more easily perfused with an infiltrating anaesthetic solution[89].

ii Pathology. Any alteration in the density and structure of maxillary bone beyond those of a physiological nature, such as those changes induced with medication either increasing or decreasing bone mineralization, density and porosity, intentionally or as a side effect, will also determine the ease or difficulty with which the infiltration of local anaesthetic can progress. Additionally: Developmental, Metabolic, Dysplastic, Neoplastic or Infective changes in bone could alter the direction and duration of infiltration anaesthesia.

A thorough intra-oral clinical exam together with the use of an appropriate pre-operative radiograph (where and when indicated) will be able to draw attention to many if not all of the relevant pathological conditions, but only if they are established to a degree that can be radiographically detected. We should remember that pathological bone changes can take several weeks until they develop to a level that can be detected with use of X-rays. Prior to these radiographically detectable changes, metabolic changes could affect the action of a local anaesthetic. It is the decrease in pH of infected tissues; lower than pH 7.4 favouring the water soluble but not the lipid soluble phase of the local anaesthetic which explains the difficulty in achieving anaesthesia if the tissue is inflamed or infected, but not yet abscessed[77].

iii Psychology. As already mentioned, maxillary infiltrations are easy to perform. However, they are difficult to perform well. Your technique frequently involves introducing a needle into the most sensitive part of the patient's mouth, towards the upper incisors or into the palate and unlike the IANB, the maxillary infiltrations are often not only in full view of the patient but directly in their line of sight. The most important factors from a patient perspective are that the dentist neither hurts them, nor gives them painful injections. Nonetheless, in order to provide dentistry that is painless, a local anaesthetic has to be injected using a cartridge, with a syringe, and of course... ...

The dreaded needle.

This leads us once more to that problem we have already discussed; the fear of needles (or if you want to impress your examiners/irritate your study partners in the BDS, MJDF or MFDS exams: trypanophobia) and the risk of vasovagal syncope either during or in the immediate aftermath of your injection[90]. More than half of all medical emergencies occurring in dental practice occur in conjunction with local anaesthetic use. The impact in terms of morbidity and mortality has been mentioned previously[6,7 and 91].

When considering consent, compliance and the comfort of your patient, the palatal infiltration has been noted to be the most painful and even an unnecessary measure when used to provide anaesthesia for the simple non-surgical extraction of upper teeth[92]. It might even prove possible to avoid distressing a patient by using adjuncts such as topical anaesthesia, or pressure, if palatal infiltration anaesthesia is needed. Or we may choose to entirely avoid palatal anaesthesia, if an articaine buccal infiltration with its demonstrated property of higher tissue diffusion when compared to lidocaine is chosen and so minimize the adverse psychological impact on the patient from using a painful (and demonstrably unnecessary) anaesthetic[93].

The techniques for maxillary local anaesthesia

With any dental local anaesthetic, we must minimize the risk of an accidental intravascular injection. It is fundamentally safety critical that aspiration prior to injection is carried out. It has been observed that very fine needles, those lower than a 30 gauge, not only demonstrate an increased difficulty in aspirating blood or tissue fluid, there is an increased risk of their breakage, when compared to the wider bore needles with gauges in excess of 25 to 27. Nearly all (99%) of needle breakages were with 30 Gauge or narrower needles[94].

In addition to these problems, there is no discernible difference in pain sensation for the patient when using either long, short, large bore or narrow gauge needles[95]. From a safety point, the only critical factor in producing a painless injection technique and minimizing the risk of a vasovagal syncope is the slow rate or low speed with which the local anaesthetic is injected.

From simple to complex, the techniques we can use for dental anaesthesia are: Topical Application, Infiltration Injection, Field Anaesthesia, Block Anaesthesia and finally: Regional Anaesthesia.

Often in the maxilla, the simple infiltration of 1ml of local anaesthetic into the buccal mucosal tissues is sufficient to cover most periodontal procedures and many minor restorative eventualities:

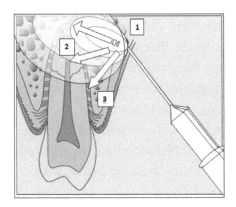

1. Infiltration anaesthesia is achieved when a solution is deposited supra-periosteally at the buccal side of the alveolus.
2. However, there are disadvantages; infiltration will only achieve pulpal anaesthesia when the anaesthetic solution diffuses through cortical bone.
3. If there is a localized infection this can track along the injection path and in such circumstances, any anaesthesia achieved will be limited in terms of duration and anatomical extent.

However with dentistry that is more involved such as simple extractions and surgical procedures in soft tissues, the nerve block techniques in the maxilla are useful.

Before we consider these in detail, it is important to remind ourselves of the origin and destinations of the second division and the branches of the Trigeminal Nerve, The Maxillary Nerve (CNV_2):

I.   The Maxillary Nerve (the Second Division of the Fifth Cranial Nerve or CNV_2) arises from the Trigeminal Ganglion, located in Meckel's cave in the Petrous part of the temporal bone. CNV_2 is a sensory nerve lying between the CNV_1 (the Ophthalmic Division) and the CNV_3 (the Mandibular Division) of the Trigeminal Nerve. CNV_2 supplies afferent sensory fibres from the maxillary teeth, the skin between the palpebral fissures, the oral cavity, the nasal cavity and the maxillary sinuses.

II.   The Maxillary Nerve initially appears as a flattened plexiform band that exits from the middle cranial fossa through the Foramen Rotundum in the Sphenoid Bone. From here the CNV_2 assumes a more cylindrical profile as it passes into the Pterygopalatine Fossa.

III.   The Pterygopalatine Fossa is a cone-shaped depression deep to the Infratemporal Fossa, lying on the posterior aspect of the maxilla and is located between the Pterygoid Process and the Maxillary Tuberosity, close to the apex of the orbit. The Pterygopalatine Fossa forms an indented area medial to the Pterygo-Maxillary Fissure leading into the Spheno-Palatine Foramen and it communicates with both nasal and oral cavities, the Infratemporal Fossa, the orbit, the pharynx, and the middle cranial fossa.

IV.   The CNV_2 lies in the Pterygopalatine Fossa with its combined branches of the Greater Petrosal Nerve with preganglionic parasympathetic fibres and the Deep Petrosal Nerve with its postganglionic sympathetic fibres. A Pterygopalatine Ganglion can be found suspended from the CNV_2. From this fossa, the CNV_2 passes laterally above the posterior aspect of the mandible and then enters the orbit via the Inferior Orbital Fissure. From here, one branch runs along the orbital floor in a groove to pass forward in the Infra-Orbital Canal, from the Inferior Orbital Foramen with Inferior Palpebral, Lateral Nasal and Superior Labial terminal branches, providing a sensory supply to the maxillary aspect of the patient's face. The infraorbital branch of the terminal third of the maxillary artery and the maxillary vein accompany these branches of the CNV_2 along their routes.

V. The remaining main branches of the CNV_2 supply three distinct anatomical areas:

i. Within the cranium: The Middle Meningeal Nerves provide sensations for the meninges.

ii. In the Pterygopalatine Fossa: The Infra Orbital Nerve passes through Infraorbital canal, the Zygomatic nerve gives off both the: Zygomatico-Temporal and Zygomatico-Facial nerves from the Inferior Orbital Fissure. Nasal Branches and Nasopalatine nerves arise from the Sphenopalatine foramen. The Posterior Superior Alveolar (PSA) nerve arises from the Pterygopalatine Fossa. Additionally, the Palatine nerve with Greater Palatine and Lesser Palatine branches, with an additional Naso palatine nerve are found here. Lastly from the Pterygopalatine Fossa, the Pharyngeal nerve is seen.

iii. If we return along the Inferior Orbital Canal, both the Anterior Superior Alveolar (ASA) and Middle Superior Alveolar (MSA) Nerves are seen along with an Inferior Orbital Nerve.

The ASA is a fairly large nerve branch and just before departing from the Infra Orbital Foramen it descends on the anterior wall of the maxillary sinus dividing into branches supplying the maxillary incisors and canines. The ASA also communicates with the MSA nerve. A nasal branch, which passes through a very narrow canal in the lateral wall of the inferior meatus will supply the mucous membrane of the anterior part of the inferior meatus and the floor of the nasal cavity, sending communicating branches to the sphenopalatine ganglion. Dental considerations for these nerves are important. The ASA usually innervates all anterior teeth, loops backwards to join the MSA forming a maxillary superior dental plexus as can be seen below:

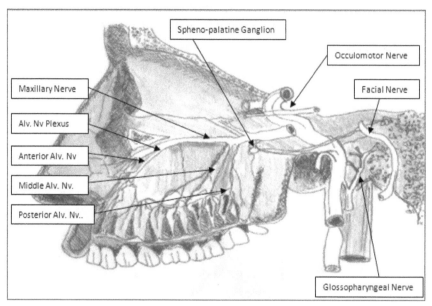

The ASA, MSA and PSA branches of the Maxillary Nerve (CNV$_2$)

Starting from the front and working to the back of the mouth, the following techniques can be used to anaesthetically block the three main branches of the Maxillary Alveolar Nerves:

The Anterior Superior Alveolar (ASA) Injection. The ASA will provide anaesthesia from the midline; the upper central and lateral incisors extending to the lateral aspect of the canines. Their periodontal ligaments, alveolar bone, supporting periosteum and surrounding buccal soft tissues will be covered

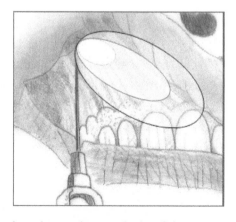

by the ASA. <u>This injection is introduced into the vestibule of the upper labial and buccal mucosa</u>. Following a check aspiration, the slow administration at a depth of 5 mm; 1.0 mL of local anaesthetic should prove to be adequate to provide pulpal anaesthesia after 2 ½ to 3 ½ minutes. In cases where anaesthesia has not occurred, excluding the usual cause of infection or inflammation, the presence of collateral or midline crossover innervations will be responsible and the administration of a contra-lateral local anaesthetic might prove to be effective in blocking supply from these additional nerve fibres.

The Middle Superior Alveolar (MSA) Injection. The MSA provides local anaesthesia from the distal aspect of the maxillary canine, to the premolars, around to the mesio-buccal aspect of the maxillary first molar. In addition and as wih the previous technique, the periodontal ligaments, alveolar 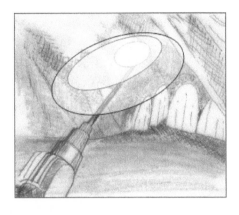 bone, supporting periosteum and surrounding buccal soft tissues will be covered by the MSA. The MSA injection is introduced into the apex of the buccal vestibule lateral to the maxillary second premolar. The tip of the needle is aimed towards the root apex of the upper second premolar. When administering an MSA, the mucosa is only penetrated to a depth of 5mm up to a maximum of 10 mm. Again 1mL of local anaesthetic is sufficient and should be slowly injected following your aspiration check. Of some anatomical importance in many patients, the MSA nerve is absent and this area can be covered by anaesthetizing the ASA and with the following injection:

The Posterior Superior Alveolar (PSA) Injection. The PSA will provide local anaesthesia for the maxillary molars. However, the mesio-buccal aspect of the first molar will be covered by the MSA or extended branches of the ASA and possibly some branches of the PSA too. Once more, as for the ASA and the MSA, the PSA will cover the periodontal ligament, alveolar bone, supporting periosteum, and surrounding buccal soft tissue adjacent to the teeth innervated by the PSA. Whereas the MSA injection is administered at the root apex of the second premolar: The PSA is given at the apex of the disto-buccal vestibule at a point just behind the malar process. The PSA is inserted to a depth of 10mm to 15 mm, with your needle being inserted distally and superiorly at approximately 45 degrees to both the mesio-distal and bucco-lingual planes. As with 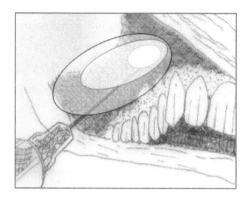 the previous two injections, a volume of 1ml should prove to be sufficient for the PSA to provide effective local anaesthesia.

In addition to these maxillary block techniques, we might consider a palatine infiltration. These are painful injections, due to the tightly adherent keratinized palatal mucosa. As a result, they are seldom used to reduce dental pain, especially if either a buccal infiltration or nerve block with articaine has been used or a proper amount of time is allowed before work commences. Nevertheless, the palatal infiltration is effective in reducing the discomfort associated with rubber dam clamps, minor periodontal procedures or other minor techniques.

Given the tightly adherent mucosa in the palate, while there is a rich vasculature, the risk of haematoma from a palatal injection is remote. Nevertheless, should you choose to use local anaesthetic palatally, the following techniques are useful:

The Nasopalatine Block. (NPB) The Nasopalatine Nerve supplies the palatal tissues and teeth of the premaxilla, chiefly the upper central incisors, the lateral incisors and potentially the canines too; however this will depend on the precise location of the roots of these teeth, relative to the nasopalatine foramen. The Nasopalatine Nerve exits the maxilla from the nasopalatine foramen deep to the incisive papilla, located posterior to the central incisors. The NPB is always going to be an uncomfortable and for paediatric patients, a distressing injection. There are two methods you might consider using:

1. The multiple approach. 1/3 mL of local anaesthetic can be introduced in the anterior labial midline of the maxilla close to or around the labial frenum. After one minute, with the needle perpendicular to the soft tissues, a second but deeper penetration can be achieved to 5mm and more local anaesthetic can now be introduced into or around the incisive papilla. If the patient can 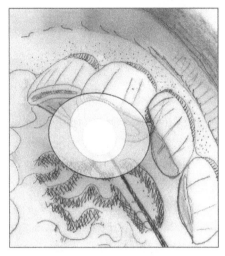 tolerate this, you will see defined blanching of the nasopalatine area. Following this, further anaesthetic is introduced but this time, deeper than 5mm and towards (but not into) the nasopalatine foramen, where following clear aspiration another 0.3mL can be safely injected as you feel the needle against the maxillary bone.

2. The single injection. can be introduced into the incisive papilla. If choosing this approach, after using topical anaesthetic with a cotton bud, be sure to continue applying pressure to the midline of the anterior palate with the cotton bud, to distract or counteract the effect of the pain of the injection. After a clear aspiration, 0.3mL of local anaesthetic can be slowly introduced around or towards the nasopalatine foramen. Again a depth of 5mm should prove sufficient and within 1 to 2 minutes the effects of the local anaesthetic will take effect.

For both the multiple and single approach, the easiest way to apply this technique, is to come close to the nerve from the side and not directly in the midline (see above illustration). The NPB is unique in dentistry as it is the only block that acts bilaterally as it can locally anaesthetise from the canine to canine in the maxilla: 13 to 23 (UR 3 to UL 3).

The Greater Palatine Block (GPB). The Greater Palatine Nerve carries sensory fibres from the Pterygopalatine ganglion and parasympathetic fibres from both Greater and Deep Petrosal Nerves (supplying the minor salivary glands in the palate). The end-fibres of the Greater Palatine and Naso Palatine Nerves intertwine to supply the: Gingival, periodontal connective and dental tissues of the upper arch. Blocking these nerves will anaesthetize the tissues of the

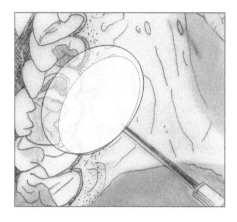

hard palate from the distal aspect, all the way forward to the canine and laterally to the midline palatal septum.

The foramen from which the Greater Palatine Nerve emerges into the oral cavity can be felt as a depression in the posterior area of the hard palate. This depression presents as a soft spot most commonly found half way between the gingival margin and the midline of the palate, on a line drawn from the distal aspect of one second molar to the midline. This can be found 5 mm to 1 cm ahead of the junction of the hard and soft palate.

As with all injections, when administering the GPB, aspirate first and only when safe to proceed, then insert your needle to a depth of 5mm until contact is made with the palatal bone and slowly introduce 0.5 mL of local anaesthetic.

From a safety point, when performing the GPB, be very careful not to penetrate the greater palatine foramen to a significant degree, if at all. However, if an intentional CNV_2 block is planned and you wish to anaesthetize: All the maxillary teeth their periodontal tissues, the hard and the soft palate, the sinuses, and extra orally: one side of the nose, an entire orbit, the upper cheek, the lower eyelid, and the remainder of the one side of the patient's face, then the Greater Palatine Foramen is the ideal place to introduce a local anaesthetic, with the desired effect of blocking CNV_2 if that is intended[96]. If it is not and most dentists in general practice do not need such profound anaesthesia which constitutes a regional block, then please be very careful with the depth, the delivery and the dose used when considering a GPB.

The key factor is the CNV_2 can be located some 30mm deep to the entrance of the Greater Palatine foramen. With anything less than this, you are in fairly safe territory. However some 1 in 7 of your patients will have a clinically significant degree of anatomical variation in the Maxillary Nerve and depth alone may not confer absolute protection from an inadvertent CNV_2 block[97].

In addition to the distress, with the risk of a vasovagal syncope, there is once more the risk of the accidental vascular injection with haematoma or systemic circulatory effect that may cardiovascularly compromise the patient if an anaesthetic containing epinephrine is used.

At the time of writing the most recent assessment of the Greater Palatine canal, using post-mortem samples has demonstrated not only a great variation in the pathway and multiple branching of the Greater Palatine nerve, but the entire CNV_2 and its relationship to the Maxillary artery being highly variable too. Your knowledge of these variations may have important implications for improving the safety of anaesthesia and those dental procedures performed in and around the palate, the maxilla and the upper dentition[98].

Mandibular local anaesthesia

Having considered maxillary local anaesthesia in some detail, we will now move on to consider mandibular local anaesthesia. Many if not all of the safety factors for maxillary local anaesthesia can also be applied to mandibular local anaesthesia. Before going on to describe the techniques available, a brief revision of the nerve supply of the mandibular region would be prudent.

The CN V$_3$

It is of course the Mandibular Division (CNV$_3$), the largest division of the Trigeminal Nerve that provides both a sensory and a motor supply to the oral and dental tissues associated with the mandible. In common with the Ophthalmic Division (CNV$_1$) and Maxillary Division (CNV$_2$), the CNV$_3$ arises from the Trigeminal Ganglion located in Meckel's Cave (near to the apex of the Petrous part of the Temporal Bone). The CNV$_3$ departs from the skull via the Foramen Ovale located in the greater wing of the Sphenoid bone. The Foramen Ovale can be found to the outside and just behind the Foramen Rotundum (from where CNV$_2$ emerges), but to the inside and just in front of the Foramen Spinosum, from where the Middle Meningeal Artery the Middle Meningeal Vein, and the Meningeal branch of the CNV3: The Mandibular Nerve re-enters the cranium. From here, CNV$_3$ begins its interesting journey reporting sensational events and controlling masticatory motion to and from the sensory and motor cortices respectively.

Exiting the skull, the CNV$_3$ motor root gets a head-start from the CNV$_3$ sensory root but soon reunites with it below the Foramen Ovale in the Infratemporal Fossa. Here, the CNV$_3$ passes down from the skull between the Tensor Veli Palatini to the inside and the Lateral Pterygoid on the outside, throwing out a sensory Meningeal branch, a motor nerve branch to the Medial Pterygoid and motor supply to the Tensor Tympani and the Tensor Veli Palatini muscles.

After this, CNV_3 divides into two trunks, a small one to the front and a large one to the rear. Both of these trunks are mixed sensory-motor nerves. Firstly the small anterior trunk provides sensory input from the Long Buccal Nerve supplying the cheek and the first and second mandibular molars. There is a motor output to the four masticatory muscles: the Masseter, the Temporalis (with Sphenomandiularis), the Medial and the Lateral Pterygoids.

While the facial muscles of expression are "spoken-for" by the Facial Nerve (CNVII), the CNV_3 "answers-to" the masticatory muscles, as these arise from the First Pharyngeal Arch, whereas the CNVII and muscles of facial expression come from the Second Pharyngeal Arch.

There is also a Buccal Branch of the Facial Nerve and this provides motor supply to the Buccinator Muscle, although both motor and sensory buccal nerves (from two different embryonic origins are present in the facial musculature). Additionally, the CNVII derived Buccal Nerve supplies a sensory branch to the patient's cheek too.

Moving on to the large posterior trunk of CNV_3, there is a motor output to the Mylohyoid (which comes off the Inferior Alveolar Nerve just before it enters the Mandibular Foramen. This branch also supplies the Anterior Belly of the Digastric.

The three nerve branches remaining from CNV_3's posterior trunk are:

1. The Auriculotemporal Nerve. This nerve departs from CNV_3 and interestingly forms something like the eye of a needle through which the Middle Meningeal Artery passes thread-like, before the nerve reunites.

After this, the nerve passes between the Sphenomandibular Ligament and the neck of the mandible. At this point, a supply to the Parotid Gland departs from the nerve, which then turns upwards, outwards and forwards before passing over the Zygomatic arch but deep to the Superficial Temporal Artery to supply the earlobe and temple.

This superior root of the Auriculotemporal nerve is purely sensory and earlier in its journey, fibres of this branch passed straight through the Otic Ganglion without stopping (or synapsing).

The Otic Ganglion located below the Foramen Ovale in the Infratemporal Fossa lies medial to the CNV_3 and contains synapses for the Parotid Gland's parasympathetic supply from the Glossopharyngeal Nerve (CNIX).

The sensory branches supply the outside of the ear drum, the earlobe and temporal regions....after all it is the Auriculotemporal nerve and it mostly does what it says. There are additional branches which provide the main sensory supply to the TMJ together with masseteric and deep temporal nerves too.

As stated, those nerve fibres which stopped to synapse in the Otic Ganglion form an inferior root carrying postganglionic fibres to the Parotid Gland. These parasympathetic fibres originate from the Glossopharyngeal Nerve (CN IX) and are transported into the CNV_3 via the Tympanic Nerve. On their way to join CNV_3, the CNIX fibres feed into a plexus of nerves in the inner ear. From here the Lesser Petrosal nerve then synapses in the Otic Ganglion.

Postganglionic sympathetic fibres are picked up and carried along on this nerve together with their arterial supply.

At this stage in the Mandibular nerve's journey we have a neural complex comprising a combination of postganglionic parasympathetic nerve fibres and postsynaptic sympathetic nerve fibres.

All together this forms the inferior root of the Auriculotemporal nerve which provides the Parotid Gland with its secretomotor supply. Even though the Auriculotemporal nerve is not the target for dental anaesthesia, it is worth knowing something about its anatomical path to be aware of and understand the following three clinical matters:

i. **The Auriculotemporal nerve is the main nerve supply to the TMJ**. As the Auriculotemporal nerve passes posteriorly to the condyles of the mandible, nerve injury is unfortunately a common occurrence, not only from participation in contact and non-contact sport, but also on those occasions when TMJ surgery is indicated. Injuries to the TMJ innervation can result in anaesthesia or paraesthesia not only to the jaw joint but to the entire auriculo-temporal territory supplied by this nerve.

ii. **Parotid gland injury, pathology and surgery** can also give rise to complications should Auriculotemporal nerve fibres become incorrectly reattached. Given the complex input to this nerve, it becomes easier to understand the peculiar presentation of Frey's Syndrome. This syndrome although relatively rare, is characterised by inappropriate cheek perspiration, rather than salivation when the Parotid gland is stimulated. This is due to the severed parasympathetic fibres reconnecting to the sympathetic nerve plexus supplying the sweat glands of the cheek and face.

iii. **The Pleomorphic Salivary Adenoma (PSA)** is one of the most common oral neoplasias and this most frequently occurs in the Parotid Gland. Considering the current increase in use of mobile phones with the attendant risks to sensitive tissues from radiation in the electromagnetic spectrum, the question of whether an increase in injury, pathology and surgery to the Parotid Gland will in time give rise to an increase in Frey's Syndrome would be an important question to ask[99].

The next two nerves arising from the CNV_3 are the Lingual Nerve and the Inferior Alveolar Nerve and you will already be aware of the safety critical issues when working close to these nerves:

2. The Lingual Nerve provides a sensory secreto-motor supply, achieving this by carrying fibres from The Facial Nerve (CNVII). These relay taste sensations via the Chorda Tympani, from the anterior $2/3^{rd}$ of the tongue, while the posterior $1/3^{rd}$ of the tongue is supplied by the Glossopharyngeal Nerve (CNIX). The lingual nerve lies beneath the <u>Lateral Pterygoid muscle</u>, medial to and in front of the <u>Inferior Alveolar Nerve</u> and is joined to this nerve by a branch which may cross over the <u>Internal Maxillary Artery</u>.

The above noted <u>Chorda Tympani</u> also carries parasympathetic fibres to the <u>Submandibular Ganglion</u>, which is suspended from the Lingual Nerve by two very fine twig-like nerves.

Passing lateral to the Medial Pterygoid and positioned against the medial aspect of the Mandibular Ramus, the Lingual Nerve crosses over both the Superior Pharyngeal Constrictor and the Styloglossus muscles to run along the inferio-lateral margin of the tongue. Between the Hyoglossus and the Submandibular Salivary Gland, the Lingual Nerve runs towards the mandibular midline crossing over Wharton's duct of the Submandibular Salivary Gland. Located just below the tongue and just below the surface of the oral mucosa, the Lingual Nerve eventually terminates as the Sub-Lingual Nerve.

We have already covered Lingual Nerve injuries caused most frequently either by surgery or local anaesthetic (Articaine) use. Overall, these risks have been quantified by the Royal College Surgeons (England) as: 2% Temporary Injury and 0.2% Permanent Injury[100].

With these risks in mind, avoiding the use of Articaine for an IANB, keeping away from a lingual approach towards the wisdom tooth, favouring coronectomy, rather than outright extraction and lastly referring to a surgical specialist are the cautious and prudent options to avoid or at least reduce the risk of injury to the lingual nerve when operating on lower wisdom teeth[101,102,103].

Whatever options are explained and whichever procedure is decided upon, given the significant risk of an injury that may carry negative consequences for the patient in terms of pain, discomfort and their psychological well being, within your consenting process and in accordance with the ideals of Montgomery Consent, the risk of a Lingual Nerve injury must be clearly explained to the patient.

This brief revision of the origins, the destination and function of the Lingual nerve should assist in your safety critical consenting process and in upholding your clinico-legal responsibilities.

3. The Inferior Alveolar Nerve (IAN). From a dental point, this is the nerve we are really interested in when using local anaesthetic in the lower arch. Just a little bit higher than the area where we apply local anaesthetic but not long after departing from the CNV_3, the IAN travels down a groove on the medial surface of the mandibular ramus, just behind the lateral pterygoid muscle where it gives off a motor branch to Mylohyoid and then another motor branch to the Anterior Belly of the Digastric.

Both the nerves to Mylohyoid and the Anterior Belly of the Digastric also have a sensory element[104]. The mesial root of the mandibular first molar and the chin can be innervated by branches from the nerve to Mylohyoid. In addition to these nerves, there is an incredible range of variation not only with the IAN but throughout the entire path of the CNV_3. Communications have been noted between the Auriculotemporal nerve and the IAN, between the Mylohyoid nerve, the Lingual nerve and the Auriculotemporal nerve[105,106].

Furthermore, communications between IAN and the Lateral Pterygoid have also been documented and the presence of these anatomical variations could provide one explanation for the failure rate in IAN Block being recorded as 20% to 25%[104,107 108]. This percentage could indicate that some 3/4 of those attending the dentist have a textbook anatomy of their head and neck, or alternatively up to 1/4 of all dental professionals (Including ourselves) need to revise our knowledge of anatomy!

After these variations, the IAN disappears down the mandibular foramen and into the mandibular canal, from where it assumes a predictable and purely sensory role.

While in the mandibular canal, the nerve supply to all the lower teeth from the molars to the premolars is taken care of. An Inferior dental plexus also gives off small gingival and small dental nerves to the buccal segment teeth. Moving forward to the bucco-labial area where the 1st and 2nd Premolars are or should be, unless an orthodontist has been exercising their powers of arch contraction or premolar extraction, the Mental Foramen marks the other end of the Mandibular Canal.

Emerging from this foramen, the sensory supply to the lower lip and chin can be found in the form of the Mental Nerve. Meanwhile back inside the mandible, the IAN continues on its sensory way becoming the Incisive Nerve delivering the sensory output from the Canines and Incisors.

In common with the Lingual Nerve, there is a risk of injury to the Inferior Alveolar Nerve (IAN). However, while the former is at risk from its exposed position and morphology, the latter is more at risk from cutting and compression as it lies inside an unyielding canal within dense mandibular bone. As with lingual nerve injuries, the effect on the patient could be catastrophic and so the risks do need to be carefully and clearly explained in your consenting phase of treatment for the lower arch as it is for the upper arch. If Montgomery Consent is the keystone in the arch of your treatment planning, it follows that the foundation upon which this arch is built will be your thorough and intimate knowledge of the origin, the destination and the function of the Trigeminal Nerve, especially its Mandibular Division: CNV_3

> **Regular review and revision with the aid of an anatomy textbook is time well spent.**
> **If you work in the UK, this should form part of your Enhanced CPD for the GDC.**

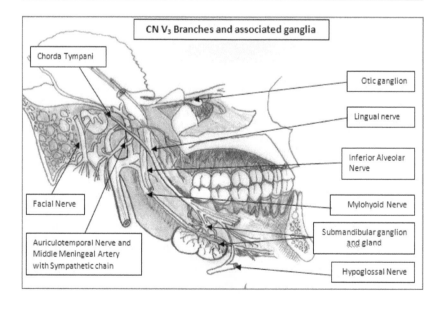

CN V₃ Branches and associated ganglia

Chorda Tympani

Otic ganglion

Lingual nerve

Inferior Alveolar Nerve

Facial Nerve

Mylohyoid Nerve

Submandibular ganglion and gland

Auriculotemporal Nerve and Middle Meningeal Artery with Sympathetic chain

Hypoglossal Nerve

This small diagram shows the relationship of the Otic Ganglion to the root of the Trigeminal Nerve (CNV) within the Infratemporal Fossa. As previously mentioned the Middle Meningeal Artery can be seen passing through the Auriculotemporal Nerve like a thread through the eye of a needle. In

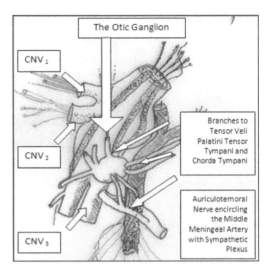

anatomical terms, this is a slightly unusual arrangement. While arteries usually carry a sympathetic supply in their walls, the Auriculotemporal nerve does not supply the Middle Meningeal Artery. Nevertheless, in addition to a somatosensory input, it carries the CNIX parasympathetic output to the Parotid Gland.

The following illustration shows the Maxillary and Mandibular nerves: (CNV$_2$ and CNV$_3$) from their lateral aspect, in addition the Chorda Tympani's connections from the CNVII to the CNV Lingual Nerve and onto the Submandibular ganglion can be seen.

The Chorda Tympani transmits both inhibitory (pain) and stimulatory (taste) sensations from the anterior 2/3^{rds} of the tongue.

You will remember this fact well, as the Chorda Tympani has earned something of an unfortunate reputation, being the subject of (in)-appropriate undergraduate anatomy class humour. It would of course be indecorous to repeat that joke here.

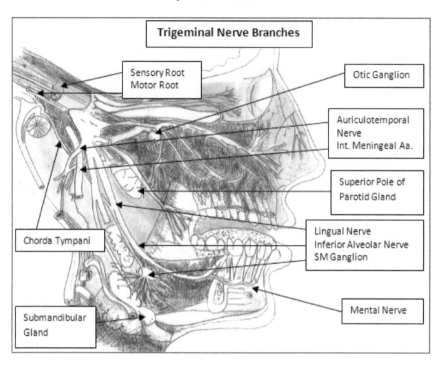

Trigeminal Nerve Branches

Sensory Root
Motor Root

Otic Ganglion

Auriculotemporal
Nerve
Int. Meningeal Aa.

Superior Pole of
Parotid Gland

Chorda Tympani

Lingual Nerve
Inferior Alveolar Nerve
SM Ganglion

Mental Nerve

Submandibular
Gland

The techniques for mandibular local anaesthesia

The Inferior Alveolar Nerve Block. (The IANB).

From the previous descriptions in this section and the two diagrams illustrating the path and relations of the CNV3, it is not surprising that the Inferior Alveolar Nerve Block (IANB) carries the highest risk of an intravascular injection accident and so aspiration prior to injection is mandatory.

However, once successfully sited, the IANB will anaesthetize all of the mandibular teeth from the wisdom teeth to the central incisors. Not only will one side of the lower dental arch be anaesthetized, all of the intra-oral soft and connective tissues from the premolars anteriorly including the gingiva and periodontium will be included in the side to which this block has been applied. In addition, the extra-oral tissues around the chin and lower lip will be involved when an IANB is used and the patient reporting symptoms of numbness in these areas is a good indication that your IANB has been successfully delivered.

The technique we know today as the IANB was first described by William Stewart Halsted and Richard John Hall around 1884/5[109]. In essence, with correct application, the IANB is not so much a block, it might be more accurately termed an oral regional anaesthetic[110].

The IANB is delivered from a **27 Gauge 32 mm** needle and not with the narrower and shorter 21mm or 25 mm needles frequently used for upper arch anaesthesia. Although there are techniques advocating the use of shorter needles and there are those who describe bending the needle at its hub to gain better access to the IAN before it enters the mandibular foramen. However, given the risk of precipitating a fatigue fracture, coupled with the hazards and complexities associated with recovering fractured needles, such methods cannot be considered to be either sensible or safe[111].

The IANB technique.

The patient is asked to open their mouth, but not wide open, while jaw support is given by your hand or that of your dental assistant. An approach is made from the opposite corner of the mouth from just above the level of the opposite premolars.

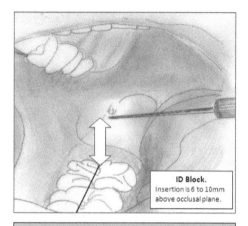

ID Block.
Insertion is 6 to 10mm above occlusal plane.

Your syringe is positioned across the occlusal plane of the lower arch towards the soft tissues of the opposite side approximately 15mm above the mandibular occlusal plane. There is evidence to suggest that at this increased level

Height from the occlusal plane is critical for the IANB to be safe in avoiding vasculature and being successful in targeting the intended nerve.

(normally the height is 6 to 10 mm; there is a greater than 10% increase in IANB anaesthesia being successful[112].

As stated above and from a safety point: The height separation from the occlusal plane is critically important in avoiding the vasculature associated with the IANB and also in avoiding delivery of anaesthetic to an area below or beyond where the IAN has entered the inferior alveolar canal.

Your anaesthetic needle is advanced through the mucosa and soft tissues to a depth of 25 mm until the bone of the mandible is contacted, then it is withdrawn by 1 to 2 mm only. Insertion is never to the needle hub for the reasons given before and at such a level you will have gone past your target point. It is essential to leave around 1cm of the needle showing.

Should metal fracture occur, the exposed end of the broken needle can be gripped with set of Spencer-Wells needle holders and will be easily retrieved from the patient's mucosal tissues.

The alternative is an urgent visit to your local hospital A and E unit, an emergency appointment with your maxillofacial surgical colleagues and a general anaesthetic procedure to recover the needle. I am sure you can appreciate such an outcome being well beyond a nightmare for your patient and more than a professional inconvenience for yourself.

For the IANB, the point of entry can be defined as 6 to 10mm above the occlusal plane, between the tendon of the Temporalis muscle anteriorly and the Pterygomandibular raphe posteriorly.

After a clear aspiration is demonstrated, up to 1.5 mL of local anaesthetic can then be safely and slowly injected into the area around and above the lingula, where both the IAN and the Lingual Nerve are located.

Should you choose to specifically target the Lingual nerve then following the deposition of 1mL to 1.5mL, the remaining contents of the anaesthetic cartridge (some 0.5 mL or 0.7mL) can be administered at a depth 1cm superficial to that depth just above the periosteum around the Lingula, where the IAN was previously placed.

With so many variations in the distribution of CNV_3 its accessory and collateral innervations, unsurprisingly numerous techniques have evolved to capture this nerve within a net of local anaesthesia. While mastery of the IANB will only come from your knowledge of head and neck anatomy, there are times when an alternative technique to capture more than one nerve is needed. The two alternative techniques we might consider using in dental practice are the Gow-Gates and the Vazirani-Akinosi:

Firstly:

The Gow-Gates technique is an open mouth technique which can capture the following nerves[112-113]:

I. Inferior Alveolar Nerve (IAN)
II. Auriculotemporal Nerve
III. Lingual Nerve
IV. Buccal Nerve
V. Mylohyoid Nerve

If placed accurately; repeated injections are not needed, the Gow-Gates technique is useful for the needle phobic patient and for those patients undergoing sedation procedures where time is always crucial. An accurately placed Gow-Gates nerve block will leave the patient with a profoundly deep and effective local anaesthesia after only one injection and do so in a very short period of time.

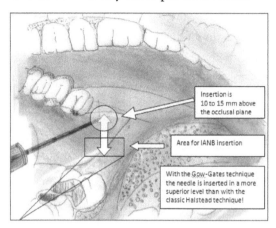

Insertion is 10 to 15 mm above the occlusal plane

Area for IANB insertion

With the Gow-Gates technique the needle is inserted in a more superior level than with the classic Halstead technique!

With this technique, the patient is instructed to open their mouth as wide as possible. This encourages the condyle to rotate/translate forward and downward on their articular eminences.

The needle is placed in front of and to the side of the condyle, just below the insertion of the lateral pterygoid.

By placing the fingers of one hand on the patient's condyle, you can gently pull at the corner of their mouth and retract the soft buccal cheek tissues with your thumb. In your other hand the syringe is introduced from the opposite canine with the needle directed towards the distobuccal cusp of the second molar.

The mucosa is penetrated to a depth of 25 mm with the end point just below and to the outside of the head of the condyle. When mandibular bone is contacted, aspiration must demonstrate that no vascular tissues have been compromised and then following this, after withdrawal of 1 to 2 mm, the local anaesthetic is then very slowly introduced.

Although the Gow-Gates is a block technique, local anaesthetic is placed superior to the division of the CNV_3 in the upper area of the Pterygomandibular space and the local anaesthetic then diffuses onto the nerves achieving its effect by infiltration.

Secondly:

The Vazirani-Akinosi closed mouth nerve block. Is the technique which is of particular use when patients cannot or will not open their mouths, either through trismus, trauma or trepidation particularly when they are undergoing conscious sedation.

As useful as this technique is, it must never ever be used forcefully on the patient who refuses treatment. It is sometimes the case that during a dental sedation procedure, a patient will resolutely clamp their mouth shut, only to open it when the effects of a local anaesthetic take hold.

I. With respect to this issue, it is wholly inappropriate to force, or attempt to force the patient's mouth open while they are sedated in an effort to introduce a local anaesthetic.

II. It is also inadvisable to increase the dose of an IV or RA sedative agent to achieve a result which can be accomplished easily and safely with patience and the use of an appropriate local anaesthetic technique.

III. When handling any sharp instrument, an uncooperative patient is a dangerous patient.

IV. Not only are they dangerous to themselves, they are dangerous to your colleagues and to you.

V. When faced with such difficulties, it is better to modify your treatment plan, accordingly downgrading the extent of dentistry that you wish to achieve within the scope of consent that has been obtained but might no longer be maintained.

The Vazirani-Akinosi block will anaesthetize the IAN, the Lingual, the Long Buccal and the Mylohyoid nerves[114]. It is administered while the patient's jaw is closed, ideally when in a resting position and not with the masseter clenched as this can present quite an insurmountable barrier to the needle. As with the IANB and the Gow-Gates technique, **a 27 or 25 Gauge needle of 32 mm length** is used. However with the

Vazirani-Akinosi block, this is introduced at an even higher level than with the previous two techniques. This time the needle is inserted parallel to the maxillary occlusal plane at the apex of the buccal vestibule.

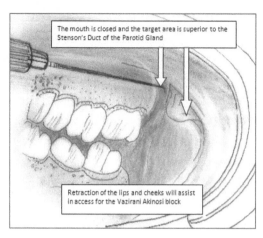

The mouth is closed and the target area is superior to the Stenson's Duct of the Parotid Gland

Retraction of the lips and cheeks will assist in access for the Vazirani Akinosi block

Your needle will be directed towards the mandibular ramus and if there is any deflection then it is towards the ramus itself, rather than towards the vulnerable vasculature in the Parotid gland and other soft tissues. Penetration to a depth of some 25mm or approximately half way along the mandibular ramus is required. One difficulty we have with the Vazirani- Akinosi technique is the blind nature of its delivery. There is no end point in bone from which we can retract before delivering the local anaesthetic. Despite this, we must still aspirate before drug delivery and with a 32mm needle, the boss or needle hub should be no deeper in the patient's mouth than the distal aspect of the upper first molar. If you or one of your colleagues has previously extracted this tooth, then placing the needle boss against the mesial buccal aspect of the second molar is the absolute limit of penetration with this technique.

Variations of Halsted, Gow-Gates and Vazirani-Akinosi

As mentioned there are possibly as many variations of the IANB as there are anatomical pathways of the IAN. Most of these techniques are variations on the three classic techniques: The Halsted IANB, the Gow-Gates and the Vazirani-Akinosi. The only thing they have in common: They are all named after those who first described the technique. As of 2014, there are an additional seven techniques to choose from, each with only a slight variation from the previous one! Each new method is stated to be better than the others. Despite such claims, each of these new techniques has shortcomings. Should you be interested in these new methods, the following is a brief summary of what is available:

1. The Thangavelu technique 2012, with this procedure the needle is advanced, inserted and repeatedly moved around the IAN. This sounds painful and it probably is. To begin with, the distance between the upper and lower arches is divided in two. An imaginary line is drawn on this plane and 6mm to 8mm above this, your needle is advanced into the mucosa. Once in the mucosa and against the bone, the syringe is now moved to form an angle from the opposite canine towards a point up to 10mm behind the anterior border of the mandibular ramus. The needle is then repeatedly inserted, withdrawn then reinserted to a depth of 21 to 24 mm... Surprisingly despite this somewhat inelegant approach, the author's report no complications and the stated failure rate is only 1 in 20[115]. This is a lot better than the previously noted 1 in 4 for Halsted's IANB. Critically thinking about this method, it cannot be anything other than exceptionally traumatic for the periosteum, the vasculature and the patient's nerves.

2. Not satisfied with tearing up the periosteum and turning the IAN into a pin cushion, Thangavelu and colleagues didn't give up and returned with a variation on the above technique. This time abandoning their triangles and geometry, instead, relying on some good old anatomy, Thangavelu recommended using the internal oblique ridge of the mandible as a reference point. Their technique is to place your thumb over the retromolar area and the edge of the internal oblique ridge. Insert your needle 6-8 mm above the midpoint of the thumb and 2 mm behind the internal oblique ridge. The syringe is directed into this area from the opposite side at the lower premolars. Penetration of the needle to 15-20 mm should touch the mandibular bone and the lingual nerve. Once more success is reported to be 95%[116]. If you don't manage to give yourself an inoculation injury or anaesthetize your thumb using this

technique, then well done. Persevering with this technique could result in tearing the lingual nerve. If you feel the urge to try this out, then make sure your thumb and the patient's lingual nerve are well out of the needle's way first.

3.   The Boonsiriseth technique from 2013. Take one 30mm needle and place a rubber stopper at a point beyond which you do not wish to penetrate the patient's soft tissues. Place the syringe along the occlusal plane of the same side you wish to anaesthetize and then slowly introduce the needle into the mucosa, up to the depth of the rubber stopper. The needle should not contact the bone of the mandibular ramus. The two critical factors here are the angle and the depth to which the needle will penetrate those deeper soft tissues which are vulnerable to trauma. The advantages of this technique include a possible reduction in the pain described by the patient and more importantly a claimed reduced risk of nerve trauma. However, with this technique: Positive aspirations were noted once in every twenty injections, possibly due to the vasculature lying in the path of the needle[117].

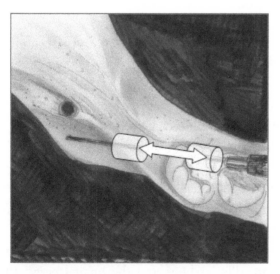

The problems with this technique are the rubber stopper can move up or down the needle and a deeper than anticipated penetration can result, with risk of tissue damage.

The insertion angle; although away from the IAN and the lingual nerve, it is towards deeper tissues, thus the risk of a vascular injection accident with systemic complications is increased.

With this technique, a 30mm needle inserted in this angle could cause havoc with the vasculature in the pterygomandibular space and with this in mind, perhaps this technique is better left in the library and not attempted in the clinic.

4. Moving on from the risk of deep tissue trauma and needle stick injuries, in 2011 Palti and co-workers described a method of placing wires along anatomical landmarks in dried mandibles and the point at which they intersected could be used to indicate where you might accurately place a needle to intercept the IAN[118]. It might not come as a surprise to learn this method has been stated to require some more work before it could be unleashed on unsuspecting patients. Perhaps the only ones who might be interested in placing wires in patient's mouths are orthodontists and they never seem to use anaesthetics anyway. When they ask others to do so, a significant number of incorrect extractions are then caused from administrative errors in: their/your/our referral letters.

Back to the drawing board with this technique...

5. For those patients with coagulation defects, a sensible safety critical approach was described by Galdames, Lopez and Matamala in 2008. With this technique, local anaesthetic solution is deposited in the retromolar triangle. This area is bounded by the medial surface of the mandibular ramus, the distal surface of the lower third molar and the temporal crest supero-distally. In the retromolar triangle there is a vascular anastomosis of the Buccal Artery perfusing the IAN with arterioles as it lies in the Inferior Alveolar Canal. It has been proposed that infiltration perfusion of this area will lead to IAN anaesthesia. However the time to onset of anaesthesia was noted to be over 10 minutes and the success rate was very low at 72%[119]. From a safety point, this technique will certainly reduce the risk of an intravascular injection accident, but it will require time and thus patience until a sufficient level of anaesthesia can be reached to enable dental treatment to proceed. While this approach

is useful for those patients with coagulation defects, one might also ask with such risks; what level of dental surgery would one reasonably undertake that could require such a degree of anaesthesia in the first place?

6. In the anterior border of the mandibular ramus there is a space between the Medial Pterygoid and the tendon of Temporalis. Injecting directly into this Pterygomandibular space has been described by Takasugi and co-workers as a safe means of achieving IAN anaesthesia. Insertion of the needle to a depth of 10mm, above the occlusal plane by 10mm and at a point lateral to the Pterygomandibular raphe, with the syringe being positioned at an angle from the contralateral mandibular molar has been stated to reduce the risk of injury to both the IAN and the Lingual nerve while decreasing the chances of a vascular injection accident. Precise positioning of the needle with this technique is facilitated with Computerised Tomography. Despite the use of such highly accurate imaging, only a 75% success rate has been reported[120].

Radiographic imaging has also been used to demonstrate that diffusion of local anaesthetic solution in the Pterygomandibular space occurs both rapidly and extensively to the IAN and Lingual nerve, doing so without the direct involvement of any large blood vessels[121].

The results from these six recent studies confirm that even with modern research methodologies utilizing the latest imaging techniques, the rate of success versus the risk of complications for an accurately placed IANB, as originally described by Halsted and Hall in 1884/5, then refined by Jorgensen and Hayden in 1967 is still the best technique with which to achieve safe lower arch dental anaesthesia[122 123]. However, even when properly administered, the failure rate of the Halsted IANB has been stated by Malamed to be some 15% to 20%[96].

If we consider these modern attempts at neuro-regional anaesthesia, they depend on your recognising intra and extra oral anatomical landmarks for success. Looking at in another way, all of these studies are a group effort at improving the success rate of the IANB. Its lack of success arises from a variation in the anatomy of neurovasculature closely associated with the mandibular ramus and indeed variation in the form of the mandible itself. When these factors are coupled with a working knowledge of clinically oriented anatomy that needs to be quite literally, if not actually, at your fingertips every day (and it often isn't), it becomes easy to see why the IANB has the highest failure rate of all dental injections.

We must also keep in mind that clinical anatomy is not static, it is dynamic and when the patient's mouth is neither open, nor closed, but somewhere in-between, with a syringe and needle thrust amid the dental arches, the relationship of the IAN and the lingual nerve to anatomical reference points becomes entirely unpredictable. For all these reasons, the IAN becomes a difficult nerve to block and the IANB will also have a high risk rate for vascular accidents too.

As if these obstacles were not enough to deal with, the numerous minor nerve branches accompanying the CNV_3 will continue their supply from the mandibular teeth after delivery of anaesthetic to the main trunk of the IAN has taken effect. Such collateral nerve supply is often the reason for an IANB failing to give pulpal anaesthesia.

When everything is considered, it is quite remarkable if we think of Halsted in 1884 discovering, developing then describing what has become the IANB and doing so without the advantageous means that benefit modern researchers. Halsted's achievements are even more outstanding when we consider he was self-medicating with morphine while in the grip of an addiction to cocaine!

Additional Techniques

The Lingual Nerve Block. On its own, this block will anaesthetize the floor of the mouth and tongue from the third molar anteriorly to the midline. When performing the IANB, the Lingual nerve is frequently involved too. So the object of this nerve block is your ability to solely target the lingual nerve without the IAN. It is more often the case, that the IAN is anaesthetized but not the lingual nerve with any injection in this area. As the Lingual nerve is positioned more superficially than the IAN, in theory any anaesthetic deposited to a depth of only 10mm, but in the same location as the IAN, should encircle this nerve giving the required anaesthetic effect, without affecting the IAN (too much). In reality, this is seldom the case and both the IAN and the Lingual nerve will be both affected.

The Long Buccal Nerve Block. This can achieve anaesthetizia by injecting to a depth of 3mm to 5mm into the distal aspect of the buccal vestibule just medial to the coronoid notch and opposite the second or the third lower molars. Local anaesthetic placed here will anaesthetize the periodontium, the gingiva and the buccal soft tissues on the lateral aspect of the mandibular molars. Very little anaesthetic is actually required for this infiltration and you could or should usefully apply the remaining 0.25ml after giving an IANB to anaesthetize the Long Buccal nerve providing additional anaesthetic cover when working in the lower arch.

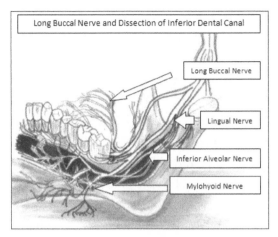

Long Buccal Nerve and Dissection of Inferior Dental Canal

Long Buccal Nerve

Lingual Nerve

Inferior Alveolar Nerve

Mylohyoid Nerve

The Long Buccal Nerve arises from the Anterior Branch of the Mandibular Nerve.

Passing downwards and forwards between the two heads of the Lateral Pterygoid, it emerges into the oral mucosa on the anterior border of the Masseter. From here it crosses the ramus level with the occlusal plane close to the second or the third molar giving a sensory supply as seen in this illustration.

Mental and Incisive Nerve Blocks

The Mental and Incisive Nerves are the terminal branches of the Inferior Alveolar Nerve and can easily be anaesthetized at the mental foramen located between the apices of the mandibular premolars. Please note: Following orthodontic extractions these reference points for the mental nerve will be altered. In cases such as this, which are increasingly frequent, the mental foramen can be accurately located with a periapical radiograph. Whereas the mental nerve exits from its foramen dividing into three branches (one ascending and two descending) providing sensations for: The lower lip, the chin, the bucco-labial mucosa around the incisors, the canines and the pre-molars; the incisive nerve remains in the mandible giving a sensory supply to the lower incisors and their gingival tissues. Of particular interest in almost 20% of your patients: the Incisive canal and its nerve terminate in the mandibular midline and so a cross-over or bilateral innervation of the lower incisors will be present[124]. In developmental terms this may be an elegant example of a natural safety mechanism or innate system-redundancy. Such duplication ensures that should one set of nerves become damaged or disconnected through injury or illness, then another set of nerves remains intact to give a basic sensory input.

For the one in five of our patients with such cross-over innervations, a bilateral injection to ensure adequate anaesthesia when working on the lower incisors will be helpful. The Incisive nerve will also have some communication with sensory branches of the Facial nerve. Given the supply of the major salivary glands (through the CNVII and the Chorda Tympani), feedback from the incisors and other teeth when chewing on something requiring more saliva to aid mastication, stimulation of the salivary glands from additional neural communication across the embryonic arch territories would be an advantageous natural development.

While an IANB should cover the territories supplied by both the Mental and the Incisive nerves, there will be many occasions when anaesthesia localized to the anterior mandibular arch is needed and in these instances a Mental or Incisive nerve block should be considered. However it must be noted that the lingual soft tissues of those teeth supplied by the Mental and Incisive nerves will not be covered by a block of these nerves and supplemental periodontal infiltration anaesthesia may be required.

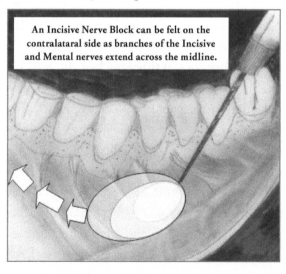

An Incisive Nerve Block can be felt on the contralataral side as branches of the Incisive and Mental nerves extend across the midline.

The technique for the Mental and Incisive blocks is almost identical. A 25mm short needle of 25 or 27 Gauge is introduced into the mucobuccal sulcus in close proximity to the Mental Foramen. The needle tip is passed into the mucosa to a depth of only 5 mm or so, with the bevel facing mandibular bone. As always a negative aspiration is required. After this, 0.5mL to 1mL of anaesthetic can be slowly delivered. The block to the Incisive nerve differs from that to the Mental Nerve, in that application of finger pressure for 2 minutes is needed to ensure the anaesthetic will directly enter the Mental foramen and thus block the Incisive nerves.

The buccal soft tissues will be excluded from an IANB, whereas the lingual soft tissues will not be covered by a block to the Mental nerve.

The previous pages contained relevant safety related information on the techniques to achieve local anaesthesia in the upper and the lower arches. In addition to these basic procedures for infiltration and block anaesthesia, the following techniques can be usefully deployed. These can be used equally in the upper or the lower arch.

1. Intraperiodontal or Intraligamentary infiltration. Some 0.2mL of local anaesthetic can be introduced into the periodontal tissues to achieve pulpal anaesthesia. If you choose to utilize this technique, then deliver the local anaesthetic at a very slow rate, as any injection into the periodontal tissues is noted to be disproportionately painful for the patient.

2. Intraseptal or gingival papillary injection. Again some 0.2mL of local anaesthetic can be infiltrated in the gingival tissues between the teeth. Your needle should enter the soft tissues until the bone is contacted, with the needle pointing towards the apex of the tooth you wish to work on. As always a slow infiltration is less painful than a rapid forceful injection. Nevertheless, some considerable pressure needs to be applied to deposit sufficient local anaesthetic.

3. The intraosseous injection. At one time this was a very fashionable technique, principally due to the immediacy with which local anaesthesia sets in. In recent times, its popularity seems to have diminished, possibly due the steps involved with this technique: Next to the tooth you wish to work on, a small hole is trephined

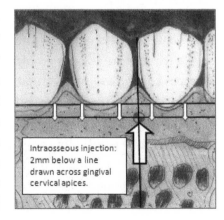

Intraosseous injection: 2mm below a line drawn across gingival cervical apices.

through (the buccal) mucosa, into the cortical plate towards the deeper cancellous alveolar bone. Into this hole, a small bore needle can deposit local anaesthetic at a slow rate and without the pressures needed for the previous two techniques. Specific sighting requirements are needed for trephination: One line is drawn horizontally along the gingival margins of the teeth and another line is then drawn from the apex of the interdental papilla. The hole is then drilled 2 mm apical to the perpendicular intersection of these two lines. Care should be taken to avoid using this technique anywhere near the area of the Mental foramen. The amount of anaesthetic is relatively small, in the range of 0.2mL to 1.0mL and as stated very little pressure is needed with the onset of anaesthesia being immediate. Depending on the solution used, the duration of pulpal anaesthesia could be from 15 to 45 minutes.

4. Intrapulpal injection. This is the perhaps the very last technique you will revert to using. The intrapulpal approach is useful for endodontic procedures. Perhaps an IANB has failed to provide adequate anaesthesia for a root canal procedure in the mandibular molars. Following exposure of the pulp chambers the only measure left is to inject local anaesthetic directly into the root canals themselves. Alternatively, following the removal of the contents of all root canals, a paradoxical pain remains and for the patient; symptoms such as these can be more than unsettling. Still having pain between appointments after all the bothersome nerves have been removed can lead to a loss of confidence in your abilities to complete the work.

Even though seemingly all the contents of all the root canals have been extirpated, the problem could be something as simple as an accessory mesio-lingual canal, which may provide sensations back through another nerve route, other than the IAN. Placing the local anaesthetic directly into the pulp chamber or the nerve canal itself can be horrendously painful for the patient. Nevertheless, the relief is almost instantaneous as 0.2mL to 0.5mL of local anaesthetic being injected directly onto the nerve itself will provide the opportunity to extirpate the last remnants of the previously hidden canal.

Should the symptoms still persist after an intrapulpal injection and there are no further canals in the tooth, the pain may be from a longitudinal split or fracture that has not been identified from your pre-operative Peri-Apical radiograph.

Perhaps the last point (no pun intended) to make about injections; is on the ideal dose to achieve the best results for the patient. We have previously considered the doses of local anaesthetic that are considered safe from the manufacturers and the doses recommended by clinicians and have found there is a difference between these two authorities. As a reminder, the following guidelines are a summary of the safe limits we should observe for the two most commonly used dental local anaesthetics in the UK[79,125]:

Children	
2% Lidocaine	4.4mgs/Kg Body Weight Maximum Safe Dose. This is 1/10th of a Cartridge/Kg.
3% Prilocaine	6.6mgs/Kg Body Weight Maximum Safe Dose. This is 1/10th of a Cartridge/Kg (For Children younger than five the above doses are halved).
Adults	
2% Lidocaine	10X 2.2mL Cartridges or 500mgs total dose.
3% Prilocaine	8X 2.2ml Cartridges or 600mgs total dose.

Conceivably another approach reconciling these differences is needed and one that will determine the ideal dose that achieves the best result for our patients. The results of recent clinical research actually indicate we should be using even lower doses:

In the upper arch, for lidocaine delivered by infiltration, a minimum volume of 0.6mL was found to be effective[46]. When a comparison was made with increased volumes; a faster onset of local anaesthesia and prolonged negative response to an electronic pulp test was observed with volumes of 0.9mL up to 1.2mL of lidocaine.

> ### For maxillary anaesthesia doses of less
> ### than one cartridge are effective.

In the lower arch, for lidocaine delivered via an IANB, doses of 1.8mL to 3.6 mL were found to be effective in producing anaesthesia in over 4 out of 5 cases[86].

> ### For mandibular anaesthesia doses of up
> ### to two cartridges are effective.

If an infiltration or an IANB is not effective after two cartridges, then alternative techniques such as those methods discussed in this chapter can be used. For all of us; whether specialist, or student: Working in the upper arch or the lower arch, if you have used three cartridges in three attempts and there is no effective anaesthesia, regardless of the dose limits from the manufacturers, or those limits set by clinical specialists, then: **STOP**

Something is clearly not working. Remember, in nature most things occur in fives, however when people get involved, trouble always come in threes.

After three cartridges or three attempts at local anaesthesia by persisting in a course of action that isn't working, not only is there a problem, trouble could be just round the corner.

There is no point in putting yourself or your patient through the agony of injections that repeatedly fail to provide anaesthesia:

From our clinical experience in practice we would respectfully advise:

> ### After three failures in Local Anaesthesia:
> ### Do not proceed
> ### Doing so could lead your patient and yourself into trouble.

References to Local Anaesthetic Safety

1. Weinstein P, Milgrom P. Kaufman E, Fiset L and Ramsay D. Patient perceptions of failure to achieve optimal local anaesthesia. General Dentist 1985; 33: 218-220.

2. Ingle JI and Bakland LK. Endodontics. 5th ed. Hamilton: BC Decker; 2002. Preparation for Endodontic Treatment; p. 385.

3. Matthews R, Drum M, Reader A, Nusstein J and Beck M. Articaine for supplemental buccal mandibular infiltration anesthesia in patients with irreversible pulpitis when the inferior alveolar nerve block fails. J Endod. 2009; 35:343–6.

4. Khan AA, Owatz CB, Schindler WG, Schwartz SA, Keiser K and Hargreaves KM. Measurement of mechanical allodynia and local anesthetic efficacy in patients with irreversible pulpitis and acute periradicular periodontitis. J Endod. 2007; 33:796–9.

5. Sokolowski C J, Giovannitti J A Jr and Boynes SG. Needle phobia: etiology, adverse consequences, and patient management. Dent Clin North Am. 2010 Oct; 54 (4):731-44.

6. Accurso V, Winnicki M, Shamsuzzaman AS, Wenzel A, Johnson AK and Somers VK. Predisposition to vasovagal syncope in subjects with blood/injury phobia. Circulation. 2001 Aug 21;104 (8):903-7.

7. Hamilton JG. Needle Phobia - A Neglected Diagnosis. Journal of Family Practice 41. 1995 August (2): 169–175 Review.

8. Shabani DB, Fisher WW. Stimulus Fading and Differential Reinforcement for the Treatment of Needle Phobia in a Youth with Autism. Woods DW, ed. Journal of Applied Behavior Analysis. 2006;39(4):449-452.

9. Jones K.M, Friman P.C. A case study of behavioral assessment and treatment of insect phobia. Journal of Applied Behavior Analysis. 1999; 32:95–98

10. Ditto B, Wilkins JA, France CR, Lavoie P and Adler PS. On-site training in applied muscle tension to reduce vasovagal reactions to blood donation. J Behav Med. 2003 Feb; 26 (1):53-65.

11. Arrowsmith J and Campbell C. A comparison of local anaesthetics for venepuncture. Archives of Disease in Childhood 2000. 82 (4): 309–310.

12. Sawyer J, Febbraro S, Masud S, Ashburn MA and Campbell JC. Heated lidocaine/tetracaine patch (Synera, Rapydan) compared with lidocaine/prilocaine cream (EMLA) for topical anaesthesia before vascular access. Br J Anaesth. 2009 Feb;102(2):210-5.

13. Pearse RM et al. European Surgical Outcomes Study (EuSOS) group for the Trials groups of the European Society of Intensive Care Medicine and the European Society of Anaesthesiology. Mortality after surgery in Europe: a 7 day cohort study. Lancet 2012; 22; 380 (9847): 1059–1065.

14. Buck N, Devlin HB and Lunn JN (Eds). The Report of the Confidential Enquiry into Perioperative Deaths 1987. The Nuffield Provincial Hospitals Trust/King's Fund, London 1987.

15. Jenkins K and Baker AB. Consent and anaesthetic risk. Anaesthesia 2003; 58: 962–984.

16. Tiret L et al. Complications relating to Anaesthesia in infants and children: a prospective survey of 40 240 anaesthetics. Br J Anaesth 1988; 61(3);263–269.

17. van der Griend BF et al. Postoperative mortality in children after 101,885 anesthetics at a tertiary paediatric hospital. Anaesthesia and analgesia 2011; 112(6) 1440–1447.

18. Confidential enquiry into Maternal and Child health: Saving Mothers' Lives. Reviewing maternal deaths to make motherhood safer: 2003–2005. Seventh Report of the Confidential enquiries into Maternal Deaths in the United Kingdom, London. CEMACH 2007. (www.cemach.org).

19. Menon DK. Editor. White S. Risks associated with your anaesthetic. Section 14. Death or Brain Damage. 2013. Information for Patients. The Royal College of Anaesthetists. London England. Available online from: http://www.rcoa.ac.uk/system/files/PI-Risk14_2.pdf
Accessed April 2016.

20. Shojaei A and Haas D. Local anaesthetic cartridges and latex allergy: A literature review. Jnl of Canadian Dental Assocn. 2002; 68: 622-626.

21. Mikesell P, Nusstein J, Reader A, Beck M and Weaver JA. A comparison of articaine and lidocaine for inferior alveolar nerve blocks. Jnl Endodontic 2005; 31: 265-270.

22. Reader A, Nusstein J and Drum M. Chapter 1 Clinical Factors Related to Local Anaesthesia in Successful Local Anaesthesia for Restorative Dentistry and Endodontics. 2011; Ch.1 1-3.

23. Lacouture C, Blanton PL and Hairston LE. The anatomy of the maxillary artery in the infratemporal fossa in relationship to oral injections. Anat Rec 1983; 205:104A.

24. Malamed SF. Medical Emergencies in the Dental Office. 4th ed. St Louis: Mosby; 1993. 304-334.

25. Taghavi Zenouz A, Ebrahimi H, Mahdipour M, Pourshahidi S, Amini P and Vatankhah M. The Incidence of Intravascular Needle Entrance during Inferior Alveolar Nerve Block Injection. Journal of Dental Research, Dental Clinics, Dental Prospects. 2008;2(1):38-41.

26. Blanton PL and Jeske AH. ADA Council on Scientific Affairs; ADA Division of Science. Avoiding complications in local anaesthesia induction: Anatomical considerations. Jnl of Am Dent Assoc. 2003; 134:888–93.

27. Laskin DM. Diagnosis and treatment of complications associated with local anaesthesia. Intl Dent J 1984; 34: 323-337.

28. Ngeow WC, Shim CK and Chai WL. Transient loss of power of accommodation in one eye following inferior alveolar nerve block: Report of two cases. Jnl. Can Dent Assoc. 2006 Dec; 72(10):927-31.

29. Chisci G, Chisci C, Chisci V, and Chisci E. Ocular complications after posterior superior alveolar nerve block: a case of trochlear nerve palsy. Int J Oral Maxillofac Surg. 2013 Dec; 42 (12):1562-5.

30. Magliocca KR, Kessel NC, Cortright GW and Arbor A. Transient diplopia following maxillary local anesthetic injection. Oral Surg Oral Med Oral Pathol Oral Radio Endond. 2006; 101:730–3.

31. Crean SJ and Powis A. Neurological complications of local anaesthetics in dentistry. Dent Update.1999; 26: 344–9.

32. Panarrocha-Diago M and Sanchis–Bielsa JM. Ophthalmic complications after intra-oral local anaesthesia with articaine. Oral Surg Oral Med Oral Pathol Oral Radiol Endond. 2000; 90:21–4.

33. Pragasm M and Managutti A. Diplopia with local anaesthesia. National Journal of Maxillofacial Surgery. 2011; 2(1): 82-85.

34. Rishiraj B, Epstein JB, Fine D, Nabi S and Wade NK Permanent vision loss in one eye following administration of local anaesthesia for a dental extraction. Int Jnl. Oral Maxillofac Surg. 2005 Mar; 34 (2):220-3.

35. Hochman MN, Friedman MJ, Williams W and Hochman CB. Interstittial tissue pressure associated with dentinal injections: A clinical study. Quintessence International. 2006; 37: 469-476.

36. Versloot J, Veerkamp JS and Hoogstraten J. Assessment of pain by the child, dentist and independent observers. Paediatric Dentistry 2004; 26: 445-449.

37. Cohen SP. Compassion fatigue and veterinary health team. Vet. Clin. North America Small Animal Practicr 2007; 37: 123-124.

38. Kanaa M Meechan J, Corbett I and Whitworth J. The speed of injection influences efficacy of inferior alveolar nerve blocks: A double blind randomized controlled trial in volunteers. Jnl of Endodontics. 2006; 32: 919-923.

39. Sultan J. Towards evidence based emergency medicine: Best BETs from Manchester Royal Infirmary. Effect of warming local anaesthetics on pain of infiltration. Emerg. Med. Jnl 2007; 24: 723-725.

40. Sultan J. Towards evidence based emergency medicine: Best BETs from Manchester Royal Infirmary. The effect of warming local anaesthetics on pain of infiltration. Emerg Med Jnl. 2007; 24: 791-793.

41. Oikarinen VJ, Ylipaavalniemi P and Evers H. Pain and temperature sensations related to local analgesia. Intl Jnl Oral Surg. 1975; 4: 151-156.

42. Volk RJ Gargiulo AV. Local anaesthetic cartridge warmer- First in, first out. Ill. Dent. Jnl 1984; 53: 92-94.

43. Brunetto PC, Ranali J, Ambrosano G, et al. Anaesthetic efficacy of 3 volumes of lidocaine with epinephrine in maxillary infiltration anaesthesia. Anaesth. Prog. 2008; 55: 29-34.

44. Mason R, Drum M, Reader A, Nusstein J, and Beck MA. A prospective randomized double-blind comparison of 2% lidocaine with 1:100,000 and 1:50,000 epinephrine and 3% mepivicaine for maxillary infiltrations. Jnl of Endodontics 2009; 35: 1173-1177.

45. Katz S, Drum M, Reader A, Nusstein J, and Beck M. A prospective randomized double-blind comparison of 2% lidocaine with 1:100,000 epinephrine 4% Prilocaine with 1:200, 000 epinephrine and 4% Prilocaine for maxillary infiltrations. Anaesthetic Prog 2010; 57: 45-51.

46. Malamed S. Handbook of Local Anaesthesia ed 5th Edition St Louis: Mosby, 2004.

47. Lai TN, Lin CP, Kok SH et al. Evaluation of mandibular block using a standardized method. Oral Surg, Oral Med, Oral Path, Oral Rad, Endod. 2006; 102: 462-468.

48. Clark K, Reader A, Beck M and Weaver J. Anaesthetic efficacy of an infiltration in mandibular anterior teeth following an inferior alveolar nerve block. Anaesth. Prog. 2002; 49: 49-55.

49. Vreeland DL, Reader A, Beck M, Myers W and Weaver J. An evaluation of volumes and concentrations of lidocaine in human inferior alveolar nerve block. Jnl Endod 1989; 15: 6-12.

50. Hersh EV, Hermann DG, Lamp CJ, Johnson PD and MacAfee KA. Assessing the duration of mandibular soft tissue anaesthesia. Jnl of Am Dent Assocn. 1995; 126: 1531-1536.

51. Andrew D, Matthews B. Properties of single nerve fibres that evoke blood flow changes in cat dental pulp. The Journal of Physiology. 2002; 542 (Pt 3):921-928. Available online from: http://www.ncbi.nlm.nih.gov/pmc/articles/PMC2290436/#b3 Accessed April 2016.

52. Cadden SW, Lisney SJW, Matthews B. Thresholds to electrical stimulation of nerves in cat canine tooth-pulp with Aβ, Aδ and C-fibre conduction velocities. Brain Research. 1983; 261:31–41.

53. Fernandez C, Reader A, Drum M and Nusstein J. A prospective, randomized, double-blind comparison of bupivicaine and lidocaine for inferior alveolar nerve blocks. Jnl of Endodontics. 2005; 31: 499-503.

54. Mikesell P, Nusstein J, Reader A, Beck M and Weaver J. A comparison of articaine and lidocaine for inferior alveolar nerve blocks. Jnl Endod. 2005; 31: 265-270.

55. Berde CB and Strichartz GR. Local anaesthetics. In: Miller RD, Eriksson LI, Fleisher LA, et al, editors. Miller's Anaesthesia. 7th ed. Philadelphia, Pa: Elsevier, Churchill Livingstone; 2009.

56. Katzung BG and White PF. Local anaesthetics. In: Katzung BG, Masters SB, Trevor AJ, editors. Basic and Clinical Pharmacology. 11th ed. New York, NY: McGraw-Hill Companies Inc; 2009.

57. Becker DE, Reed KL. Local Anesthetics: Review of Pharmacological Considerations. *Anesthesia Progress*. 2012;59 (2):90-102. Available online from:
http://www.ncbi.nlm.nih.gov/pmc/articles/PMC3403589/
Accessed April 2016.

58. Routledge PA, Barchowsky A, Bjornsson TD, Kitchell BB and Shand DG. Lidocaine plasma protein binding. Clin Pharmacol Ther. 1980 Mar; 27(3):347-51.

59. Scott DB, Jebson PJR, Braid DP, et al. Factors affecting plasma levels of lignocaine and prilocaine. Brit J Anaesth. 1972; 44: 1040–1049.

60. Thomson PD, Melmon KL, Richardson JA, Cohn K, Steinbrunn W, Cudihee R and Rowland M. Lidocaine pharmacokinetics in advanced heart failure, liver disease, and renal failure in humans. April 1973 Ann. Intern. Med. 78 (4): 499–508.

61. Perusse R, Goulet J-P and Turcotte, J-Y. Contraindications to vasoconstrictors in dentistry: Part I. Oral Surg Oral Med Oral Pathol 1992; 74: 679–686.

62. Meechan JG, Parry G, Rattray DT and Thomason JM. Effects of dental local anaesthetics in cardiac transplant recipients. Br Dent J 2002; 192: 161–163.

63. Meechan JG. The effects of dental local anaesthetics on blood glucose concentration in healthy volunteers and in patients having third molar surgery. Br Dent J 1991; 170: 373–376.

64. Sunada K, Nakamura K, Yamashiro M, et al. Clinically safe dosage of felypressin for patients with essential hypertension. Anesth Prog 1996; 43: 108–115.

65. Ash-Bernal R, Wise R, Wright SM. Acquired methemoglobinemia: a retrospective series of 138 cases at 2 teaching hospitals. Medicine Baltimore 2004. *83 (5): 265–273.*

66. Barker SJ, Tremper KK and Hyatt J. Effects of methaemoglobinemia on pulse oximetry and mixed venous oximetry. Anesthesiology. 1989 Jan; 70(1): 112-7.

67. Benz EJ. Disorders of hemoglobin. In: Longo DL, Kasper DL, Jameson JL, et al., editors. Harrison's Principles of Internal Medicine. 18th ed. New York, NY: McGraw Hill; 2012.

68. Feiner JR, Bickler PE and Mannheimer PD. Accuracy of methaemoglobin detection by pulse CO-oximetry during hypoxia. Anesth. Analg. 2010 Jul; 111(1): 143-8.

69. I P Corbett, J C Ramacciato, F C Groppo and J G Meechan. A survey of local anaesthetic use among general dental practitioners in the UK attending postgraduate courses on pain control. British Dental Journal 2005. 199, 784-787. Available online from: http://www.nature.com/bdj/journal/v199/n12/full/4813028a.html
Accessed April 2016.

70. Daubländer M, Muller R and Lipp MDW. The incidence of complications associated with local anaesthesia in dentistry. Anesth Prog 1997; 44: 132–141.

71. Ramacciato JC, Ranali J, Volpato MC, Groppo FC, Flório FM and Soares PCO. Local anaesthetics use by dentists profile. *J Dent Res* 2002; 81(Spec Iss B): 491

72. Haas DA, Lennon D. A 21 year retrospective study of reports of paresthesia following local anesthetic administration. Jnl Can Dent Assoc. 1995; 61:319–330.

73. Garisto GA, Gaffen AS, Lawrence HP, Tenenbaum HC and Haas DA. Occurrence of paraesthesia after dental local anaesthetic administration in the United States. Jnl Am Dent Assoc. 2010; 141:836–844.

74. Hillerup S, Jensen RH, Ersboll BK. Trigeminal nerve injury associated with injection of local anesthetics: needle lesion or neurotoxicity. J Am Dent Assoc. 2011; 142:531–539.

75. Hillerup S, Bakke M, Larsen JO, Thomsen CE and Gerds TA. Concentration-dependent neurotoxicity of articaine: an electrophysiological and stereological study of the rat sciatic nerve. Anesth Analg.2011; 112:1330–1338.

76. Pogrel MA, Schmidt BL, Sambajon V and Jordan RC. Lingual nerve damage due to inferior alveolar nerve blocks: a possible explanation. Jnl. Am Dent Assoc. 2003 Feb; 134(2):195-9.

77. Berde CB and Strichartz GR. Local Anaesthetics. In Miller RD, Eriksson LI, Fleisher LA, et al: Miller's Anaesthesia. 7th ed. Philadelphia, Pa: Elsevier, Churchill Livingstone; 2009.

78. Scott DB, Jebson PJR and Braid DP, et al. Factors affecting plasma levels of lignocaine and prilocaine. Brit J Anaesth. 1972; 44: 1040–1049.

79. Mitchell L and Mitchell DA in Mitchell and Mitchell Oxford Handbook of Clinical Dentistry. Chapter 13. Analgesia Anaesthesia and Sedation pp584-585. 5th Edition. Oxford. Oxford University Press. 2010.

80. Dionne RA, Goldstein DS and Wirdzek PR. Effects of diazepam premedication and epinephrine-containing local anaesthetic on cardiovascular and catecholamine responses to oral surgery. Anaesth Analg. 1984; 63: 640–646.

81. Hersh EV, Giannakopoulos H, Levin LM, et al. The pharmacokinetics and cardiovascular effects of high-dose articaine with 1 : 100,000 and 1 : 200,000 epinephrine. J Am Dent Assoc. 2006; 137: 1562–1571.

82. Gandy W. Severe epinephrine-propranolol interaction. Ann Emerg Med. 1989; 18:98–99.

83. Foster CA and Aston SJ. Propranolol-epinephrine interaction: A potential disaster. Plast Reconstr Surg.1983; 72:74–78.

84. Kennedy M, Reader A, Beck M and Weaver J. Anaesthetic efficacy of ropivacaine in maxillary anterior infiltration. Oral Surg Oral Med Oral Pathol Oral Radiol Endodon. 2001; 91:406–412.

85. Petersen J.K, Luck H, Kristensen F and Mikkelsen L. A comparison of four commonly used local analgesics. Int J Oral Surg. 1977; 6: 51–59

86. Brunetto PC, Ranali J, Bovi Ambrosano GM, de Oliveira PC, Groppo FC, Meechan JG and Volpato MC. Anaesthetic Efficacy of 3 Volumes of Lidocaine With Epinephrine in Maxillary Infiltration Anaesthesia. Anaesthesia Progress, 2008 55 (2), 29–34.
Available online from:
http://www.ncbi.nlm.nih.gov/pmc/articles/PMC2424013/
Accessed May 2016.

87. Jorgensen N.B and Hayden J. Sedation, Local and General Anaesthesia in Dentistry. Philadelphia, Pa: Lea & Febiger; 1973. pp. 35–47

88. Nusstein J, Wood M, Reader A, Beck M and Weaver J. Comparison of the degree of pulpal anaesthesia achieved with the intraosseous injection and infiltration injection using 2% lidocaine with 1:100,000 epinephrine. Gen Dent. 2005; 53:50–53

89. Reader A, Nusstein J and Drum M. Chapter 3 Maxillary Anaesthesia. in Successful Local Anaesthesia for Restorative Dentistry and Endodontics. 2011; Ch. 3 66-67.

90. Reed KL, Malamed SF and Fonner AM. Local Anaesthesia Part 2: Technical Considerations. Anaesthesia Progress. 2012; 59(3): 127-137.

91. de St. Georges J. How dentists are judged by patients. *Dent Today.* 2004 23:96, 98–99.

92. Isik K, Kalayci A and Durmus E. Comparison of Depth of Anaesthesia in Different Parts of Maxilla When Only Buccal

Anaesthesia Was Done for Maxillary Teeth Extraction. International Journal of Dentistry. 2011; 2011: 575874.

93. Fan S, Chen WL, Yang ZH and Huang ZQ Comparison of the efficiencies of permanent maxillary tooth removal performed with single buccal infiltration versus routine buccal and palatal injection Oral Surg Oral Med Oral Pathol Oral Radiol Endod. 2009 Mar; 107(3): 359-63.

94. Malamed SF, Reed KL and Poorsattar S. Needle breakage: incidence and prevention. *Dent Clin North Am.*2010; 54: 745–756.

95. Delgado-Molina E, Tamarit-Borras M, Berini-Aytes L and Gay-Escoda C. Evaluation and comparison of 2 needle models in terms of blood aspiration during truncal block of the inferior alveolar nerve. *Jnl. Oral Maxillofac Surg.* 2003; 61: 1011–1015.

96. Malamed SF. *Handbook of Local Anaesthesia.* 5th edition. St Louis: The CV Mosby Co; 2004.

97. Reed KL, Malamed SF, Fonner AM. Local Anesthaesia Part 2: Technical Considerations. Anaesthesia Progress. 2012; 59 (3):127-137. Available online from:
http://www.ncbi.nlm.nih.gov/pmc/articles/PMC3468291/
Accessed June 2016.

98. Hafeez NS, Ganapathy S, Sondekoppam R, Johnson M, Merrifield P and Galil KA. Anatomical Variations of the Greater Palatine Nerve in the Greater Palatine Canal. *J Can Dent Assoc 2015; 81:f4. Available online from:*
http://www.jcda.ca/article/f14
Accessed June 2016.

99. Levis AG, Minicuci N, Ricci P, Gennaro V and Garbisa S. Mobile phones and head tumours. The discrepancies in cause-effect relationships in the epidemiological studies - how do they arise? Environmental Health. 2011;10:59.
Available online from: http://www.ncbi.nlm.nih.gov/pmc/articles/PMC3146917/
Accessed June 2016.

100. Royal College of Surgeons (England), Get Well Soon; Wisdom Tooth Extraction. What to Expect After the Operation (2016).

Available Online From:
http://www.rcseng.ac.uk/patients/recovering-from-surgery/
wisdom-teeth-extraction
Accessed June 2016.

101. Meechan JG. The use of the mandibular infiltration anaesthetic technique in adults. Jnl Am Dent Assoc. 2011 Sep; 142 Suppl 3:19S-24S.

102. Robinson P and Smith KG. Lingual nerve damage during lower third molar removal: a comparison of two surgical methods. Br Dent J. 1996 Jun 22; 180 (12):456-61.

103. Robinson PP, Loescher AR and Smith KG. The effect of surgical technique on lingual nerve damage during lower 3rd molar removal by dental students. Eur Jnl Dent Educ. 1999 May; 3(2):52-5.

104. Khalil H. A basic review on the inferior alveolar nerve block techniques. Anaesthesia, Essays and Researches. 2014;8(1):3-8.
Available online from: http://www.ncbi.nlm.nih.gov/pmc/articles/PMC4173572/
Accessed June 2016

105. Thotakura B, Rajendran SS, Gnanasundaram V and Subramaniam A. Variations in the posterior division branches of the mandibular nerve in human cadavers. Singapore Med J. 2013; 54:149–51.

106. Siessere S, Hallak-Regalo SC, Semprini M, De Oliveira-Honorato R, Vitti M and Mizusaki Iyomasa M, et al. Anatomical variations of the mandibular nerve and its branches correlated to clinical situations. Minerva Stomatol. 2009;58:209–15.

107. Kim SY, Hu KS, Chung IH, Lee EW and Kim HJ. Topographic anatomy of the lingual nerve and variations in communication pattern of the mandibular nerve branches. Surg Radiol Anat. 2004; 26:128–35.

108. Thangavelu K, Kannan R, Kumar NS, Rethish E, Sabitha S and Sayeeganesh N. Significance of localization of mandibular foramen in an inferior alveolar nerve block. J Nat Sci Biol Med.2012; 3:156–60

109. López-Valverde A, De Vicente J and Cutando A. The surgeons Halsted and Hall, cocaine and the discovery of dental anaesthesia by nerve blocking. Br Dent J. 2011 Nov 25; 211(10):485-7

110. Phillips WH. Anatomic considerations in local anaesthesia. *Jnl Oral Surg.* 1943; 1:112–121.

111. Rifkind JB Management of a broken needle in the pterygomandibular space following a Vazirani-Akinosi block: case report. Jnl Can Dent Assoc. 2011; 77.

112. Watson JE. Appendix: some anatomic aspects of the Gow-Gates technique for mandibular anaesthesia. *Oral Surg Oral Med Oral Pathol.* 1973; 36: 328–330.

113. Gow-Gates GA. The Gow-Gates mandibular block: regional anatomy and analgesia. Aust Endod J. 1998 Apr; 24 (1):18-9.

114. Reed KL. Advanced techniques of local anaesthetic injection. *Gen Dent.* 1994; 42: 248–251.

115. Thangavelu K, Kannan R and Senthil-Kumar N. Inferior alveolar nerve block: Alternative technique. Anaesth Essays Res. 2012; 6:53–7.

116. Thangavelu K, Sabitha S, Kannan R and Saravanan K. Inferior alveolar nerve block using the internal oblique ridge as landmark. SRM Univ J Dent Sci. 2012; 3:15–8.

117. Boonsiriseth K, Sirintawat N, Arunakul K and Wongsirichat N. Comparative study of the novel and conventional injection approach for inferior alveolar nerve block. Int J Oral Maxillofac Surg. 2013; 42:852–6.

118. Palti DG, Almeida CM, Rodrigues Ade C, Andreo JC and Lima JE. Anaesthetic technique for inferior alveolar nerve block: A new approach. J Appl Oral Sci. 2011; 19: 11–5.

119. Suazo-Galdames IC, Cantin-Lopez MG and Zavando-Matamala DA. Inferior alveolar nerve block anaesthesia via the retromolar triangle, an alternative for patients with blood dyscrasias. Med Oral Pathol Oral Cir Buccal. 2008; 13:E43–7

120. Takasugi Y, Furuya H, Moriya K and Okamoto Y. Clinical evaluation of inferior alveolar nerve block by injection into

the pterygomandibular space anterior to the mandibular foramen. Anaesth Prog. 2000; 47:125–9

121. Okamoto Y, Takasugi Y, Moriya K and Furuya H. Inferior alveolar nerve block by injection into the pterygomandibular space anterior to the mandibular foramen: Radiographic study of local anaesthetic spread in the pterygomandibular space. Anaesth Prog. 2000; 47:130–3

122. Matas R. The story of the discovery of dental anaesthesia by nerve blocking: Achievements of William Steward Halsted. Surgery 1952; 32: 530–7.

123. Jorgensen NB and Hayden J. Premedication, local, and general anaesthesia in dentistry. London: Kimpton, 1967.

124. Mraiwa, N. Presence and course of the incisive canal in the human mandibular inter-foraminal region: Two-dimensional imaging versus anatomical observation. Surg Radiol Anat 2003; 25:416-423.

125. Mitchell L and Mitchell DA in Mitchell and Mitchell Oxford Handbook of Clinical Dentistry. Chapter 3 Paediatric Dentistry pp78-79. 5th Edition. Oxford. Oxford University Press. 2010.

Sedation Safety

Conscious sedation and dentistry today

So far in this chapter, we have covered the basics of drug safety; looking into the actions and the interactions of the drugs you can use as a dental professional. Moving on from this, the actions of those drugs we prescribe with the interactions of drugs commonly prescribed by our medical colleagues was explained. Digging deeper into the subject of drug safety, in the preceding section we then looked into the most commonly used dental local anaesthetics.

In this section we will move away from drug safety and the administration of medicines in clinical practice and briefly look into the drugs and procedures used for conscious sedation in dentistry. Before doing so it must be emphasised that until very recently this area of dentistry was firmly rooted in the domain of the general dental practitioner. However, following the publication of reports into both training and quality assurance in this area of dental practise, it seems almost inevitable that conscious sedation will become, if not part of specialist dental practise, then one that may well be practised exclusively by specialists. From a safety perspective, such a move is justifiable and this short section will touch on the basic safety concepts of sedation. For a more detailed appreciation of conscious sedation in dentistry, you must refer to the latest regulations and evidence based guidelines as and when they are released and updated.

For most of your patients, the use of a local anaesthetic is immensely helpful if not to eliminate, then to reduce to a manageable level the pain associated with many dental procedures. However, there are still a few but a significant number of patients requiring further means to achieve a standard of dentistry that is free from pain and anxiety. Frequently, many of these patients suffer from systemic medical conditions, while other patients although fit and well; are possessed of a real fear of dentistry. It is our professional responsibility to ensure all such patients can be treated in a dental clinic to the same standard as those patients who do not require the additional measures of conscious sedation which we will discuss in this section.

In 2015, the UK Intercollegiate Advisory Committee for Sedation in Dentistry (the IACSD) of the three Dental Faculties of the Royal Colleges of Surgeons of: Edinburgh, Glasgow and England, together with the Royal College of Anaesthetists released their document:

Standards for Conscious Sedation in the Provision of Dental Care[1].

The intention of that publication was to create a: UK National Standard for Conscious Sedation superseding the following three documents:

i.   Conscious Sedation in the Provision of Dental Care (2003)[2]
ii. Standards for Conscious Sedation in Dentistry (2007)[3]
iii. Conscious Sedation in Dentistry (2012)[4]

Less than one year after the IACSD publication, in April 2016, the Chief Dental Officers of the UK intervened to request that the Scottish Dental Clinical Effectiveness Program (SDCEP) review the findings of the IACSD. Advice was requested from the SDCEP to ensure any revisions of the IACSD document as deemed necessary might then be utilized to achieve the following aims:

1. To reduce the risk to patients.
2. To develop the provision of dental sedation in the NHS.
3. To invest in future training of dental graduates who might then be able provide safe effective conscious sedation.

The overarching principle running through all of these publications, interventions and recommendations is that conscious sedation must be safe. The most recent document from the IACSD is effectively based on the publication:

Safe Sedation Practice for Healthcare Procedures[5]

This publication was in turn based on the National Institute for Health and Care Excellence (NICE) document:

Sedation in Children and Young People.[6]

These six publications span a decade documenting safety in dental conscious sedation, but despite this, there still remains throughout: Europe, North America and beyond, some very real differences in the rules, regulations, requirements and rationale supporting the provision of conscious sedation in dentistry. Not only are such differences global, they are to be found between and within the national regions of the UK as well. Even though there are such variations and there is a need to obey the rules implemented on a regional basis if not a national basis, safety will always be of paramount importance in this area of dentistry as it should be for all areas of dentistry.

Due to the somewhat unsettled nature of the recommendations in the UK, the default position is to revert to the previously accepted and well founded guidelines published in the ten year advent of the IACSD document. Whereas in the wake of the 2015 publication, the dental professional undertaking sedation will in future act on the recommendations of the CDO's report in response to the findings of the SCDEP.

With respect to all of the above, the ability to use conscious sedation in dentistry and to do so safely will always be a valuable means to assist you and your colleagues in providing a service that is free from pain and anxiety. In the UK, conscious sedation will be available in the general dental practice setting, but training will be more structured than at present, perhaps as stated above; becoming a specialized activity. Building on this, teaching and mentoring will become mandatory for all members of the sedation team as the dental profession embraces a more safety critical approach not only for conscious sedation but across the entire spectrum of dental practice.

As noted, the purpose of this section is to provide a background and a review of some basic safety concepts in conscious sedation. If you are already experienced in either providing conscious sedation or are working in a team doing so, then this section may provide a useful method of revision to complement your mandatory CPD. This is currently set at a level of 12 hours, specifically dealing with conscious sedation.

An essential part of this CPD must include medical emergencies with training in both Paediatric and Adult Immediate Life Support (the PILS and the ILS) with measures taught to a level in advance of those methods and techniques for the basic or the core CPD in Medical Emergencies we have covered in Chapter 1 and those measures specified by the GDC.

On the other hand, if you or your dental practice does not provide conscious sedation, preferring instead to refer to specialists or those dental clinics dedicated to a conscious sedation service, reading this section will give you a better understanding of what is involved in this field of dentistry. Taking this a little further, a foundation might be formed upon which further clinically oriented knowledge can be built. Should you then choose to develop an interest and clinical skills in this area or attend one of the many courses organised in the regional or national area where you practice, time spent reading this section will be time well spent.

In the UK it is the Society for the Advancement of Anaesthesia in Dentistry (SAAD); the second largest dental professional association in the UK (the British Dental Association (BDA) being the largest) that organises courses in conscious sedation in dentistry and advises on the best standards that we must maintain for clinical safety when sedating patients.

Following publication of the above noted IACSD standards document, all dentists, doctors and those dental professionals who have no previous experience of providing conscious sedation for dentistry must now undertake appropriate training before working in an independent clinical setting providing conscious sedation. All training programmes for those beginning conscious sedation after 2015 must include clinical experience that is supervised by a recognised person who themselves have undergone an approved program of conscious sedation training. In addition to these requirements, all new training courses must be externally validated.

In the UK, those courses based in universities or those courses organised by post-graduate dental deaneries are considered to be IACSD compliant. Whereas other courses leading to independent clinical practice, including those run by private providers, must now be accredited to the IACSD standard. The accreditation process requires the beginner in conscious sedation to be supervised by an approved clinician who is an experienced sedationist. In addition, an appropriate number of supervised clinical cases must be completed then logged in an appropriate format that has been approved by the UK Dental Sedation Teachers Group (DSTG) before unsupervised conscious sedation can take place in practice.

Those dental professionals who gained experience prior to 2015 and are in current practice or those requiring an update-course do not require such external revalidation, nevertheless in every 5 year GDC CPD cycle, 12 hours of sedation related CPD must be undertaken.

In the UK, should you choose to provide conscious sedation in your dental clinic, while membership of SAAD and BDA is not mandatory, it is advisable.

Society and sedation

Today, and every day in dental practice, you will see and hear of patients for whom:

Firstly, their fear of the dentist and fear of your equipment, such as the needle or the drill, either on their own or coupled to the smell of a dental clinic is so off-putting that very little if any treatment can be undertaken.

Secondly, if treatment is attempted, while it may be technically finished to a text-book standard, the experience for the patient will be so deeply disturbing that the seeds of lifelong dental phobia may well be sown on the day you decided to persist with a course of action that was so simple and safe but had disastrous psychological and behavioural consequences for the patient.

Should such patients either on their own or with a good measure of encouragement from a well meaning friend, family-member, or one of your not so well meaning colleagues (as now happens more than ever) decide to make a complaint to your professional regulator... their disaster might soon become your catastrophe.

For other patients who can normally accept routine dentistry, it may well be that the more involved procedures such as surgical extractions, implant placement or even attaching orthodontic appliances, then removing them again are too much of an ordeal. For these procedures, the use of local anaesthetic will never eliminate or even reduce to a manageable level the distress to the patient as your healing hands go about their health-giving work.

In many ways it is the patient, who has not been physically hurt but whose feelings have been hurt, who could be more problematic. Frequently the patient will consent to treatment with local anaesthesia but later, after a week, or a month, or even a year, if something is not to their liking, then the smallest excuse will send them off to 37 Wimpole Street. They will allege treatment so brutal and so rough, that it was the worst dental treatment they ever had...EVER.

In reality it may have been, that during their appointment (and for whatever reason), there was an inability to complete all of the treatment and another visit to achieve this would be realistic. However, somehow somewhere, something that mattered to the patient was overlooked, either by yourself or your dental team and the experience left the patient troubled in some small but significant way. The treatment was allegedly terrible and the procedure so sadistic and cruel, the patient wrote: They won't be coming back and legal action is intimated. In years gone by, the often engaged, but not so engaging phrase:

"*YOU WILL BE HEARING FROM MY LAWYER*" (Yes sometimes in capitals too) was not so much a turn of the screw, but a harmless if somewhat offensive start to an angry letter.

Reading this meant the clinical notes could be completed, the case closed and you would get a good night sleep. It was no more than an impolite notice of the patient deciding to end their professional relationship with you.However with the passage of time; fast forward a few years and these days such a phrase while marking the end of one professional relationship, often heralds the start of another one, usually between your indemnity provider and the patient's solicitor.

Closing cases and forgetting about patients was never either adequate or responsible then and even less so now. In addition to reflecting on the appointment and the reasons for failure, you might engage in a period of learning from the shortcomings, after which implementing a schedule of further training seems very necessary to appease the public and a GDC keen for answers in their quest for transparency and their truth. In addition to all of that, something and then somebody must be seen to be blamed and then...

Punished.

The punishment from the regulator is apparently not punitive, but sentencing should be within an open arena; the very public delivery acting as some kind of deterrent.

Society and our professional regulator ingrained with such a culture will hardly be satisfied with an upholding of a duty of candour, a duty that applies not only when things go wrong, as they rarely do, but for every day when things go right. When things go wrong candour is externalised, when things go right candour is internalized in a never ending cycle of; critical reflection, audit and review. After all if we can't be honest with ourselves and each other in a professional relationship, we aren't going to be honest with our patients. Are we?

When patients are more reasonable, then technical failures, rather than behavioural ones will be easier to deal with. The complications arising may ultimately require the input from a specialist or referral to a hospital. With thorough treatment planning and case assessment, the risks of such occurrences will never be eliminated, but they will be reduced to a level while not acceptable to the person for whom the risk becomes a clinical incident, it will be manageable for an indemnity organisation who then inconveniently and not so subtly recover their costs through increased membership fees in the many years of trouble free clinical practice that follow from the causative incident.

For every case, a thorough patient assessment is critically important and for all patients their expectation that dental treatment should be completed in a manner that is both free from pain and anxiety must be met at each of their dental visits. The former can be addressed with the use of local anaesthetics and the latter with the option to use conscious sedation.

In today's practice of safety critical dentistry, the option of conscious sedation must be discussed and where necessary made available, not only for the patient who reasonably requests it, but for all patients who may benefit from its use. Such patients could be those who may come to harm if conscious sedation is not used.

The extent of harm can be anything from physical injury; should the patient become upset or distressed to such a degree that they become uncontrollable injuring themselves or others, to the harm from an anxiety state that develops into a chronic phobia. Such fears can rise to an insurmountable level, so much so that dental attendance is avoided for many years. At some point in the distant future the former patient's oral health is so degraded that their next dental attendance is their inappropriate demand that all teeth be removed under a general anaesthetic.

In the consenting process, not only must you discuss the option to use conscious sedation, you must clearly state the risks and benefits that come with its use.

It is the responsibility of the dental professional to ensure that should conscious sedation become an option, the quality and the safety of the sedation provided are protected. Such safeguarding must be present not only for those patients whose treatment is contained within one practice but also and perhaps even more so, for those patients who are referred onwards to specialist sedation dental clinics where their dental care will continue.

The referral of any dental patient for conscious sedation comes only after all the appropriate and the alternative methods of anxiety management have been clearly discussed with the patient and they fully understand what their treatment is and what their treatment pathway will involve.

In the previous chapter on medical emergencies, we have discussed the use of behaviour and physiological modification techniques such as Applied Muscle Tension (AMT) for the needle phobic patient who is prone to fainting[7]. For those patients who may tolerate the presence of a dental syringe near them but perhaps cannot bear the feelings that come from being injected, or thinking about it (does anyone?), the use of cognitive behaviour therapies with topical anaesthetic gels are possibly more appropriate than the use of the referral process.

Let's be honest here, some of your colleagues may well use the referral process as a substitute for file 13. NB file 13 is not used in root canal treatment, nor is it in a cabinet with other files supporting those rarely consulted documents from the CQC. It is of course the round one that gets emptied every night, into which some of your dental colleagues deposit notes for patients who need more than your colleagues think they can reasonably be asked to give within the NHS.

When consulting with the patient who will be referred for conscious sedation, it is beneficial for you to describe in clear and easy to understand terms those differences between local anaesthesia, conscious sedation, (either Relative Analgesia (RA) inhalational sedation or Intra-Venous (IV)) and on extremely rare occasions; if referral for a General Anaesthetic (GA) might be considered.

In addition to such descriptions in your consenting and referring process, you should clarify how the sedation will be achieved. Whatever else you do, don't tell the patient or a parent that they or their child will be put to sleep. For those of you, who have read, studied for and passed the MFDS and MJDF exams, you will remember the now infamous OSCE (Objective Structured Clinical Exam) question, based on a true story about the parent who was discussing the merits of referring their child for a sedation procedure to a hopeful exam candidate, who then clearly explained:

"If we can't give your son a local anaesthetic, we can send him to hospital to be put to sleep."

The response from the parent was:

"Put to sleep?....What do you mean put to sleep? You mean put to sleep like our pet dog?"

Your use of clear unequivocal terms, is vital, please don't use euphemisms in your exams or in real life[8].

A simple approach will help the patient to understand what is available and how their treatment can be successfully completed.

As noted previously, if you are the dental professional who is referring your patient, you must be satisfied that the standards and level of care under which the conscious sedation is being delivered are in accordance with those standards of your professional regulator. A further point must be made and that is the duty of both the referring practitioner and the registered professional, who provides the sedation (whether they are medically or dentally qualified), is to both encourage and to guide the patient towards continuing their dental care, so that any treatment securing the patient's oral health is thought of as an investment in health that will be maintained after the sedation appointment.

Failing to do these things may not necessarily result in an enquiry from your regulator. However failing to ensure continuity of care is arguably far worse. While you will not be failing yourself or your profession, you will be failing in your duty of care for your patient. If the patient cannot or will not maintain your work in good order, then why do the work in the first place?

While such measures may not be necessary for your adult patients, they will be required for the child patient needing conscious sedation. By ensuring continuity of care by the patient and for the patient, you will be ensuring the investment of your time and your professional skills together with those of your colleagues will not be wasted.

Referring patients for conscious sedation

When referring a patient for conscious sedation the following data must be present in your letter:

> I.   The reasons and justification for the use of conscious sedation.
> II.   An outline of the dental treatment being requested.
> III. An up to date and complete medical history.
> IV.   An up to date and relevant dental history
> V.   The scope and extent of sedation treatment with the total number of visits estimated.

An indication should be made whether your referral is for a single procedure or whether the patient is being referred for all further treatment. A copy of the referral letter should be kept and a note of all discussions with the patient should be retained.

In the UK, the GDC have published guidelines for conscious sedation in dentistry. The use of conscious sedation must be patient centred as indeed any procedure should be. In these times of clinical practice following the findings and the recommendations from the report of Sir Robert Francis into the failings of the Mid Staffordshire Hospital Trust, many of the changes that will apply to the medical and nursing profession can and must be applied equally to the dental profession.

The final report from Sir Robert Francis concluded with the previously noted duty of candour, to be open and honest when things go wrong. In addition, the recommendation was made that professionals in primary care have a fundamental role and an important responsibility on behalf of their patients to monitor the specialist or specialised services they receive in primary or secondary care.

The following safety based proposals have been adapted from those recommendations published as part of the response of the Royal College of General Practitioners (RCGP) to the Francis report[11]. While these proposals were drawn up with the medical professional in mind, they can be applied in the same way for any health care worker including the dental professional:

I. The dental professional needs to review the quality of referral services provided, in particular assessing treatment outcomes.

II. Internal systems are needed that enable the dental professional to flag any patterns of concern.

III. The dental professional has a responsibility to their patients to keep them informed of the standards of services and providers of those services and to inform patients of the choices available.

IV. The dental professional will have an ongoing responsibility for their patients. Such a responsibility does not end when the patient is referred to hospital or to the specialist providing conscious sedation.

V. The dental professional referring patients for conscious sedation are in effect the commissioners of this service and should take advantage of this position to ensure patients get dental care that is both effective and safe.

These proposals are straightforward enough and when we think about it, the process of referral from primary care to secondary care is the same whether it is from the medical practice to hospital or from within the dental clinic from one colleague to another, who will then provide the conscious sedation.

Sedation referral and consent

In the UK, without doubt most dentistry and almost all medicine is conducted within the NHS. In addition to the above proposals, the RCGP recommended a culture that places the patient first while sharing information throughout the patient's NHS care pathway would ensure the lessons learned from the Mid Staffordshire enquiry and the reports that were published could be implemented and invested in future care that would be far safer than that delivered previously.

In dentistry arguably the most important area to implement these changes is with the use of conscious sedation. This can be in the primary care setting, the referral centre, or the dental hospital environment.

The reasons for this are that conscious sedation is the only area in dentistry where those patients who have mental capacity, elect to have this capacity reduced to a level allowing dental treatment to proceed and as a result of this the patient becomes vulnerable.

Such is the extent of safeguarding, not only must the patient be secure and made medically safe while the procedure is taking place, the security and safety extend to the recovery period too.

Perhaps this is best expressed in the words of James Badenoch QC who concisely assures us that[12]:

> *"There is a duty to safeguard the patient's body and brain."*

In dentistry we must accept these words and the duty to protect encompasses the time of treatment, the recovery period and extends to cover any consequence that a diminished capacity following sedation may have on a patient, their relatives and their dependents too.

Just before getting into the RA and IV methods of dental conscious sedation we might consider the following ideas on consent not only as they apply to conscious sedation in particular but to dentistry in general:

Those dental patients attending with pain, discomfort, or disease, will quite naturally be anxious and in a state of stress, therefore:

> **Communication, Co-operation, Capacity and Capability to Consent is Commonly Compromised**

Gaining, then maintaining consent for treatment

Before any treatment can begin, consent must be obtained and during treatment it must be maintained. If a patient does not object to treatment beginning or they are compliant during treatment itself, then traditionally this is a strong indication that consent has been granted or it is implied. However this in itself does not mean the consent is valid. For consent to be valid, the three factors underlined below need to be fulfilled:

I.   The patient must have <u>capacity</u>, to be able and be capable of making the decision to undergo treatment.

II. The patient must be <u>informed</u> receiving all relevant data to reach the decision that the treatment option chosen is the most appropriate for them.

III. The decision to receive treatment is <u>voluntary</u> and can be withdrawn at any time.

When obtaining and maintaining consent from a patient, we must be certain the patient understands the benefit of accepting the treatment with the risks involved, together with the risks of not accepting treatment and the option to choose an alternative. Should another form of treatment be available and reasonable, then the benefits and risks of the alternative must be explained to the patient in the same reasonable balanced way the first and subsequent options were presented.

In the UK, depending on which country you are working in, the age of legal capacity, ie the age at which a person can enter into any form of agreement (including dental treatment) is different. In Scotland this age is 16 years old, whereas in England Wales and Northern Ireland it is 18 years old. However, as is usual with clinical matters, things are not so straightforward. Whereas the laws across the UK set the age limits for legal capacity, this can be qualified in so far as a contractual arrangement can be made by the person younger than 16 if it is not unreasonable and such contracts are commonly entered into by those of a similar age.

It should be noted this may well apply to the young person who wishes to become tattooed, pierced or acquire some form of body modification, but peculiarly it seldom applies to dental treatment. With those patients younger than 16, it would most often be the parent or legal guardian who makes the definitive decision on the dental treatment that can and will take place.

With almost all matters in dentistry and especially the treatment of a minor with conscious sedation, it is the parent or the legal guardian who holds some if not all of the responsibility for the young person and it is the parent or the legal guardian who can significantly contribute to the decision to accept or to reject dental treatment.

The extent of such parental contribution depends on the child's maturity together with their ability to understand what is involved with the treatment that is being proposed.

It was Lord Denning, in 1969 in the appeal case of Hewer v Bryant who said:

"The legal right of a parent to custody of a child ends at the 18th birthday and even up till then, it is a dwindling right which the courts will hesitate to enforce against the wishes of a child, and the more so the older he is. It starts with a right of control and ends with little more than advice."[13]

This now famous dictum cleared the way forward for the case that has possibly made the greatest contribution to the acceptance of the idea of children's rights, which you will remember from your pre-qualification studies as the case of Gillick in the 1985 House of Lords.

In that judgment it was Lord Scarman who commented:

"...it is not enough that the child should understand the nature of the advice which is being given: the child must also have a sufficient maturity to understand what is involved."[14]

Lord Scarman went further adding:

"The parental right yields to the child's right to make their own decisions when the child reaches a sufficient understanding and intelligence to be capable of making up their own mind on the matter requiring decision."[14]

The decisions in those two cases reasserted the concept of the limitations in the rights and the responsibilities of parents. The essence being judgment is based more on the facts surrounding the individuals at the time of the events in question and less on applying the law as it stood at the time of the events in question.

Furthermore, while Lord Denning stated the level of parental control decreased inversely to the extent of the individual child's capacity and this is the fundamental principle leading to Gillick competence, it must be noted, there have been appeal cases which do not embrace these ideas in full, in so far as a child who is competent can consent to accept treatment, there are no equivalent rights empowering the very same child to refuse treatment[15,16,17].

It must be stated these rights and responsibilities are to <u>protect the child and not the adult</u>. In so far as gaining consent is concerned, all of these cases ensure that if the case law is adhered to, then the dental professional (you) will be in a safer position regarding valid consent, should an allegation of unauthorised contact with a child be made and <u>such an allegation can be made by anyone</u>.

While the parent and child hold concurrent rights to consent for treatment, neither party can veto a decision of the other if that decision is made in the patient's best interest. Either the competent child or the competent adult (and sometimes both together) are the key holders who can unlock the door to allow a procedure to go ahead[17].

This is the basis for Gillick competence. Young patients less than 16 years old are only able to consent for any procedure or treatment if they are Gillick or more specifically Scarman competent to do so. However in the UK there is a default assumption that patients younger than 16 years old do not possess either the maturity or the understanding to consent for dental treatment and therefore a responsible adult parent or guardian will assent or grant permission to the dental professional to proceed with treatment.

The obvious reason for this is while the winds of puberty are sweeping teenagers into adulthood they clearly will not be capable of reaching a decision that would be either sensible or safe while in a state of hormonal turbulence.

With those patients who are around 16 and 17 years of age, they are more settled (hormonally at least) and are likely to behave as younger adults rather than older children. As a result, they will most likely be Gillick competent. If they agree to dental treatment, then for sure they have capacity to consent. If on the other hand and for whatever reason they don't, then clinical manoeuvring that is subtle and sensitive will always be more successful than the battle of egos arising from the head on approach and that is only guaranteed to alienate everyone watching from the side lines in a state of disbelief or horror.

By 18 years old a line has been drawn between childhood and adulthood and your patient can consent to accept or refuse to consent for treatment[18] [19] [20].

Legal guardianship

With the younger patients the order of precedence for parental responsibility and legal guardianship is as follows:

I. Birth mother unless an adoption order has removed this.

II. Surrogate mother unless a parental or court order removes this.

III. Biological father if married to the birth mother either at the time of birth or subsequently.

IV. Birth father if the child was born after 1st December 2003.

V. If the father is neither biological nor married to the mother, the father does not have parental responsibility; however joint responsibility can be applied for.

Following the immediate family members, the order of precedence for legal guardianship is:

I. Adoptive parents with an adoption order.

II. Guardians with responsibility following the death of a parent or other responsible person.

III. Special guardians consenting for a child but the birth parents do maintain some rights.

IV. Local authorities with arrangement orders also having parental responsibilities.

V. Lastly: foster carers, but they will seldom hold parental responsibilities.

It is possible that more than one person can have responsibility and should any doubt arise it is important that consent has been obtained from the correct person, the persons or individual officer within an organisation, such as a local authority who is authorised to hold a Child Arrangement Order. While anyone from the above groups can determine the treatment plan for a patient, the person holding legal responsibility must have the capacity both legal and mental to give consent.

The 2005 Mental Capacity Act (MCA)

For adults who lack capacity, it is the **2005 Mental Capacity Act (MCA)** that provides clear principles and a framework guiding everyone working with or caring for those people aged 16 or over who are not capable of making their own decisions.

In such circumstances, consent is specific to one procedure, one appointment, a treatment plan or course of action.

Should there be any changes in what is intended, then any permission obtained is non transferrable and new consent specific to the altered proposal must be obtained.

There are five key principles underpinning the MCA[21]:

I. **There is a presumption of capacity** – every adult has the right to make his or her own decisions and must be assumed to have capacity to do so unless it is proved otherwise. This means that you cannot assume that someone cannot make a decision for themselves just because they have a particular medical condition or disability.

II. **Individuals being supported to make their own decisions** – a person must be given all practicable help before anyone treats them as not being able to make their own decisions. This means you should make every effort to encourage and support people to make the decision for them. If lack of capacity is established, it is still important that you involve the person as far as possible in making decisions.

III. **Unwise decisions** – people have the right to make decisions that others might regard as unwise or eccentric. You cannot treat someone as lacking capacity for this reason. Everyone has their own values, beliefs and preferences which may not be the same as those of other people.

IV. **Best interests** – anything done for or on behalf of a person who lacks mental capacity must be done in their best interests.

V. **Least restrictive option** – someone making a decision or acting on behalf of a person who lacks capacity must consider whether it is possible to decide or act in a way that would interfere less with the person's rights and freedoms of action, or whether there is a need to decide or act at all. Any intervention should be weighed up in the particular circumstances of the case.

Mental capacity is the ability to make a decision. If a patient is to make a decision that is valid then they must be able to understand the relevant details long enough to allow the decision to be made and then their decision needs to be communicated in a way that is clearly understood and not ambiguous allowing those who will enact that decision to be certain this is the correct course of action to take.

Once more the MCA is helpful in providing a two stage test for mental capacity for our patients. The following staged questions can be applied to determine if capacity is present:

1. Does your patient have an impairment or disturbance in the functioning of their mind at the time of your consultation? If so, then what is the diagnosis and how will this affect the person?
2. If an impairment or disturbance of the mind can be documented, does this mean the person is unable to make the decision for treatment required of them at this time?

The second stage or question presents a functional aspect to the test of capacity.

If your patient is unable to:

I. Understand the information that is relevant to the decision.
II. To retain the information to make a decision.
III. Balance the information to reach their decision.
IV. Understand the risks and benefits of making or not making the decision.
V. Communicate their decision.

Then your patient lacks the capacity to consent for treatment.

It is extremely important to recognize there are many conditions and indeed situations that can adversely impact on a patient's mental functioning so their capacity is; if not entirely removed then it could be significantly impaired. We have already discussed needle phobia and it is accepted that anxiety displayed by the phobic dental patient in the waiting room may result in our finding them in a state of terror, or shock with loss of capacity; but this is clearly only temporary.

Take them out of the dental surgery and their capacity soon returns. This temporary loss of capacity must be borne in mind when undertaking the consenting process and should a request for conscious sedation or any dental treatment be made, we must ensure the patient is in a fit mental state to understand the material risks and benefits as well as the appropriate alternatives for any dental procedure we might consider offering.

While a request for conscious sedation is simple and clear enough, it is the consent for the dental treatment while the patient is being sedated that may be scrutinized afterwards. With respect to the 5th principle of the MCA:

Is the least restrictive option being offered and considered?
Perhaps the patient may actually have wished for a conservative approach eg: root treatment and crowning rather than a surgical procedure eg: extraction. However with their capacity reduced or removed, the permission for extraction may have been well intentioned but did it come with a consent that was valid?

With these circumstances, before the patient can co-operate and their capability and capacity to consent is achieved, we must be able to communicate our intentions with the treatment options for the patient. If the ability to communicate orally is compromised, then pictures and sign language can be used instead. If confusion still remains after using these measures, rather than asking assistance from family members, the professional skills of carers, social workers and translators should be sought and as much time as is needed must be given until a well-founded decision is reached.

That decision must be accepted, but perhaps more importantly than this; the route to achieving it should be documented in the patient records. If your patient lacks capacity and there is firm evidence to support this, above anything else in accordance with the MCA, there is a legal obligation to act in the patient's best interests. Such best interest decisions will not be made on your own but will involve the patient's family members, social and key workers, nursing and support staff, but only if there is no conflict or competing interests between them, each other and your patient. With such cases, an Independent Mental Capacity Advocate (IMCA) could be appointed, but their input will most often not be required for routine dental procedures even those requiring conscious sedation. Instead, their input will be reserved for those more serious and significant events such as surgical interventions with GA.

For those dental procedures involving conscious sedation, both the treatment plans and the consent must be in writing. Where a health authority or care provider such as the UK NHS mandates that specific forms are to be used for conscious sedation, then: <u>There is no substitute and the approved forms must be completed</u>. Included in these will be sufficient space to discuss any alternatives, with the risks and the benefits for the patient to either have or not to have the procedure. The risks must be explained in a clear way so that the reasonable person would understand them and would wish to know about them.

The duty to disclose and discuss material risks

In addition, there may be risks specific to your procedure and these should be both comprehensively and clearly explained to your patient. While explaining the risks you must also consider if there are justifiable reasons why you would wish to consider withholding information from the patient. You must then ask, by doing so will this affect the decision of the patient to accept or to reject one option and favour another?

In the process of gaining consent you have a clear duty to disclose those material risks that may give rise to adverse outcomes. This follows from Lords: Steyn, Hope and Walker, who in the 2004 judgment of Chester v Afshar stated:

> *"It is a basic principle of good medical practice that adults should consent on a fully informed basis to surgery, so they are aware of all the risks."*[22.]

Lord Steyn further reinforced this opinion by quoting Professor Ronald Dworkin:

> *"The value of autonomy derives from the capacity it protects: the capacity to express one's own character- in the life one leads. Recognizing an individual right of autonomy makes self-creation possible. It allows each of us to be responsible for shaping our lives according to our own coherent or incoherent - but, in any case, distinctive - personality. It allows us to lead our lives rather than be led along them, so that each of us can be, what we have made of ourselves. We allow someone to choose death over radical amputation or a blood transfusion, if that is his informed wish, because we acknowledge his right to a life structured by his own values."*[23.]

The ascendency of Scarman and demise of Diplock

Prior to this school of thought and sitting at the opposite end of the legal spectrum was the view held by Lord Diplock. In the 1985 appeal case of Sidaway, Diplock stated that any breach in the duty of care should be determined by use of the Bolam test; whether the actions of a doctor (or a dentist) were in accordance with the practices accepted as proper by a body of responsible and skilled medical (or dental) opinion... To decide what risks the existence of which a patient should be voluntarily warned and the terms in which such a warning, if any, should be given, having regard to the effect that the warning may have, is as much an exercise in professional skill and judgment as any other part of the doctor's comprehensive duty of care to the individual patient and expert medical evidence on this matter should be treated in just the same way.[24 25.]

Somewhat arrogantly Diplock went even further than this, stating the kind of training that a judge will have undergone at the Bar would make it natural for him to say (correctly): It is my right to decide whether any particular thing is done to my body and I want to be informed of any risks there may be involved of which I am not aware from my general knowledge as a highly educated man of experience, so that I may form my own judgment as to whether to refuse the advised treatment or not....

Essentially Diplock was saying our patients who are neither judges nor professional people, somehow have fewer rights! This over-egging of the legal pudding reveals the extent to which Diplock was socially and perhaps psychologically removed from normalcy. What is more disturbing than the breathtaking arrogance of Diplock was that for 30 years, following Sidaway, his opinion of: There being no obligation to provide patients with unsolicited information about risks was unequivocally accepted by the medical and dental professions as being an appropriate way to approach patients with a view to obtaining their consent.

Despite Diplock and the ruling in Sidaway, courts in the UK lower than those of the Lords and Appeals, together with those throughout the Commonwealth began to tacitly reject Diplock's adherence to the Bolam test. Instead we find that their approach was closer to that of Lord Scarman who in opposing Diplock stated that:

> *"If therefore, the failure to warn a patient of the risks inherent in the operation which is recommended does constitute a failure to respect the patient's right to make his own decision, I can see no reason in principle why, if the risk materializes and injury or damage is caused, the law should not recognize and enforce a right in the patient to compensation by way of damages."*

From Scarman the following points have been taken and have been applied to the process of gaining consent:

I. If the patient comes to harm.

II. For the reason that a risk that was concealed then materializes.

III. A risk that a considerate clinician exercising reasonable care would have revealed.

IV. The reasonable patient knowing of this risk would avoid the procedure and thus the harm.

V. The patient has not granted consent and a cause of action based on negligence can follow.

Montgomery Consent

Following from this and many other cases, by 2015 our approach to consent had become far less paternalistic and more patient centred. This socio-legal shift culminated in the decision of the UK Supreme Court in the case of Montgomery v Lanarkshire Health Board to reverse the decisions made by two Scottish Courts (where it was awkwardly decided that Bolam should be adhered to and Diplock followed) and uphold an appeal. The final decision in this case now completely removes any further reliance on Sidaway.

The judgment in Montgomery stated:

> "....patients are now widely regarded as persons holding rights, rather than as the passive recipients of the care of the medical profession."[26]

The difference in opinions between the ruling of the Scottish Courts and the Supreme Court is one clear example of how far behind the times the law had fallen and reliance on 30 year old dictums must be questioned. It is no longer acceptable and perhaps it never has been, to unequivocally accept either legal advice or a judgment. Such tardiness in the law has permitted certain courts to maintain at best a problematic imbalance between patients and clinicians by the courts reliance on outmoded and outdated rulings.[27]

In their rulings in Montgomery, Lord Kerr and Lord Reed also pointed to significant shifts in the behaviour and attitudes of patients with respect to the provision of healthcare. Today patients increasingly access information from wider sources, joining patient support groups and receiving information from healthcare providers now constitutes a normal part of the patient experience in the clinical encounter.

The move away from such paternalism does come with the caveat of therapeutic exception. Information which may compromise the decision of the patient to undergo treatment, or to receive information; that if revealed, would be detrimental to the patient's health can be withheld. However, therapeutic exception is an extremely narrow concept and it should not be used to subvert the principle of consent in those circumstances where the patient is liable to make a choice which may be contrary to their best interests.[28].

For Nadine Montgomery and her son Sam, this landmark ruling enabled them to make a successful claim for damages. While this will never restore the potential to realise a future free from the tragic consequences from a birth so traumatic Sam was starved of oxygen for 12 minutes resulting in cerebral palsy affecting all of his limbs and nerve damage causing paralysis of one arm, it might make the cost of Sam's care more bearable.

For all of us, the case of Sam and Nadine Montgomery has changed the way we will both obtain and maintain consent. The extensive shadow that Bolam has cast over the way we practice has been lifted and the views of Diplock banished. In contrast to many judgments, the Montgomery ruling will be retrospective. As a result, it has been stated there will be rich pickings ahead[27].

Rather than focussing on the rich pickings, what we must learn from Montgomery is that obtaining and maintaining consent is critically dependent on the language we use to communicate the nature and extent of the risks the patient will face if they choose to undergo a procedure.

The use of words must clearly explain the risk that a reasonable person would attach significance to and thereby come to a decision that is balanced.

In dentistry our patients are fortunate that procedures which carry a substantial risk of grave consequences are seldom if ever undertaken. Nevertheless, with conscious sedation in addition to the elected loss of capacity, more invasive surgical procedures will take place. As a result the patient will be placed at a potentially greater risk when compared to those lesser measures which can be undertaken with local anaesthetic while the patient retains capacity.

Before we subject our patients to conscious sedation, as with all procedures in dentistry, we must fully involve them in their treatment decisions and provide unbiased evidence helping them to reach and support their choice of treatment.

If we do so, then we will be upholding not only the modern enlightened approach to patient care but those foregoing principles that have contributed to Montgomery consent.

Conscious Sedation: Relative Analgesia with N_2O

The safest and perhaps the simplest forms of conscious sedation we can use in dentistry are: Inhalation Sedation and Relative Analgesia (RA). With both techniques, the gases used are Oxygen (O_2) and Nitrous Oxide (N_2O). Not less than 30% Oxygen can be delivered from the machines approved for use in dentistry in the UK and it should be noted that while premixed 50% O_2 and 50% N_2O (Entonox or Nitronox) is most commonly used in emergency medicine, pre-hospital care and childbirth, the use of any such premixed gases are not approved for use in dentistry.

With inhalation sedation, a constant gas concentration is used, whereas with RA, the gas concentration can be continuously altered throughout the procedure in response to the patient's level of consciousness. RA is preferable to inhalation sedation as this technique allows the operator the flexibility to titrate the N_2O in response to the patient's needs, so they can be adequately sedated, but not over-sedated while receiving dental treatment. With this technique, as noted: A variable mixture of not less than 30% Oxygen but no greater than 70% Nitrous Oxide is delivered via a nasal mask to the patient.

Success with this form of conscious sedation is not only dependent on the sedative and analgesic effects of the gases, the patient needs to be treated in a calm manner and within an environment that is calming. From experience, if the patient attends for treatment in a state of agitation or has an aggressive and impatient temperament, this technique seldom works. Or if it does, it seldom works for a period of time that is sufficient to allow a dental procedure to be completed. Or worse still, the concentration of N_2O required for conscious sedation rapidly rises to the maximum one can safely use and even then the chances of success are limited.

While there are safety measures restricting the maximum concentration of N_2O we might use, any tendency towards using high levels of N_2O that verge dangerously towards those gas concentrations required for general anaesthesia cannot ever be considered to be safe practice. Nevertheless, with the correct patient selection, RA is both safe and effective with almost no side effects and it is especially useful for those adults requiring the simplest of dental treatments or the most minor of surgical procedures.

For those children for whom IV sedation with a benzodiazepine is not suitable, RA provides a useful means whereby they can readily accept dentistry in an outpatient day care setting, without the need for a lengthy period of waiting following referral to a specialist secondary care clinic for treatment.

Contraindications to the use of RA

Although RA with N_2O and O_2 is inherently safe and with those machines approved for use in dentistry, there is after many years still a 100% safety record, there are certain patients for whom the use of RA could <u>potentially</u> lead to clinical and legal complications:

1. Patients with psychiatric conditions. The use of any drug (or gas) that has a disinhibitory effect must only take place with the input and guidance of the medical psychiatric specialist who has prescribed the medication for the patient, together with input from the patient's mental health services team. Although the dental care for many patients who are in this category will take place in a hospital, a specialist centre, or other secondary care clinic, increasing numbers of such patients are now being looked after in community clinics. Very often these patients find their way to a general dental practice in search of treatment. Their route to your door is either through referral from a colleague or of the patient's own volition. As with any patient, your access to an up to date, accurate and comprehensive medical history is vitally important before embarking on any treatment either with or without the use of RA or other sedative agent.

2. Pregnant patients in their first trimester. These patients should not routinely have any elective dental treatment. Except for maintenance of oral hygiene, all other forms of dentistry should be avoided wherever possible during pregnancy. The question of N_2O use during pregnancy is based on the adverse effects noted from chronic exposure. However, the use of RA for a single appointment should present no risk for the mother and unborn child in cases where emergency dental treatment for an anxious or phobic patient is simply unavoidable and not using RA would mean the mother would suffer more distress than if N_2O; the safest of sedative agents were not to be used at all. A retrospective analysis of three studies covering nearly 6000 pregnant patients exposed to N_2O (as an essential component of GA techniques) revealed no adverse outcomes for the mother or more importantly for the child[29,30,31]. For the pregnant patient who is apprehensive and <u>requires urgent dental care, RA with N_2O should be regarded as the first choice of sedative</u>[32,33]. Any evidence of complications developing during pregnancy will mean your involvement in consultation with the obstetrics and gynaecology team looking after your patient, but given the results from the three studies cited above, this would be a rare occurrence.

3. Patients with gastro-intestinal tract obstructions. For dental patients with bowel obstructions, strictures or those having had recent surgery such as colostomy or ileostomy, while N_2O is not absolutely contra-indicated, supportive guidance from the patient's general medical practitioner or specialist gastro-enterologist would be advisable. The occurrence of painful bowel distension has been documented and studied in surgical patients exposed to N_2O. Although the dose and period of exposure would be far greater than with RA used in dentistry, nevertheless N_2O will diffuse into body cavities, resulting in a doubling of the occurrence of moderate or severe but in almost all cases, distension of the bowels that is painful[33].

The main reason for this clinical presentation is the higher gas partition co-efficient of nitrous oxide when compared to inspired air which is 78% nitrogen. Thus N_2O can easily enter into and leave the gas filled spaces in the patient's gastrointestinal tract. (We will return to consider this phenomenon in some more detail below)

4. Patients with airway obstruction. Patients with a deviated nasal septum, nasal polyps, Upper Respiratory Tract Infections, (URTIs) allergic rhinitis, or severe sinusitis may be unable to adequately inhale or exhale N_2O/O_2 with the nasal masks used in dental RA. Furthermore, should their Eustachian tubes become blocked, or the communication from the pharynx to the middle ear be significantly reduced, then once more due to the greater gas partition co-efficient of N_2O/O_2, (compared to air), this may lead to pressure increases within both the middle and inner ear, contraindicating the use of RA for the following reasons:

The volume and pressures of N_2O can become dangerously high within the middle ear if the patency of the Eustachian tubes are compromised by inflammation or any traumatic or pathological obstruction. Rupture of the tympanic membrane would be a disastrous outcome as a result of administration of nitrous oxide. Even if the ear drum is not compromised, upon completion of the procedure with RA, with a reduction in concentration of N_2O and increase in concentration of O_2 a negative pressure may develop to such an extent in the middle ear that postoperative nausea and vomiting may be experienced by your patient as a result of *otitis media*[34][35].

Similar painful after-effects may be experienced when N_2O in dental RA is administered to patients with sinusitis. As an aside, but for the same reasons as noted above, the expansion of gas bubbles of N_2O and O_2 in the orbital structures of the eye following retinal surgery (where gasses have been deliberately introduced intra-ocularly) may have serious consequences for the patient, should there be any further unintended pressure increases. Of particular note and thus importance; in the UK, every year, some 8,000 vitreo-retinal procedures are conducted using medical gases introduced into the orbit to reattach retinas. There has been a recent case reporting the devastating consequences of N_2O use after ophthalmic surgery, resulting in irreversible blindness. For patients undergoing any form of eye surgery, before considering the use of RA and N2O in dentistry, it would be prudent to consult with the patient's medical practitioner and their ophthalmic specialist[36].

Setting the rare but devastating complications of ocular surgery to one side and returning to airway obstruction, the more common complications of COPD will be considered on the next page.

COPD and the use of RA

Patients suffering from Chronic Obstructive Pulmonary Disease (COPD) rely on incipient hypoxia to drive their respiration. Taking this into consideration, some authorities do suggest that dental RA with N_2O is far from ideal. Their reasoning being, not only is the patient's hypoxemic driver in an already depressed state, because relatively high O_2 concentrations are delivered together with N_2O in RA, this may (theoretically) remove any remaining stimulus for the patient's hypoxemic drive to continue working.

In opposition to this, another school of thought advises that we follow the principles of moderate sedation and where necessary, the patient can always be instructed to breathe more deeply while undergoing RA. Both points of view can be reconciled should you choose to visit any Medicine of the Elderly (MOE) Unit in the UK NHS. There you are sure to find many patients with COPD who are being kept alive, awake and quite vital, with O_2 delivered in anything from 2 Litres per minute up to 10 to 15 litres per minute.

COPD is an unfortunately common condition with some 5% of the world's population affected to a lesser or a greater degree. Mostly those over 40 years, smokers, or those with industrial, occupational or recreational exposure to pollutants, irritants or tobacco smoke suffer from COPD.

It shouldn't come as any real surprise for you to read that in the UK, COPD prevalence can be mapped across a North: South socio-economic divide; almost 3% in the North against some 1% in the South. The incidence of COPD is seemingly static, but with a prevalence that is not only increasing it is linked to the increased rate of tobacco smoking seen in economically depressed areas. While the incidence for COPD may have peaked, the number of people affected remains high and this presents a major challenge for health services, especially for those of us who serve the most socially deprived patients and communities[37].

Respiratory Failure

The presence of COPD, especially if it is undiagnosed is worthy of consideration for those patients who request either RA or IV sedation. In addition to COPD, we frequently see Respiratory Failure: this can be either Type 1 or Type 2:

Type 1 Respiratory Failure. In such cases the patient has normal blood CO_2, but lowered levels of O_2 this is a result of a Ventilation/Perfusion (V/Q) mismatch. With respect to V/Q ratios, the air going into and coming out of the lungs is not matched by blood flow into and out of the lungs and the causes can be:

i.   Insufficient O_2 in the air
ii. V/Q mismatch from a pulmonary embolism.
iii. Pneumonia or Acute Respiratory Distress Syndrome: O_2 cannot diffuse into the blood stream.
iv. Arterio-venous shunting with oxygenated blood mixing with non-oxygenated blood.
v.   Alveolar hypoventilation from respiratory muscle weakness, but this may lead to a Type 2 respiratory failure.

Type 2 Respiratory Failure. In such cases the patient has increased blood CO_2, together with lowered levels of O_2 this is a result of inadequate alveolar ventilation. In other words gaseous exchange is not adequate and the patient in Type 2 Respiratory failure will be building up increased levels of CO_2, the causes are:

i.   Increased airway resistance from COPD Asthma or suffocation.
ii. A reduced ability to breathe effectively due to medication, TIA, CVA or morbid obesity.

iii. Decrease in alveolar area due to chronic bronchitis.

iv. An inability to use the muscles of respiration due to paralysis, medication or other neuromuscular condition.

v. Skeletal deformity such as extreme kyphosis or a malformed chest cavity.

We will return to this topic to consider the V/Q ratio and lung function in greater detail in the next section.

5. Patients with poor vitamin B 12 uptake. Nowadays this is less frequently caused by dietary deficiencies such as those arising in or associated with vegetarians or vegans, but more commonly as a result of Intrinsic Factor (IF) deficiency that is linked to an auto-immune disorder such as Pernicious Anaemia. This can be associated with Hashimoto's Thyroiditis and Adrenocortical Insufficiency. Alternatively, the presence of antibodies directed against Gastric Parietal Cells, responsible for releasing IF, that binds to Vitamin B 12 or anti IF antibodies in the patient's serum, effectively mean: although Vitamin B12 is present in the diet, there is no possibility of it being efficiently absorbed. In other cases, the effective absorption of Vitamin B 12 is significantly reduced in patients with Crohn's Disease, Coeliac Disease or in those patients who have undergone ileostomy, gastrectomy or who have had radiation therapy to the GI tract. For any patients in the above noted groups, it has been noted that the use of N_2O may be contraindicated.

However, these concerns have only been raised with chronic exposure to N_2O and with doses far in excess of those used in dental RA. The reasons for such concerns are that N_2O has the ability to irreversibly oxidize the cobalt atom of vitamin B12, thus reducing the activity of B 12-dependent enzymes such as methionine and thymidylate synthetase. These enzymes are vital in the synthesis of myelin and nucleic acids. If these metabolic pathways are interrupted, N_2O derived toxicity can result. However, the minimum concentration and the length of exposure to N_2O at which such effects become clinically significant have not as yet been determined. Of interest, N_2O exposures within the doses and durations used for GA procedures are certainly capable of inducing megaloblastic changes in bone marrow cells after 24 hours. After some 4 days, these effects continue with Agranulocytosis being noted.[38] Despite these worrying haematological signs, animal studies have so far failed to determine if there are any harmful reproductive effects following N_2O exposure.[39.]

Taking these concerns one stage further, it has also been suggested as N_2O affects the production, the differentiation and the function of leukocytes. On this basis, it might not be advisable to provide RA for patients who are either taking immuno-suppressant medication or who are immuno-compromised. However such concerns may be based on theoretical extrapolation rather than practical consideration; in so far as work in the dental clinic is concerned, in contrast to the dental school laboratory; the benefit of N_2O for the anxious patients far outweighs the risks for the nervous lab rat.

The use of an active N_2O scavenging device during dental procedures is capable of reducing, if not entirely eliminating any significant risks to the patient and to the practitioner from N_2O exposure and the toxicity effects noted above. We must recognize that the proper use of scavenging equipment is only one of several methods we might utilize to reduce N_2O accumulation in the dental clinic and surrounding environment[40].

Even though there are patients for whom RA with N_2O may be contra indicated; from the five groups above, you can see that RA with N_2O is both relatively simple and in most cases exceptionally safe. Before proceeding to look at the mechanism of how this form of conscious sedation works, it would be prudent to revise the physiology of the respiratory system in some more detail and then return to look at V/Q ratios, before considering the effects of N_2O on the patient.

I. O_2 is quite insoluble in plasma and tissues, while in the blood some 97% of all O_2 is carried by Haemoglobin (Hb).

II.   When the demand for O_2 rises due to muscle activity, an increase in temperature or a decrease in tissue pH, then Haemoglobin releases O_2

III. If the level of O_2 in the lungs decreases when your patient becomes breathless, more air is inhaled and thus the balance in the level of O_2 is regained.

IV.   In contrast to O_2, the transport of CO_2 by Haemoglobin is minimal. CO_2 is carried in red blood cells, but only after it has been hydrolysed by Carbonic Anhydrase to form Bicarbonate.

V. H^+ ions are released from Haemoglobin in the lungs combining with Bicarbonate ions to form CO_2 which is then exhaled.

One quarter (25%) of all CO_2 is combined with Hb to form Carbamino-Hb (from which CO_2 is exhaled) while 5% of all CO_2 remains dissolved in blood and is not released into the lungs. Therefore it takes only a very small increase in the partial pressure or PCO_2 (the concentration of CO_2 dissolved in blood) to cause an increase in respiratory rate. This can be achieved without any decrease in the partial pressure or PO_2 levels.

Of considerable importance in those patients with COPD and type 2 Respiratory Failure: The effect of an increase in PCO_2 but lowered PO_2 is not enough to maintain adequate levels of PO_2 even with an increased respiratory rate.

**With such patients, additional O_2 will be needed
to maintain sufficient respiration:**

I.   The physiological control of respiration from O_2 levels is crude, whereas the physiological control of respiration from CO_2 is extremely precise.

II. In such cases, increased respiration or hyperventilation will not increase the PO_2.

III. Increasing PO_2 can be achieved by: Increasing the O_2 concentration by using supplemental Oxygen (as noted above).

IV. O_2 carriage can be improved by increasing the Haemoglobin concentration in the patient's blood either through Iron supplements or with whole blood transfusion.

V.   Increased PO_2 also results from increasing the blood flow through the lungs by raising the cardiac output.

As you can see from the above summary, adequate lung function is essential to supply O_2, remove CO_2 and thus balance the pH of plasma since $CO_2 + H_2O \rightarrow H_2CO_3$ with carbonic acid playing a pivotal role in maintaining the acid: base balance of blood.

With contraction of the diaphragm and accessory muscles of respiration: the Pectorales Major and Minor, the Sternocleidomastoids and Platysma, negative pressure develops in the patient's lungs and air will be drawn in. Of note in COPD, the involvement of the accessory muscles of respiration become critically important to aid breathing. While inspiration is an active event, expiration is in the main a passive event, as the muscles of respiration are in a relaxed state. However with coughing and in asthma, it is the rapid contraction of the internal intercostal muscles that are responsible for creating the positive pressure wave associated with forceful expiration.

Lung function and physiology

Together with skeletal muscle activity, there are three physiological mechanisms occurring in the lungs during respiration:

1. Ventilation: Air flow into and out of the lungs.

Ventilation or V is the amount of air going into and leaving the lungs. This is measured in litres per minute. Ventilation is controlled both subconsciously from the patient's brain stem and consciously from the patient's motor cortex. With such involuntary and voluntary inputs acting on the patient's ability to breath their ventilation can be carefully controlled. In addition to these control pathways responding to CNS chemo-receptors, there are PNS chemo-receptors too:

i. Chemoreceptors in the Carotid and Aortic bodies respond to changes in both CO_2 and H^+ in blood, in addition in the airways and connective tissues of the lungs there are similar receptors finely responding to changes in CO_2 and H^+ concentrations.

ii. Mechanoreceptors in the chest wall respond to physical changes in the length of muscles. These receptors forming part of the efferent motor pathways control ventilation and so ensure arterial CO_2 levels are very finely determined.

Ventilation is controlled by these effector pathways which ascend to the CNS or descend in the spinal cord to the phrenic nerves supplying the intercostal and abdominal muscles. The overall effect of these pathways is to ensure the patient's arterial CO_2 levels are very finely controlled.

2. Perfusion: Blood flow into and out of the lungs.

Perfusion or P is the amount of blood being pumped out of the heart and into the lungs. This is also measured in litres per minute.

Blood flows from the pulmonary circulation into the capillaries around the alveoli. A decrease in perfusion leads to dead spaces in the lungs and CO_2 levels may rise. In response, an increase in ventilation can counteract this compensating for higher CO_2 levels. However, with reduced perfusion, the O_2 levels will decrease and if this is to be counteracted, an increase in the O_2 concentration in air is then required.

3. Diffusion: The efficient exchange of gasses in the lungs.

This depends on Ventilation (V) and Perfusion (Q) being balanced according to physiological needs, but this is not necessarily in a state of precise chemical equilibrium. In the resting state the average V/Q values are:

4 litres per minute of air enter and leave the lungs /5 litres per minute of blood flows into and out of the lungs. This gives a V/Q ratio = 0.8.

The V/Q ratio is the balance between:

Ventilation: O_2 entering with CO_2 leaving the alveoli and:
Perfusion: O_2 leaving with CO_2 entering the alveoli.

The V/Q ratio is an important factor in the concentrations of Alveolar (PA) levels of O_2 and CO_2 and arterial (Pa) levels of O_2 and CO_2.

A decrease in the V/Q ratio can come from either lowered ventilation or raised perfusion, the effect is both PA O_2 and Pa O_2 decrease and PA CO_2 and Pa CO_2 increase.

An increase in the V/Q ratio results in an increase in PA O_2 and Pa O_2 with a decrease in PA CO_2 and Pa CO_2

V/Q mismatches can occur in response to positional, physiological and pathological changes. Of particular importance to dentistry with the use of N_2O and RA sedation, is the possibility of a V/Q mismatch. V/Q mismatches are naturally present between the apices and the bases of the lungs. When your patient is standing or sitting upright the bases of the lungs will be more perfused and less ventilated, when compared to the apices, while lying down the lung bases will be more ventilated and less perfused. This V/Q mismatch comes from the effects of gravity and the patient's heart being positioned central to the apices and bases of their lungs. When the patient is in the supine position, the V/Q ratio becomes more evenly balanced throughout the lungs.

As noted, V/Q mismatches can also occur in response to pathological conditions. If pulmonary blood flow decreases as a result of circulatory restriction or embolism, then the V/Q ratio increases. With a pulmonary embolism, a low V/Q ratio arises and blood will be shunted to other areas of the lungs that are more effectively ventilated and perfused. Those areas that are not perfused but ventilated then become <u>alveolar dead spaces</u>.

If on the other hand, the effective ventilation decreases but perfusion continues as normal, (for example, from an FBAO entering and impacting into patient's right main bronchus), the V/Q ratio significantly diminishes, the $Pa\ O_2$ drops and $Pa\ CO_2$ rises as a <u>physiological shunt</u> is now taking place.

If blood reaches the lungs but then leaves the lungs with no ventilation, perfusion does not occur and the arterial blood gas levels will soon resemble those of venous blood.

In contrast to a physiological blood shunt, an <u>anatomical blood shunt</u> occurs when a shortened circulation occurs if blood crosses directly from the right to the left ventricle with no intervening pulmonary circulation.

The most common causes of such shunting can be from ventriculo-septal defects such as those in Eisenmenger's Syndrome where a left to right shunt reverses after the compensatory hypertrophy in the left ventricle is matched, then surpassed by a reactive hypertrophy in the right ventricle. This unusual cardio-myo-pathology is often associated with Down's syndrome. From a safety perspective we must be aware of the possibility this condition might be present in our patients who have Down's syndrome.

<u>With both physiological and anatomical</u>
<u>shunts $Pa\ O_2$ falls and $Pa\ CO_2$ rises.</u>

Returning to other pathological conditions such as COPD, the V/Q ratios will not be consistent throughout the lungs. In our patients suffering with COPD there is destruction of both alveolar and capillary tissues. This leads to the creation of the above noted dead spaces in the lungs with some lung tissue being (i) over-perfused while other lung tissues are (ii) under-perfused.

i. With the first of these: While the V/Q ratio remains low, adequately oxygenated blood is not leaving the pulmonary circulation to enter the systemic circulation for the benefit of the patient.
ii. With the second of these the high V/Q ratio means oxygenation is sufficient but blood is simply not entering then leaving the pulmonary circulation so exchange of CO_2 with O_2 has not taken place in the pulmonary circulation.

From this brief description of COPD, you can understand that both hypoxia and hypercapnia will be seen. Your patients with COPD will be able to compensate for such a problem, but only to a certain degree, but this will eventually prove to be ineffective as the COPD is an invariably degenerative condition with a life limiting and life ending outcome.

With a low V/Q ratio, hypoxic vasoconstriction can decrease perfusion to allow normalization of the V/Q ratio. Thus $Pa\,O_2$ will rise and $Pa\,CO_2$ will fall. But it must be remembered that the circulation will already be in a diminished and thus a compromised state.

A summary of lung patho-physiology

In summary 1:

I.   A low V/Q ratio will impair the pulmonary gas exchange, causing low Partial Arterial pressure of oxygen (Pa O_2).

II. The elimination of CO_2 is also impaired.

III. A rise in the Partial Arterial pressure of carbon dioxide (Pa CO_2) is seldom observed, as this leads to respiratory stimulation and the resultant increase in alveolar ventilation then rapidly returns Pa CO_2 to normal physiological values.

IV. This clinical picture is seen in chronic bronchitis, asthma and acute pulmonary oedema.

V.   It is also seen in those patients with chronic hepatic syndrome due to morbidly high blood pressures in the hepato-portal circulation.

With a high V/Q ratio broncho-constriction can reduce the ventilation to match the compromised perfusion. Thus the overall effect of alveolar dead spaces will decrease and the respiratory effort to ventilate these areas will be decreased.

In summary 2:

I.   A high V/Q ratio will both decrease the PACO$_2$ and increase the PA O_2.

II. This finding is most commonly seen with pulmonary embolism due to an obstruction in blood flow to an area of the lung.

III. Thus ventilatory efforts are inefficient and blood will not be adequately oxygenated.

IV. A high V/Q ratio is also seen in emphysema, due to loss of capillary supply to alveolar surface area, there is proportionally more ventilation available per perfusion area.

V.   The loss of surface area across which gas exchange can take place leads to a decreased Pa O_2

It is certain that disruption of these physiological processes will lead to respiratory failure, because of this: From a safety perspective, it is incredibly important that these physiological and pathological processes are fully understood to reduce, if not remove the risk and prevent the harm from occurring that leads towards respiratory failure. This understanding must form the foundation of your working knowledge for RA. For the avoidance of doubt:

Respiratory Failure is defined by:

I.   The Pa CO_2 rising above 40.5mm Hg.
II. The Pa O_2 falling below a level: $100.1 - 0.303$ x Age of Patient (in years)

From the aforementioned definitions, respiratory failure will be diagnosed in the specialist hospital environment from the analysis of arterial blood gasses and not in the dental clinic from your clinical observations. Nevertheless, when using RA, you must be vigilant to the risk of the patient's physiological processes giving rise to the possibility of a pathological progression towards respiratory failure.

The pharmacokinetics of nitrous oxide

In common with those drugs discussed in the previous sections, N_2O is:

I.   Introduced.
II. Absorbed.
III. Distributed.
IV. Metabolized then:
V.   Eliminated.

However unlike drugs which are either injected or ingested, N_2O is inhaled and therefore the continued absorption and distribution will be dependent on a pressure gradient being maintained. When the pressure of the inspired gas equals the pressure of the gas in the alveoli, equilibration occurs and absorption into the tissues will result. It is this pressure gradient of N_2O in the tissues, plasma and blood which is responsible for driving N_2O across the blood-brain barrier and once in the CNS, the sedating effects of RA will be observed.

As N_2O is a simple molecule, its solubility is low and its absorption is the highest of all anaesthetic agents.

Another way to quantify this property is by using the partition co-efficient values for N_2O. These ratios are an indication of the ability of an anaesthetic to cross tissue membranes. With one of the lowest blood: gas partition co-efficient values: 0.47 (this is 30 X more than Nitrogen alone and inspired air has 78% Nitrogen) and the lowest of all blood: adipose tissue partition co-efficient values: 2.3; the ease with which N_2O can rapidly cross from the alveolar membranes into the blood stream: where it neither combines with haemoglobin nor undergoes biotransformation and from there to cross the blood brain barrier to act in the CNS, can be more easily appreciated[40].

With such properties some 90% of N_2O equilibration is reached within 10 minutes from first inhalation. Another property of N_2O is the absolute safety with which it can be used in RA.

Another way to qualify this property is by use of the Minimum Alveolar Concentration (MAC), which is the percentage of the anaesthetic agent required which will cause anaesthesia (the non-response to a surgical stimulus) in 50% of those patients exposed to an inhaled anaesthetic. Interestingly the N_2O MAC is 104%. Essentially at normal atmospheric pressures ie: sea level N_2O cannot induce a state of surgical anaesthesia.

The MAC is a measure of a healthy volunteer patient's response to a given dose of anaesthetic and incremental increases in MAC cannot be used to predict physiological responses in your patient's respiratory, cardiovascular or other organ system's functioning. It must be stressed that your patient will most likely not be a healthy male volunteer aged 18-35 and they will most likely have a relevant medical and medication history that <u>must</u> be taken into account when considering the use of RA with N_2O.

Despite the simplicity and safety of RA with N_2O, you must be both aware and wary of those nervous patients with pre existing respiratory, cardiac, hepatic and renal conditions and those who are taking any medication that may interact with N_2O.

All inhalation sedative agents exert some physiological effects on a patient's respiratory function.

With respect to this, while not altering blood pressure or heart rate, N_2O will cause a decrease in tidal volume, due to the CNS sedation of all skeletal muscle function, including those used to control breathing and thus an increase in respiratory rate will be observed in your patient being sedated with N_2O and O_2. The overall effect is that net ventilation remains unaltered. Unlike other inhalation anaesthetics, N_2O does not lower the intrinsic tone of skeletal muscles[41][42].

While N_2O has a low potency but a high MAC, in those patients who are elderly, or young, taking opioid medications, who have COPD, or any other condition that compromises their cardiovascular fitness, the MAC to achieve quite deep sedation or even general anaesthesia can be easily reached at relatively low N_2O concentrations such as those used for dental RA, therefore:

I.   A decrease in N_2O MAC can be seen with an increase and extremes of age (the elderly inactive the infirm and the very young), with the use of recreational drugs such as cannabis, excess use of alcohol and in those patients with hypercapnia (Pa CO_2 > 90mm Hg), those with hypoxia (O_2 < 40) and those patients with severe anaemia (haematocrit <10%).

II. An increase in N_2O MAC can be seen with a decrease in age (the young healthy athletically fit), the use of recreational drugs such as cocaine or other CNS stimulants and in the chronic alcoholic whose CNS and hepatic metabolite pathways have developed a tolerance to exogenous sedatives to the degree that N_2O has almost no effect on them.

Another important factor to remember with N_2O and MAC is the concentration of gas leaving the RA machine is not the same as that concentration entering the patient's lungs. There will be a significant reduction in N_2O, mostly from the patient who relies on mouth-breathing with leakage from around the nasal mask being significant. It has been estimated that little more than 0.3 to 0.5 N_2O MAC has ever been received by dental patients. In other words; if a mix of 70% N_2O: 30% O_2 is being delivered, little more than 30% N_2O will be present in the alveoli. If it is not being actively scavenged and pumped out for the benefit of those walking past below your surgery window, then the other 40% of N_2O being dispensed will be in the dental clinic, floating around your feet[43].

In dental RA, we can now leave MAC alone, as we will only ever use one sedative agent on one patient at one appointment. In the UK, with dental RA, this will be N_2O. With the current safety critical recommendations from the SCDEP and the changes in the regulations governing dental sedation in the UK, combinations of inhalational sedative agents will no longer be used.

Another interesting phenomenon to consider with N_2O sedation is the occurrence of post-procedural hypoxia. During RA, there will be a continuous and relatively high partial pressure of N_2O in the patient's blood stream. Should there be a sudden discontinuation of N_2O delivery, then in theory, but perhaps not in practice; (at least not with the volumes and concentrations of N_2O being used in dental RA) a relatively high volume of O_2 will leave the blood stream to enter the alveoli together with the outflow of N_2O.

To avoid the risk of such diffusion hypoxia, upon completion of their dental procedure, it is customary to give the patient 100% O_2 for a few minutes. While this may have little if any physiological benefit for the patient, it does allow any residual N_2O in the RA machine to be flushed out. The benefits of this process being environmental rather than clinical[44].

The mechanism whereby N_2O exerts its sedative effect is still not clearly understood. For our purposes in dentistry, it is sufficient to suggest that protein binding on the surfaces of neuronal membranes by N_2O results in an alteration of ion flow and the transmission of signals across synapses is thus inhibited. N_2O is capable of producing a mild analgesic effect and of considerable interest is the blockade of N_2O action by the opioid antagonist naloxone. This pharmacological interaction would suggest that N_2O induces the release of encephalins that bind to endogenous opioid receptor sites and thus trigger descending nor-adrenergic (inhibitory) pathways[45]. Something of a proof for this has been provided by the estimate that 30% N_2O produces analgesia that is equivalent to 15 mgs of Morphine[40].

While N_2O on its own will not depress respiratory activity, should your dental patient undergoing RA be taking any opioid medication, then a more pronounced circulatory and thus respiratory depression can occur; as the combination of N_2O and opioids can result in an unmasking of the depressant action of low doses of N_2O. This pharmacological effect on the patient's circulatory ability must be borne in mind when considering RA for your patients who may be taking opioids and who are cardiovascularly compromised.

Against this potential for N_2O at low doses to depress the hypoxic O_2 dependent drive; during dental relative analgesia, the paient's venous return increases due to a greater contractility of venous smooth muscles following from an elevation in sympathetic tone when higher doses of N_2O are used. Arterial blood pressure remains unaffected by the concentrations of N_2O used during dental RA[40 46]. Overall when we consider the totality of clinical evidence; N_2O is a safe inhalational sedative drug. However, the following five safety principles should be followed when using N_2O for dental RA:

I. Sufficient vacuum and active N_2O scavenging devices must be used at all times.

II. Without exception, the equipment, the gas cylinders, the nasal masks, the fittings and all of the tubes must be checked before every procedure for every patient, with nasal masks being checked for size to ensure the fit is correct.

III. The patient should be discouraged from mouth breathing and talking during the procedure.

IV. Following the procedure 100% O_2 should be given to the patient for 3 to 5 minutes.

V. The clinical environment must be well ventilated with good fresh air circulation and the exhaust of exhaled N_2O must be to an external location.

Although RA with N_2O has a long history of being safely used in dentistry, there are patients for whom procedures with RA simply cannot proceed because of an inherent inability to tolerate or use a nasal mask. This may be due to a psychological or cognitive impairment or an anatomical problem such a nasopharyngeal obstruction, most commonly nasal polyps, a deviated septum, acute sinusitis or chronic rhinitis. For dentally phobic patients while RA may not be tolerable, where possible and applicable, patients should be encouraged to try dental RA before consideration is given for intravenous sedation.

Conscious Sedation: Intravenous Sedation

The use of intravenous sedative drugs may provide the means whereby routine dentistry can be safely undertaken for dentally phobic patients and for those patients attending with any of the previously discussed contra-indicatory medical conditions for whom inhalational sedation with N_2O cannot be safely used.

At the start of this section, it was mentioned that the IACSD together with the SDCEP have investigated the provision of conscious sedation in primary dental care in the UK. Although this investigation focussed on the findings for conscious sedation within the NHS, the recommendations apply equally to the private dental sector. Furthermore, the findings from the IACSD and SDCEP investigations and review may well prove to be useful for your practice of dentistry even if you work outside the UK and out-with the NHS.

One initial recommendation was to limit the numbers and the types of drugs that could be used in the dental clinic and thus multi-drug conscious sedation may continue but only within specialized dental clinics and only under the supervision of dentists with specialist training. As mentioned, one of the main reasons for this recommendation and for an investigation was to improve the safety of conscious sedation. The recommendation that intravenous (IV) conscious sedation should be limited to one drug only would seem to be a safe and a sound decision to make, but this decision does seem contrary to the findings coming from the significant advances that have been made in the clinical trials of multi-drug use for IV conscious sedation in dentistry.

In this last section together with the recommendations of the IACSD and SDCEP, we will focus on some safety principles for the most commonly used IV agent: midazolam. After dealing with this drug we will complete this section with brief notes on three other drugs still used in dental practices conducting conscious sedation and these are: fentanyl, propofol and ketamine.

Airway Assessment of the Sedation Patient

With regard to Chapter One: Medical Emergencies: **A B C D E** and for all of your patients: Protection and management of their **A**irway will always be your first and your foremost consideration. For the patient who will undergo conscious sedation, the importance of evaluating their airway; in anticipation of a medical emergency must never be overlooked or relegated to an afterthought in your sedation assessment appointment.

The management of all emergencies starts with: **A** <u>Airway</u> !!

When accepting a patient for conscious sedation, your empathic consideration of what matters to them; noted by Professor Jason Leitch in 2016 to be a **vital sign** of compassion and care is fundamental to lowering perceived professional barriers, establishing communication, building rapport, gaining, then earning: Trust from your patient.

Remember (but some too often forget), that many dental patients coming to us for sedation will have had that trust significantly eroded or entirely swept away in the aftermath of an adverse interaction with a member of our profession...leaving us to pick up the pieces.

From the outset, your patient must be made to feel as comfortable as possible. If we fail to do this during the assessment appointment, then what chance do we have of achieving this during the sedation appointment itself?

We must not forget that the sedation we deliver in dentistry is: Conscious Sedation and not General Anaesthesia and one way of achieving the best outcome is to work with a patient to find out what matters to them and so reduce their apprehensions to a workable level before, during and after the procedure.

The commonly found sources of stress arising on a daily basis in your busy surgery: *e.g:* screaming children must be removed from the clinical environment in which you are working, so the patient and their chaperone will feel as relaxed as possible, from their first to their last visit with you. The patient and their chaperone will talk about you after every appointment: So....never, never, never disregard the chaperone and be careful that your conduct towards them is respectful at all times. After all without them your patient cannot come to their appointment and leave afterwards and it is into the care of the chaperone that your patient will be placed.

In your assessment appointment, once the patient is comfortably seated, the dental procedure can be explained once more (in fact; explained as many times as is necessary) and by doing so you can maintain the consent you are seeking to obtain from the referral letter that has brought the patient to see you. In the first assessment appointment in addition to finding out what matters to the patient, further clinical signs are measured:

1. Blood pressure.
2. Resting Heart Rate.
3. Body Mass Index (BMI)

and the most important observation of all:
Airway Assessment will be completed.

The patient's airway is assessed with the (modified) Mallampati Score:

The (modified) Mallampati Classification:

Class I: Soft palate, uvula, fauces and pillars visible.
Class II: Soft palate, uvula and fauces visible.
Class III: Soft palate and base of uvula visible.
Class IV: Only the hard palate visible.

The Modified Mallampati Score

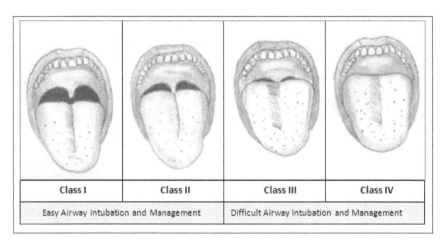

Class I	Class II	Class III	Class IV
Easy Airway Intubation and Management		Difficult Airway Intubation and Management	

The Mallampati classes I and II are associated with relatively easy intubation, whereas the classes III and IV are associated with an increased intubation difficulty.

With relevance to conscious sedation in dentistry, a recent study noted that the modified Mallampati score (as noted above) may be a useful indicator for identifying those patients for whom laryngoscopy and intubation could be easily performed, it <u>was not</u> however so beneficial in recognizing those patients for whom ventilation with a bag-mask could be effectively performed, a procedure we may need to administer in a medical emergency[47].

To support the Mallampati Score in those dental practices undertaking conscious sedation, other tests to predict the ease or the difficulty with which an airway could be maintained are therefore needed.

One such assessment that can easily be performed by the referring dentist, is the Upper Lip Bite Test (ULBT) which has been proven to be significantly more accurate than the other tests with respect to airway assessment and if necessary; management too.

However, the ULBT should be used conjunction with further evaluations and when combined, these could more reliably predict the patients for whom easier laryngoscopy, safer intubation and overall better management of their airways could be achieved, should the need arise.[48].

One such assessment is the Simplified Airway Risk Index (or SARI). This is a multivariate risk score for predicting the difficulty with which tracheal intubation can be performed. The SARI scores ranges from 0 to 12 points. The higher number of points indicates the patient's airway will be more difficult to manage in an emergency.

If the SARI score is greater than 4, this is an indication that intubation will be difficult[49]. Seven criteria are used to calculate the SARI score and the individual scores from these criteria are added to give the total SARI value:

SARI: The Simplified Airway Risk Index:

	Parameter	0 points	1 point	2 points
1.	Mouth opening	> 4 cm	<4 cm	
2.	Thyromental Distance	>6.5 cm	6 to 6.5 cm	<6 cm
3.	Mallampati	I or II	III	IV
4.	Neck movement	> 90°	80 to 90°	< 80°
5.	Underbite	Can protrude jaw	Cannot protrude jaw	
6.	Body weight	< 90 kg	90 to 110 kg	> 110 kg
7.	Previous intubation history:	No difficulty	Unsure or Unknown	Difficulty
	Score ≥ 4 = Predictor of difficult intubation			

1. **Mouth opening:** A mouth opening greater than 4 centimetres measured inter-incisally, gives a score of O, whereas less than 4cms gives a score of 1.

2. **Thyromental distance:** A thyro-mental measurement greater than 6.5 centimetres, gives a score of 0, whereas any value between 6cms to 6.5 cms has a value of 1. A measurement less than 6 cms has a value of 2.

3. **Mallampati score:** Classes I and II of the Modified Mallampati Index gives 0, whereas a Class III is given 1 and a Class IV results in a value of 2.

4. **Neck Movement:** The ability to move the neck more than 90 degrees results in a value of 0, whereas a movement range of 80 degrees to 90 degrees results in a value of 1 and a movement range less than 80 degrees results in a value of 2.

5. **Underbite:** If the patient is able to protrude the jaw enough to create an underbite a score of 0 is given if the patient is skeletal Class II, then a score of 1 is given.

6. **Body weight:** A weight below 90 kilograms results in 0. A body weight between 90 and 110 kilograms is given 1 and a weight above 110 kilograms counts as 2.

7. **Previous intubation history:** If the patient has previously been intubated without any difficulties, a value of 0 is given. If the patient has not previously been intubated, is unsure whether there were any difficulties, or there are no medical records, a score of 1 is given. If there is a positive history of intubation difficulty then a value of 2 is given.

An Intravenous Outline

There is no harm in repeating these assessments before, during and after your sedation procedure, but harm may come if those measurements which are necessary are not taken from your clinical observations.

Once these have been completed, only a few patients in true text book fashion will cheerily offer you a handy finger on which to clamp the sensor for a pulse oximeter, while extending their other hand with a healthy set of dorsal veins into which you will effortlessly introduce the midazolam via a cannula or butterfly needle.

Some patients will do all of the above without too much fuss, but in real life (the place where most of us work) most patients will not be textbook cases and a considerable amount of encouragement will be needed to overcome their resistance. Convincing your patient to offer their finger for the pulse oximeter, or an arm around which a tourniquet will be tied, while their veins are being tapped, stroked or by other physiological means; somehow persuaded to rise to the surface, so the cannula or butterfly needle can be introduced, often presents us with greater difficulties than any textbook could offer advice on how we might overcome such behavioural obstacles.

There is only one word, repeated again and again (and again) that is useful in many of these cases:

Practise, practise, practise.

After the needle has been successfully introduced and the red flashback of blood is observed in the cannula chamber, can the needle then be fully introduced into the vein, secured in place with tape and any air present is then aspirated out of the needle or tubing, before the sedative drug of choice is introduced.

The tourniquet can be released and once the patient is placed in the supine position, one to two milligrams of midazolam can be introduced. The response of the patient is monitored and after one to two minutes, further incremental doses can be administered as necessary to achieve the level of conscious sedation that is needed for the procedure to be undertaken. The following two matters are of critical importance:

Firstly, should the antagonist or reversal agent flumazenil be needed, the needle must be left in place throughout the procedure and during the immediate recovery phase in the clinic.

Secondly, the protective laryngeal reflex and swallowing ability of the patient must be maintained together with verbal responses to stimuli throughout the procedure. Any loss of these indicates over-sedation with a risk of the patient lapsing into that state of unconsciousness associated with general anaesthesia together with loss of their reflexes protecting their airway. Such over-sedation must be avoided in every procedure for all of your patients.

Throughout the procedure, both the pulse and oxygen levels must be monitored and recorded together with the concentration of midazolam being introduced. Such measurements can be noted in a log of the drug titration v time.

Intravenous Sedation Pharmacology

Moving away from this summary of the clinical procedure of intravenous sedation, applying what we have already learned:

Pharmacokinetics: Occurs to midazolam when inside the patient.
Pharmacodynamics: Occurs to the patient when midazolam is inside them.

When midazolam is injected intravenously, there is complete bioavailability as the uptake, absorption and the processes of first-pass metabolism begin. The distribution of midazolam is dependent on its protein binding and lipid solubility, whereas the excretion is dependent on both drug interaction and the patient's ability to eliminate the active metabolites of midazolam.

There are five basic principles of pharmacokinetics that apply to midazolam and indeed any of the other drugs previously considered and those drugs that are being used in dentistry for conscious sedation. These principles are defined as follows:

I.   The initial concentration of a drug: (C_o) = Dose/Volume of Distribution.

II. Volume of distribution: (Vd) = Dose/Initial Concentration.

III. The elimination constant: $(K_e) = \ln (C_1/C_2) / (t_1 - t_2)$

IV. Drug Clearance: $(CL) = Vd \cdot K_e$

V.   Half Life: $(T_{1/2}) = \ln (2) \cdot Vd/CL$

(ln is the natural logarithm)

In considering the use of any intravenous drug for conscious sedation, if safety is to remain our prime concern, the concepts supporting these five basic principles must be understood. Given that very little (if any) time in the undergraduate dental curriculum is allocated for training in conscious sedation and for the post graduate dentist; theory and practice in conscious sedation has become the preserve of SAAD and/ or specific post-graduate programs leading to qualifications in this discipline, much of the science supporting sedation could be viewed as quite challenging.

Setting the science aside, (we will return to it in a moment) and turning to the practise of IV conscious sedation, the following safety critical considerations must be adhered to:

I.   **Conscious Sedation with Midazolam must be practised rapidly and safely as defined by the NICE, the SIGN and the IACSD 2015-2016/17 National Guidelines.**

II. **The patient's response to anaesthesia, anxiolysis and analgesia must be accurately assessed.**

III. **The pharmacokinetics (I ADD ME) and any drug Interactions for midazolam should be recognized.**

IV. **The pharmacodynamics for patients in various health and disease states needs to be understood.**

V.   **The need for drug reversal with Flumazenil understood with the doses and pharmacology of this reversal agent being known.**

The bioavailability of a drug is the proportion of that drug reaching the patient's circulation after oral, inhalational, intramuscular or transdermal application, when compared to the amount of drug that is introduced by intravenous administration. By this definition, when a drug is administered intravenously, 100% is available for the patient to begin to metabolize.

Therefore IV Midazolam has 100% bioavailability.

The fundamentals of midazolam pharmacology

While we need to be aware of what midazolam will do to the patient (the pharmacodynamics), it is perhaps more important that we begin with what our patient will do to midazolam (the pharmacokinetics). Once more this is: drug distribution, metabolism and finally; elimination. While the pharmacodynamics are actual physiological, anatomical (and sometimes pathological) processes, the pharmacokinetics are mathematically modelled processes that can be illustrated for convenience in a series of graphs. These graphs have no anatomical or physiological meaning other than allowing us to understand how much of the drug that is injected will be available for the patient's target organ(s) to use.

To assist in our understanding of midazolam pharmacokinetics, the patient's body can be divided into five <u>compartments</u>; which are separate but connected (while we can disconnect these compartments in the laboratory under experimental conditions, in real life: they usually remain fairly well connected.)

I.   The first compartment into which the drug is introduced: The circulatory system.

II.   Next are the tissues and organs that are highly perfused: The heart, lungs and GI Tract

III. Then those tissues and organs that are poorly perfused: Fat and connective tissues.

IV. Following from these compartments, is the target organ for midazolam: The patient's brain.

V.   Finally, the organs of drug elimination and excretion: The liver and kidneys.

The concentration of midazolam in plasma is controlled by several exponential processes working together in each of these compartments. From the initial intravenous dose, the concentration of midazolam rapidly rises during the absorption phase then falls off during the elimination phase. The independent variable time (t) is presented on the horizontal axis and the dependent variable: Plasma Concentration is presented on the vertical axis:

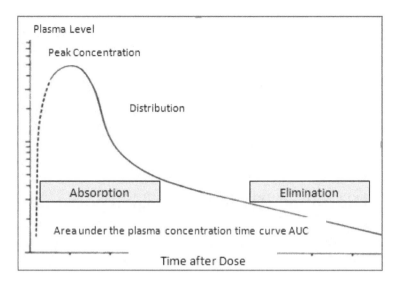

The AUC or area under the: Concentration: Time Curve, indicates the bioavailability of midazolam and when given intravenously: this is 100%. The differences in AUC and thus bioavailability between IV and oral drug administration can be seen in the next illustration:

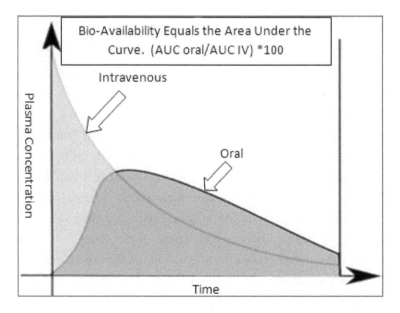

The intravenous administration of midazolam produces a predictable curve. The changes in plasma concentration and the shape of the curve are dependent on the interaction between drug redistribution in the anatomical compartments noted above and the effects of the patient's ability to firstly metabolise then eliminate midazolam. The contribution of these processes to the pharmacokinetics of midazolam depends on the duration of drug administration and the rate constant of drug elimination (K_e). Before we consider the pharmacokinetics of midazolam, it is important to look at the:

Midazolam : The pharmacological properties

1. **Class:** Midazalom belongs to the Benzodiazepine drug group. If you want to know the full name it is: 8-chloro-6-(2-fluorophenyl)-1-methyl-$4H$ imidizo [1,5-a][1,4] benzodiazepine.

2. **Structure:** An Imidazole Ring, which looks like this:

3. **Formulation:** Midazolam is water soluble and can be given orally in tablet form in doses of 5mgs or 7.5mgs, almost always with the support and guidance of the patient's general medical practitioner. However, when dispensed by a dental practitioner for conscious sedation, midazolam will be given intravenously (IV) in titrated doses from prepared concentrations of 10mgs in 5ml. A solution of 10mgs in 2ml is also available. However volumes of 0.5ml containing 1mg Midazolam are easier to administer, the ease with which titration can achieve the desired level of sedation will be easier and thus safer to work with when using a lower concentration of this drug.

4. **Doses:** As noted, doses in the range of 0.5mg to 5.0 mgs of Midazolam introduced intravenously are sufficient to produce adequate levels of conscious sedation for the dental outpatient undergoing minor procedures.

5. **Site of action:** $GABA_A$ BZ receptor in the CNS.

The pharmacokinetics of midazolam:

1. **Availability**: Orally some 27% to 44% of midazolam becomes available with first-pass metabolism.
2. **Distribution:** 90% of midazolam is protein bound with an elimination half life of 1.5 to 2.5 hours.
3. **Metabolism:** Is via the CYP3A P450 hepatic pathways, which are relatively slow. With hydroxylation and glucoronidization, the end product (α 4/α1-hydroxymidazolam) can be detected after 2 to 4 hours.
   i.   Those drugs capable of inducing midazolam metabolism are: rifampicin, phenytoin and carbamazepine.
   ii. Those drugs capable of reducing midazolam metabolism are: omeprazol and diltiazem.
4. **Excretion** is from the kidneys and those patients with renal failure will have reduced excretion rates.
5. **Total time to peak effect:** 13 minutes, there is strong sensitivity to this drug with a multiple dose effect being seen.

The pharmacodynamics of midazolam:

1. **Central Nervous System**: Midazolam has anxiolytic, amnesic and sedative properties. However in adolescents and children, paradoxical stimulation with agitation, hallucinations and euphoria can occur. The extent of such disinhibition with midazolam seen in younger patients has been termed aggressive dyscontrol, rage-reaction and has led to assaults against staff by patients. So in administering midazolam some caution is urged and controls are needed.
2. **Cardiovascular System:** Vasodilation, and a depression in myocardial function can occur.
3. **Respiratory System:** Airway reflexes will be diminished as will the response to elevated CO_2 levels, hypoxia with reduced tidal volume and respiratory rates are seen.
4. **Musculoskeletal System:** Muscle relaxation will be seen.

5. **Gastrointestinal Tract:** Diminished motility with a reduction in the risk of vomiting. This is always a bonus in the dental surgery, if not for your patient and yourself, then at least for your dental nursing colleagues.

Following the dental procedure with conscious sedation, your patient must be supervised in a dedicated recovery area by a suitably trained and qualified member of the sedation team. Monitoring of their blood pressure and pulse oximetry will continue for up to one hour in this area, although the time in recovery is usually only ten to twenty minutes.

Only when the patient is capable of walking securely unassisted *i.e*: with supervision and guidance at close hand, can they be discharged into the care of their escort who has been briefed with written instructions detailing what they can and cannot do for the next 24 hours.

Midazolam sedation can be reversed or the effects antagonized with flumazenil:

Flumazenil

1. **Class:** Flumazenil is a benzodiazepine antagonist, its full name is: Ethyl 8-fluoro-5-methyl-6-oxo-5, 6-dihydro-4H-benzo [f] imidazo [1,5-a] diazepine-3-carboxylate.

2. **Structure:** Flumazenil is an imidazo-benzodiazepine which looks like this:

3. **Formulation:** Flumazenil is given intravenously through the same cannula or butterfly needle as used for midazolam administration.

4. **Dose:** 200 µgms are given in 1 to 2 minutes. You will be aware that the elimination half life of flumazenil at 40 to 80 minutes is far less than that of midazalom at 90 minutes to 2.5 hours (as noted above). When considering the use of flumazenil, the risk of re-sedation and the increased potential for seizures must be considered.

5. **Site of Action:** The same as midazolam, flumazenil acts on the $GABA_A$ BZ receptor complex site in the CNS.

As mentioned, in addition to midazolam, there are three further drugs that a specialist anaesthetist may consider using for out-patient day care conscious sedation in the dental practice. While it is extremely unlikely that these drugs will be used by a dentist, if you are working in a team with a medically qualified sedationist, it is important that you do know something of the clinical properties of Fentanyl, Propofol and Ketamine, the indications for their use and the clinical limitations associated with these drugs.

Fentanyl: The pharmacological properties

1. **Class:** Fentanyl is a potent synthetic opioid with a rapid onset and a short duration of action. Due to very high lipid solubility, it is some 100X more powerful than morphine. Its full name is: N-(1-(2-phenylethyl)-4-piperidinyl)-N-phenylpropanamide.

2. **Structure:** Fentanyl is a phenylpiperidine or a pethidine analogue, with a structure which looks like this:

3. **Formulation:** Being particularly useful in dentistry for conscious sedation, fentanyl can be given intravenously. Fentanyl can also exert its effect after being administered intramuscularly or transdermally. Of some concern is that a narcotic effect can be seen after intranasal or inhalation use of this drug for recreational or frankly illicit purposes.

4. **Dose:** Incredibly small doses are needed to provide a clinical effect and these are in the range of: $0.25 - 0.50$ μgm/Kg body weight of the patient.

5. **Site of action:** Fentanyl exerts an effect on the μ_1 Opioid Receptors in the CNS.

The pharmacokinetics of fentanyl

1. **Availability**: While 100% will be available intravenously, remarkably over 90% will be available transdermally and orally around 33% of fentanyl will become metabolically active.
2. **Distribution:** 80% of fentanyl will become protein bound with a very rapid elimination half life of some 10 to 20 minutes.
3. **Metabolism:** As with the other sedation drugs, the hepatic CYP 450 system is involved and with fentanyl it is the CYP 3A4 group. The metabolism of fentanyl is decreased through concomitant use of the antifungal azole drugs such as fluconazole. A similar inhibitory effect could be seen with the antiviral drug ritonavir.
4. **Excretion:** Renal elimination is seen with some 10% of fentanyl being excreted in an unchanged state.
5. **Total time to peak effect:** The maximum effect is seen in only 3.5 minutes, making fentanyl particularly useful for the short out-patient procedures such as those in dental practices offering sedation.

The pharmacodynamics of fentanyl

1. **Central Nervous System**: In addition to sedation, fentanyl causes anxiolysis and analgesia, these properties make fentanyl an extremely useful all round drug for use in dentistry where multiple drug administration for conscious sedation is not considered to be best practice, however....
2. **Cardiovascular System:** Of critical concern, fentanyl use results in bradycardia, which is not ideal because of the effects on the:
3. **Respiratory System:** Together with a lowered heart rate, the patient's tidal volume will be reduced too. A reduction in respiratory rate leads to apnoea and a greatly reduced response to blood gas CO_2 with hypoxia is seen. If this isn't bad enough for you, then the patient's gag and upper airway reflexes will be diminished too.

It was all quite promising for fentanyl in dentistry until all of the above safety critical pharmacodynamic factors were considered and so its use is highly restricted in dentistry.

4. **Musculoskeletal System:** Should the patient not be too compromised by all of the above, muscle rigidity; especially of the chest muscles has been observed in patient's being sedated with fentanyl.

5. **Gastrointestinal Tract:** Having survived all of these adverse pharmacological factors, fentanyl use is also associated with increased nausea and vomiting. So dental nurses won't be too keen for this drug to be used in the dental clinic, if they are the ones who have to tidy up after you or your medically qualified seditionist have finished working with the patient!

Should you choose to use fentanyl or be part of the dental sedation team using this drug, then you must be aware of the need to have an opioid antagonist present in the clinic. The drug that you need to be familiar with is: naloxone.

Naloxone

1. **Class:** Naloxone is an opioid antagonist, its full name is (1S, 5R, 13R, 17S)-10, 17-dihydroxy-4 (prop-2-en1-yl)-12-oxa-4 azapentacyclo [9.6.1.0^{1,13}·0.^{5,17}. 0^{7,18}] octadeca-7 (18),8,10-trien 14-on2

2. **Structure:** The full name of naloxone kind of gives you some idea that it might actually have a complicated structure and it does, it looks like this:

3. **Formulation:** In case of an opioid overdose, naloxone can be administered intravenously,

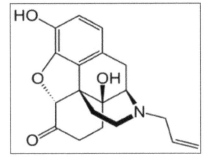

intramuscularly, or subcutaneously. Recently it has been established when an opioid overdose presents as a medical emergency, naloxone can be delivered via an intranasal atomiser[50]. Certainly, in those dental sedation clinics where opioid analgesic anxiolytic sedatives are not being used, or indeed in any general dental practice, there will always be a significant number of patients who use opioids recreationally and staff training in recognizing and treating opioid overdose not only in the clinic but in the community may well be a useful measure in harm reduction[51].

In the UK it has been noted that there is a marked socio-economic divide for those patients attending dental sedation clinics, with a greater uptake of sedation from those areas that are most deprived. Given that intravenous drug use and the recreational use of opioids follows a similar pattern, these two factors would seem to support the training of the dental team in harm prevention and harm reduction measures such as naloxone administration[52].

For those dental clinics where fentanyl is being used in sedation, the use of such devices must become part of the safety critical approach to patient care.

4. **Dose:** Via the different routes of administration, up to 10mgs of naloxone can be given at 2 minute intervals. The half life of naloxone is in the region of 30 to 80 minutes.
5. **Site of action:** Having seen that naloxone has a complicated structure; it won't come as a surprise to learn that naloxone has a complicated mode of action too. Naloxone is both a competitive antagonist exerting its effect at the MOR μ opioid receptor sites in the CNS and as an inverse agonist at the KOR and DOR opioid receptor sites in both the CNS and PNS.

What this means in clinical terms is:

If we were to administer naloxone to a patient who has taken an opioid, then reversal of the sedative effect will be seen. If a patient has not taken an opioid and naloxone is given, then a partial but not a complete block of the body's inherent response to endorphin release will be seen.

While naloxone is an incredibly useful drug in both harm-prevention and harm-reduction in the community, some caution must be exercised in its clinical use. A critical safety alert was released from the UK NHS in late2015:

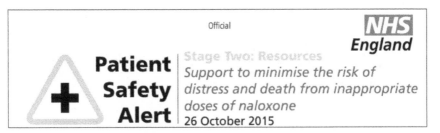

The use of naloxone can be life-saving when respiratory depression and arrest follow from an overdose of opioids. However, the use of naloxone in patients for whom it is not indicated, or in larger than recommended doses for those patients for whom it is indicated (those taking opioids), a rapid reversal of the physiological effects of pain control, leading to intense pain and distress have been observed. In these cases the stimulation of the sympathetic nervous system can be dramatically increased from a rise in cytokine levels and an acute opioid withdrawal crisis rapidly develops.

Hypertension, cardiac arrhythmias, pulmonary oedema and cardiac arrest may result from the inappropriate use of naloxone in these patients. For those elderly patients enduring palliative medical care with opioids, we must be especially vigilant when considering the use of naloxone.

Propofol: The pharmacological properties

1. **Class:** Propofol is an anaesthetic and hypnotic drug with amnesic properties too. It is a short acting medication with a rapid onset of

action. Its full name is: 2, 6-di (propan-2-yl) phenol or [di isoprophylphenol]. Propofol has **no analgesic properties** and when used in conscious sedation additional pain control measures such as local anaesthetics or opioid medication might be considered, although the use of such measures encroach on the restrictions imposed from single drug conscious sedation.

2. **Structure:** Propofol has a relatively simple structure with one phenol ring and a hydroxyl group:

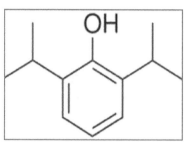

3. **Formulation:** Propofol can only be administered intravenously. Usually this is within a concentration range of 1% to 2% propofol in a suspension of 10% soya bean oil, 1.2% egg phospholipid and 2.25% glycerol with Sodium Hydroxide.

4. **Dose:** Propofol is injected intravenously in bolus doses of 0.25 to 0.50 mg/Kg body weight. If an infusion pump is to be used, then a rate of 3-4 mgs/Kg/hour is set.

5. **Site of action:** Propofol acts on the CNS $GABA_A$ and Na^+ Channels.

The pharmacokinetics of propofol

1. **Availability:** As propofol is administered intravenously, there is 100% bioavailability.

2. **Distribution:** Propofol is an incredibly highly bound drug with some 95% being bound to transport proteins.

3. **Metabolism:** As with the other intravenous sedative drugs, the hepatic cytochrome P450 pathways result in glucoronidization and hydroxylation of propofol to a series of inactive metabolites. Of interest for our needs in conscious dental sedation, the metabolism of midazolam can be significantly reduced by the concurrent administration of propofol, thus multidrug use should be avoided should the use of propofol be considered.

4. **Elimination:** Nearly half of all propofol will be eliminated through the kidneys and we must be aware of those patients who have reduced renal function or who have kidney or liver failure.

5. **Total time to peak effect.** Propofol is an extremely fast acting sedative with a maximal effect noted in only 1 to 3 minutes from administration. For this reason it has been used by those medically qualified anaesthetists conducting outpatient day care sedation procedures.

The pharmacodynamics of propofol

1. **Central Nervous System:** Propofol produces a wide range of effects including: sedation, amnesia anxiolysis and in sufficiently large doses: anaesthesia. In smaller doses such as those administered for dentistry; euphoria and hallucinations have been observed. However we must remember that propofol has no anaesthetic properties. If we are working with a medically qualified specialist anaesthetist administering propofol, then our effective use of local anaesthesia is essential.

2. **Cardiovascular System:** While propofol can induce vasodilation, propofol will block the cardiovascular mechanisms physiologically compensating for this and the patient's myocardial output will be lowered. The inhibition of a sympathetic neural output by propofol can result in blood pressure decreasing by up to 30%[53]. Of importance, propofol injections are noted to be more painful than injections with other sedative drugs. This is due to the activation of the Transient Receptor Potential Cation Channel A$_1$ (TRPA$_1$) present on the endothelium of small blood vessels. The pain of propofol injections can be reduced by adding lidocaine to the solution, but such a measure could be taken as a multidrug procedure[54].

3. **Respiratory System:** Propofol reduces the tidal volume to a level where the respiratory rate can become so depressed there is a risk of apnoea occurring. In common with the effects of fentanyl, there is a greatly reduced response to blood gas CO_2 with an added risk of hypoxia. As with fentanyl the patient's gag and upper airway reflexes

will be diminished. Should these clinical signs arise, in contrast to fentanyl or midazolam, with propofol there is no antagonist which can be given to reverse or at least control the effects of this drug.

4. **Musculoskeletal System:** Propofol has been observed to induce irregular unco-ordinated muscle activity, such dystonia and myoclonic movements are commonly seen with other hypnotic sedative drugs.

5. **Gastrointestinal Tract:** Propofol can exert an anti-emetic action.

Ketamine: The pharmacological properties

1. **Class:** Ketamine is an anaesthetic hypnotic drug with sedative analgesic and amnesic properties. On administration in the doses used in out-patient day care a trance like state can be rapidly induced, with no loss of consciousness but profound relief from pain has been observed. Its full name is (RS)-2-(2-Chlorphenyl)-2-(methlyamino) cyclohexanone.

2. **Structure:** Ketamine has 2 phenol rings and is a derivative of phencyclidine, it looks like this:

3. **Formulation:** Ketamine is quite a versatile drug and it can be given intravenously, intramuscularly, subcutaneously, orally or mucosally too via other areas that need not concern us in the dental setting. For these routes of administration, ketamine has become very versatile drug used by paramedics and favoured by recreational abusers.

4. **Dose:** injections of bolus doses in the range of 0.25 to 050 mgs/Kg body weight can be used, while infusions of 10- 20 mgs/Kg/hour are also possible for dental sedation.

5. **Site of action:** Ketamine has multiple sites of action and to date these have not been completely documented, while those sites we do know about are not fully understood. This is one of the reasons

why its use in dental sedation in the UK may be curtailed or severely restricted to specialist medical use only. Ketamine exerts its effect by non-competitively antagonizing N-methyl-D aspartate (NMDA) receptors and by negatively modulating an effect on N-acetyl choline receptors both located in the CNS. In addition to these actions, ketamine can agonise endogenous mu and kappa opioid receptors and inhibit the reuptake of serotonin. The complexity of these actions when combined is still poorly understood.

The pharmacokinetics of ketamine

1. **Availability:** Ketamine has good oral bioavailability at 30% with good absorption mucosally and intramuscularly too.
2. **Distribution:** Although some 95% of ketamine will be protein bound the half life is rapid at 11 to 16 minutes.
3. **Metabolism:** As with all the sedative drugs we have considered, the hepatic cytochromes are involved in ketamine metabolism, specifically these are: CYP3A4, CYP2B6 and CYP2C9. Ketamine metabolism can be reduced by any drug that reduces the activity of these cytochromes. Of specific relevance to dentistry, the use of azole antifungals and macrolide antibiotics by a patient may prolong the clinical effects of ketamine.
4. **Excretion:** Renal excretion can be confirmed by the presence of the metabolites; dehydronorketamine and norketamine in urine
5. **Total time to peak effect:** A very rapid onset of action is seen with ketamine with effects being observed within a minute after intravenous injection, within five minutes of intramuscular injection and up to 30 minutes via oral administration.

The pharmacodynamics of ketamine

1. **Central Nervous System:** Ketamine can rapidly induce a dissociative state with profound anaesthesia.

2. **Cardiovascular System:** In some contrast to the other sedative agents we have considered, ketamine actually elevates the blood pressure and heart rate in the patient. There will be a noticeable increase or stabilization in cardiac output when ketamine has been administered.

3. **Respiratory System:** As with the cardiovascular system, ketamine can maintain or increase the drive to ventilate and usefully from a safety point, airway reflexes are maintained as the bronchioles are dilated with ketamine use.

4. **Musculoskeletal System:** Very rarely an increase muscle tone may be seen with tonic clonic movements.

5. **Gastrointestinal Tract:** In contrast to midazolam but in common with fentanyl and propofol, ketamine can induce nausea and vomiting. While there is a risk of this occurring with ketamine use, thankfully the patient's airway will be protected. However, the real problem for dental sedation comes from the increased salivation associated with ketamine use.

The essence of IV dental sedatives:

Midazolam: Can be antagonised with Flumazenil
Fentanyl: Can be antagonised with Naloxone
Propofol: Has no Antagonist
Ketamine: Has no Antagonist

The potential pharmacokinetic competitive drug interactions we frequently note have a minimal effect. While the pharmacodynamic additive drug interactions we rarely see will have a profound effect.

For all forms of drug interaction whether minor or major, competitive or additive we must be vigilant in taking an updated medical and medicine history at every appointment and especially for those patients we assess for sedation whether: RA, or IV, with single or with multiple drugs.

Combining sedatives with analgesics may result in non linear effects with a heightened risk of co-morbidity. Adding to this, there could be an unpredictable synergy and our intended and well planned conscious sedation may rapidly descend towards or into an accidental general anaesthesia.

Lastly:

From this section you will see there is no ideal single sedation drug.

A good sedative is not a strong analgesic.

Whereas...

A strong analgesic is often a weak sedative.

But perhaps the last words in this section belong to James Badenoch QC, while a patient, he informed his anaesthetist of the following maxim, which applies to our patients too:

"If you're putting me to sleep....
... just make sure you can wake me up when you've finished!"

References to Safety in Sedation

1. The Intercollegiate Advisory Committee for Sedation in Dentistry. Standards for Conscious Sedation in the Provision of Dental Care. The Royal College of Surgeons of England 2015.
   Available online:
   http://www.rcseng.ac.uk/fds/committees/intercollegiateadvisory-committee-for-sedation-in-dentistry
   Accessed June 2016.

2. Department of Health. Conscious Sedation in the Provision of Dental Care 2003. London: UK DOH. 2003.

3. Standing Committee on Sedation for Dentistry. Standards for Conscious Sedation in Dentistry: Alternative Techniques 2007. London: Royal College of Surgeons of England and Royal College of Anaesthetists 2007.

4. Scottish Dental Clinical Effectiveness Programme. Conscious Sedation in Dentistry. 2nd edn. 2012 Dundee: SDCEP.

5. Academy of Medical Royal Colleges. Safe Sedation Practice for Healthcare Procedures. London: AoMRC; 2013.

6. National Institute for Health and Care Excellence. Sedation in Children and Young People 2010. London: NICE.

7. Holly CD, Torbit L and Ditto B. Applied tension and coping with blood donation: a randomized trial. Ann Behav Med. 2012 Apr; 43(2).

8. Laszlo J. Chapter 3: Medical Matters, OSCE Number 25 in Clinical Problems in Dentistry. page 315. Penguin Random House X-Libris Bloomington Indiana 2013.

9. General Dental Council. Standards for the Dental Team; September 2013.
   Available from:
   http://www.gdc-uk.org/dentalprofessionals/standards/pages/home.aspx
   Accessed June 2016.

10. Francis R, QC. Report of the Mid Staffordshire NHS Foundation Trust Public Inquiry 2013. UK House of Commons

Available online from:
http://webarchive.nationalarchives.gov.uk/20150407084003/
http://www.midstaffspublicinquiry.com/sites/default/files/report/
Executive%20summary.pdf
Accessed June 2016.

11. Royal College of General Practitioners. RCGP Summary The Francis Report 2013. RCGP London.
Available online from:
http://www.rcgp.org.uk/policy/rcgp-policy-areas/~/media/Files/Policy/A-Z-policy/RCGP-Francis-Report-Overview-2013.ashx
Accessed June 2016.

12. James Badenoch QC Personal communication. Easter Monday March 26th 2016.

13. Bainham A. Lord Denning as a champion of children's rights: The legacy of Hewer V Bryant. In Denning Law Journal. University of Buckingham Press Journals. pp 81-91, 2012.

14. Gillick V West Norfolk and Wisbech Area Health Authority and Department of Health and Social Security 1984 Q.B. 581.

15. R (A Minor) (Wardship: Medical Treatment) [1992] 1 Family Law Review 190.

16. W (A Minor) (Consent to Medical Treatment) [1993] 1 Family Law Review 1.

17. Douglas G. The Retreat from Gillick. Modern Law Review, 1992 55; 4, 569-576.

18. McFarlane A. Mental capacity: one standard for all ages. Family Law, 2011 41(5): 479-485.

19. Taylor R. Reversing the retreat from Gillick? R (Axon) v Secretary of State for Health. Child and Family Law Quarterly, 2007 19(1): 81-97.

20. Wheeler R Gillick or Fraser? A plea for consistency over competence in children: Gillick and Fraser are not interchangeable. British Medical Journal, 2006 332(7545): 807

21. Mental Capacity Act 2005. UK Government. Available from:
http://www.legislation.gov.uk/ukpga/2005/9/contents/section 1
Accessed June 2016.

22. House of Lords Judgments - Chester v. Afshar [2002] EWCA Civ 724; [2003] QB 356.
    Available online from:
    http://www.publications.parliament.uk/pa/ld200304/ldjudgmt/jd041014/cheste-2.htm
    Accessed June 2016.

23. Dworkin R. Life's Dominion: An Argument about Abortion and Euthanasia p224; Knopf 1993 University of Michigan.

24. Bolam v Friern Hospital Management Committee [1957] 1 WLR 582

25. Sidaway v. Board of Governors of the Bethlem Royal Hospital. 1985 AC 871

26. United Kingdom Supreme Court, Montgomery v Lanarkshire Health Board 2015 UKSC 11.
    Available online from: http://www.bailii.org/uk/cases/UKSC/2015/11.html
    Accessed June 2016.

27. Priaulx N. See ya Sidaway – informed consent: Montgomery v. Lanarkshire Health Board [2015] UKSC 11. The Law Lab @ Cardiff
    Available online from: http://sites.cardiff.ac.uk/cels/2015/03/15/see-ya-sidaway-informed-consent-montgomery-v-lanarkshire-health-board-2015-uksc-11/
    Accessed June 2016.

28. David Hart QC. UK Human Right Blog. Supreme Court reverses informed consent ruling: Sidaway is dead. Available online from:
    https://ukhumanrightsblog.com/2015/03/13/supreme-court-reverses-informed-consent-ruling-sidaway-is-dead/
    Accessed June 2016.

29. Mazze R.I and Kallen B. Reproductive outcome after anaesthesia and operation during pregnancy: A registry study of 5405 cases. Am J Obstet Gynecol. 1989; 161:1178–1185.

30. Aldridge L.M and Tunstall M.E. Nitrous oxide and the fetus: A review and the results of a retrospective study of 175 cases of

anaesthesia for insertion of Shirodkar suture. Br J Anaesth.1986; 58:1348–1356.

31. Crawford J.S, Lewis M. Nitrous oxide in early human pregnancy. Anaesthesia. 1986; 41: 900–905.

32. Santos A.C, Braveman F.R and Finster M. Obstetric anaesthesia. In: Barash P.G, Cullen B.F, Stoelting R.K, editors. Clinical Anesthesia. 5th ed. Philadelphia: Lippincott-Raven; 2006.

33. Rosen M.A. Management of anaesthesia for the pregnant surgical patient. Anesthesiology. 1999; 91: 1159–1163.

33. Akça O, Lenhardt R, Fleischmann E, Treschan T, and Greif R et al. Nitrous Oxide Increases the Incidence of Bowel Distension in Patients Undergoing Elective Colon Resection. Acta Anaesthesiologica Scandinavica 48.7 (2004): 894–898.

34. Munson E.S. Complications of nitrous oxide anaesthesia for ear surgery. Anaesth Clin North Am. 1993; 11:559–572

35. Morgan G.E, Mikhail M.S and Murray M.J. Clinical Anaesthesiology. 4th ed. New York: Lange Medical Books/McGraw Hill; 2006.

36. Yang YF, Herbert L, Rüschen H and Cooling RJ. Nitrous oxide anaesthesia in the presence of intraocular gas can cause irreversible blindness. BMJ : British Medical Journal. 2002; 325 (7363):532-533.

37. Simpson CR, Hippisley-Cox J and Sheikh A. Trends in the epidemiology of chronic obstructive pulmonary disease in England: a national study of 51 804 patients. The British Journal of General Practice. 2010; 60 (576).
Available online from: https://www.ncbi.nlm.nih.gov/pmc/articles/PMC2894402/
Accessed July 2016.

38. Nunn J.F. Clinical aspects of the interaction between nitrous oxide and vitamin B_{12}. Br J Anaesth. 1987; 59:3–13.

39. Mazze R.I, Fujinaga M, Rice S.A, Harris S.B and Baden J.M. Reproductive and teratogenic effects of nitrous oxide, halothane, isoflurane, and enflurane in Sprague-Dawley rats. Anesthesiology. 1986; 64:339–344

40. Becker DE, Rosenberg M. Nitrous Oxide and the Inhalation Anesthetics. Anesthesia Progress. 2008; 55(4):124-131.
Available online from: http://www.ncbi.nlm.nih.gov/pmc/articles/PMC2614651/
Accessed June 2016.

41. Eger E.I. Respiratory effects of nitrous oxide. In: Eger E.I, editor. Nitrous Oxide. New York: Elsevier; 1985.

42. Morgan G.E, Mikhail M.S and Murray M.J. Clinical Anaesthesiology. 4th Edition. New York: Lange Medical Books McGraw Hill; 2006.

43. Sher A.M, Braude B.M, Cleaton-Jones P.E, Moyes D.G and Mallett J. Nitrous oxide sedation in dentistry: A comparison between Rotameter settings, pharyngeal concentrations and blood levels of nitrous oxide. Anaesthesia. 1984; 39:236–239.

44. Quarnstrom F.C, Milgrom P, Bishop M.J, DeRouen T.A. Clinical study of diffusion hypoxia after nitrous oxide analgesia. Anesth Prog. 1991; 38:21–23.

45. Zhang C, Davies M.F, Guo T.Z and Maze M. The analgesic action of nitrous oxide is dependent on the release of norepinephrine in the dorsal horn of the spinal cord. Anesthesiology. 1999; 91:1401–1407.

46. Eisele J.H. Cardiovascular effects of nitrous oxide. In: Eger E.I, editor. Nitrous Oxide. New York: Elsevier; 1985.

47. Lee A, Fan LT, Gin T, Karmakar MK and Ngan Kee WD. A systematic review (meta-analysis) of the accuracy of the Mallampati tests to predict the difficult airway. Anaesthesia and Analgesia. June 2006 102 (6): 1867–78

48. Khan ZH, Mohammadi M, Rasouli MR, Farrokhnia F and Khan RH The diagnostic value of the upper lip bite test combined with sternomental distance, thyromental distance, and interincisor distance for prediction of easy laryngoscopy and intubation: a prospective study. Anaesthesia and Analgesia. 2009 Sep; 109 (3):822-4.

49. Nørskov, A K, Rosenstock C V, Wetterslev J and Lundstrøm L H. "Incidence of unanticipated difficult airway using an objective airway score versus a standard clinical airway assessment: the

DIFFICAIR trial – trial protocol for a cluster randomized clinical trial October 2013.

Available from: https://trialsjournal.biomedcentral.com/articles/10.1186/1745-6215-14-347

Accessed April 2017.

50. Doe-Simkins M, Walley AY, Epstein A, Moyer P. Saved by the Nose: Bystander-Administered Intranasal Naloxone Hydrochloride for Opioid Overdose. American Journal of Public Health. 2009; 99(5):788-791. Available online from: https://www.ncbi.nlm.nih.gov/pmc/articles/PMC2667836/

Accessed October 2016

51. Wheeler E, Jones TS, Gilbert MK, and Davidson PJ. Opioid Overdose Prevention Programs Providing Naloxone to Laypersons - United States, 2014. MMWR Morb Mortal Wkly Rep. 2015 Jun 19; 64(23): 631-5.

52. Wanyoni KL, White S and Gallagher JE. Conscious sedation: Is this provision equitable? Analysis of sedation services provided within primary dental care in England, 2012-2014. British Dental Journal Open. 2016.

53. Robinson, B; Ebert, T, O'Brien, T et al. Mechanisms whereby propofol mediates peripheral vasodilation in humans. 1997 Anaesthesiology. 86: 64–72

54. Picard P and Tramer MR. Prevention of pain on injection with propofol: A quantitative systematic review. Anesth Analg 2000 90: 963–969.

CHAPTER TWO

Medicine and Drug Safety
Verifiable CPD Questions

The first 20 questions are based on this chapter and the BNF (bnf.org) section on prescribing guidance.

1. **Any drug can produce an unwanted or an unexpected adverse reaction this should be recorded in the:**
   A. The patient's Blue Card.
   B. The patient's Yellow Card.
   C. The most recent edition of the BNF.
   D. The Medicines and Healthcare products Regulatory Agency (MHRA) Yellow Card.
   E. The dental practice incidents and accidents log book.

2. **In addition to recording an adverse drug reaction you can:**
   A. Complain to the GDC.
   B. Complain to the pharmacist where the patient obtained the medication.
   C. Get the patient or their carer to self report the incident to the MHRA
   D. If harm occurs, report an adverse reaction to the National Reporting and Learning System (NRLS)
   E. Both options C and D would be appropriate.

3. **Drug side effects are listed in order of frequency, please match the following side effects to their frequency:**
   Very Common, 2. Very Rare, 3. Common, 4. Rare and 5. Uncommon (or less common):
   A. Greater than 1 in 10.
   B. 1 in 100 to 1 in 10

C. 1 in 1,000 to 1 in 100

D. 1 in 10,000 to 1 in 1,000

E. Less than 1 in 10,000

4. **The risk of an adverse drug reaction can be reduced by:**

A. Not using a drug unless there is a good reason and do not use drugs for patients who are pregnant unless it is imperative to do so.

B. Taking a full and comprehensive medical and medication history.

C. Taking account of genetic and disease processes before prescribing.

D. Using as few drugs as possible, those that are well established and not using those that are newly released, homeopathic or experimental in any way.

E. All of the above.

5. **All drugs have the potential to cause an adverse reaction, but not all are allergic reactions. Which of the following are true or false: A reaction is more likely to be allergic if:**

A. The reaction occurred while the patient was taking the drug.

B. The drug contains adrenaline

C. The drug is known or recognized to cause such a pattern or reaction.

D. The patient has had a similar reaction to the same drug or drug class before.

E. The patient is immune-suppressed or immune-compromised.

6. **Which of the following drugs is unlikely to cause oral ulceration?**

A. ACE inhibitors.

B. NSAIDS.

C. Penicillamine.

D. Aspirin.

E. Penicillin.

7. **Which of these drugs is likely to result in a lichenoid reaction in the oral mucosa?**
   A. ACE inhibitors.
   B. NSAIDS.
   C. Methyldopa.
   D. Thiazide diuretics.
   E. All of the above can cause a lichenoid reaction.

8. **Candidiasis can be an oral complication following treatment with:**
   A. Local anaesthetic injections.
   B. Sedative drugs especially Nitrous Oxide
   C. Antibacterials
   D. Immunosuppressants
   E. Corticosteroid inhalers used in asthma.

9. **Which of the following are true?**
   A. Antibiotics cause extrinsic staining of teeth.
   B. Chlorhexidine causes intrinsic staining of teeth.
   C. We can safely prescribe tetracycline in breast feeding mothers and children up to 12 years old
   D. Tetracyclines rarely cause intrinsic staining if given to a pregnant mother from 4/9 *i.u.* onwards.
   E. All of the above are false.

10. **Osteonecrosis of the jaws may be associated with:**
    A. A poorly controlled diet.
    B. A patient taking oral bisphosphonates more so than intravenous bisphosphonates for either cancer or osteoporosis.
    C. A patient taking intravenous bisphosphonates more so than oral bisphosphonates for a patient with cancer rather than osteoporosis.
    D. Monoclonal antibodies such as *bivacizumab*.
    E. Tyrosine kinase inhibitors such as *sunitinib*.

11. **Overgrowth of the gums or gingival hyperplasia is a side effect of:**
    A. Loop diuretics
    B. Corticosteroids
    C. Phenytoin
    D. Cyclosporin
    E. Calcium channel blockers such as nifedipine

12. **Which of the following drugs are least likely to cause xerostomia?**
    A. Antihistamines.
    B. Dopamine 5HT alpha adreno-receptor antagonists such as clozapine
    C. Anticholinergic drugs such as the antimuscarinic ipratropium bromide.
    D. Antidepressants such as the tricyclic antidepressants.
    E. Serotonin and noradrenaline re-uptake inhibitors such as bupropion hydrochloride.

13. **Disturbances in taste are sometimes associated with:**
    A. Metronidazole
    B. Chlorhexidine
    C. Metformin hydrochloride
    D. Amoxycillin
    E. Acyclovir.

14. **Which of the following are true and which are false?**
    A. There is no difference between children and adults in their response to drugs.
    B. In the neonate (first 28 days of life) there is no risk from metronidazole in breast milk.
    C. Drug clearance and target organ sensitivity in the neonate is the same for the juvenile patient.
    D. Pharmacokinetics in children are the same as they are for adults.

E. When prescribing medicines for use in children we have to be aware of the risk of an adverse reaction being delayed that can subsequently affect a child's growth potential.

15. **In the following situation which answers are true? Late at night, your patient needs an urgent prescription for an antimicrobial drug; however the patient cannot attend with you but instead goes to their all night chemist who knows them well. The patient:**
A. Cannot get any medicine from the BNF without a valid prescription from you.
B. Can attend a hospital accident and emergency department where a prescription for any broad spectrum antimicrobial drug can be given to them.
C. Can be interviewed by their pharmacist and if the pharamacist is satisfied that it is impractical to obtain a prescription from yourself and the drug has been issued to the patient before, then a prescription of an appropriate non-controlled drug can be given which is the minimum dose required for the problem the patients has attended with.
D. Can obtain a private prescription from the pharmacist.
E. Can verify the details in answer C with you over the telephone, then a prescription can be issued and paid for. An NHS form FP10 D * can then be issued by you to be presented to the pharmacist by the patient after the patient attends with yourself during working hours.

* NB in the NHS in the UK when prescribing:

i.   In England an FP10 D is used.
ii. In Wales this is a WP10D
iii. In Scotland this is a GP14.

All of these forms have different titles but are subject to the same (2012) Human Medicines Regulations.

16. **When writing out a prescription, which of the following answers are false?**
    A. Provided there is a clinical requirement and a legal authority: You can prescribe anything you want from the BNF DPF and for those drugs and controlled substances not used in everyday clinical practise, you can write out a private prescription on your headed note paper.
    B. You don't need to put a child's weight down as the pharmacist can check the dose from the child's age.
    C. The drug dose per unit mass eg: mg/Kg or dose per m^2 eg: mg/m^2 should not be written out as this would only confuse the pharmacist and too much information may cause an error.
    D. You can get your dental nurse/manager/receptionist to write out prescriptions and stamp them for you.
    E. Only write out a prescription legibly in indelible ink on an NHS FP10D for those drugs normally used in everyday clinical practise.

17. **Which of the following are needed on a prescription?**
    A. Using the most appropriate values the strength and or quantity of the drug must be written in simple terms without the need for decimal points and zeros.
    B. Decimal points and zeros must be noted down to clearly denote the doses and the total values can be expressed in either cc's (cubic centimetres) or mm^3 (cubic millimetres) or any dose value you feel is needed.
    C. Abbreviations of milligrams to mgs and millilitres to mls.
    D. Nanograms and micrograms must never be abbreviated these dose values need to be fully written.
    E. Dose and dose frequency with a minimum dose interval clearly stated.

18. **Computer prescriptions are now being increasingly used in medical and dental practices. Which of the following answers apply to these prescriptions and will now appear on computer generated FP10Ds?**

   A. The name of the prescribing clinician must be clearly printed below a space for a signature to be hand written.

   B. Computer generated signatures are now permissible, so you don't need to sign these documents.

   C. The computer can print out either the proprietary drug name or the non-proprietary drug name but not both.

   D. The computer cannot write out: NO MORE ITEMS you must manually do this and remove further space on the prescription.

   E. The computer will automatically print out numbers and codes to be used for data retrieval of patient identification and you must ensure these codes are always present on the prescription form so a patient's personal details and their background can be accessed by the pharmacist, drugs companies or anyone else out with your dental practice.

19. **When writing or typing out a prescription you can:**

   A. Present the patient with a prescription for Amoxycillin to be taken just in case they need antibiotics while on holiday for a sore throat or infected thumb.

   B. Safely and certainly ignore any topical medication the patient is taking as no interactions between topically applied medicines and systemic drugs have ever been reported.

   C. Safely provide a repeat prescription after a telephone conversation with your patient as they simply do not want to pay the NHS fee for a clinical examination, for advice and assessment or for an appointment for urgent conditions.

   D. Write down as much information on the dose and about the patient as you feel is necessary to ensure there is minimum risk of a dose or drug error occurring.

   E. Hand over a prescription to a child to go to the pharmacy on behalf of a parent who does not speak English.

20. **With any medication that has been dispensed, which of the following <u>must</u> appear on the medicine packet that is presented to the patient?**

   A. The name of the patient only and no more data is needed than this.

   B. The name, the address and the date of birth of the patient, with the directions for the use of the medicine, together with the date and location of the dispensing pharmacist.

   C. Precautions for the use of the medicine including warnings such as: KEEP OUT OF SIGHT AND REACH OF CHILDREN.

   D. Information for the patient to contact the GDC if they are not happy about any aspect of their treatment.

   E. Information on where to obtain further repeat prescriptions from online or internet sources and online consulting physicians who can authorize further medications and drug treatments.

The second group of 65 questions deal with drug safety, pharmacology and physiology.

21. **Antibiotic stewardship is:**

   A. A waste of time and another meaningless directive from the NHS and the GDC we can ignore it as it is of theoretical importance only.

   B. The optimal selection, dosage, and duration of antimicrobial treatment that results in the best clinical outcome for the treatment.

   C. Something we should aim for when treatment planning and when considering the use of all antimicrobial drugs.

   D. The right drug, the right dose, the de-escalation to pathogen-directed therapy, and the right duration of therapy.

E. Can be used in connection with a referral to medical microbiology of the patient or a sample from the patient to determine the best antibiotic to use to treat the patient.

22. **DDD and DOT are abbreviations for**
    A. Dental Drug Delivery and Dentally Optimised Treatment
    B. Defined Daily Dose and Days Of Treatment.
    C. Disease Determined Drug and Drug Ordered Treatment
    D. Defined Dental Disease Dental Occlusal Trauma.
    E. Answers A and B

23. **The advantage of DDD over DOT is that:**
    A. DDD can compare the efficacy of the same treatment given to patients in different clinical settings. While the DOT will not indicate the actual doses being used.
    B. DDD are useful in comparing many different dental practices using the same drug. While DOT can compare different antibiotics.
    C. In clinical terms both DDD and DOT are useful for research but have limited practical application for practising dentists.
    D. There is no advantage of DDD over DOT they are separate entities.
    E. DDD must be used with DOT to gain the optimum result for drug treatment.

24. **Please match the following age ranges to mean weights:**

(i) Birth to 1 year, 9 (ii)1 to 3 years, (iii) 3 to 6 years, (iv) 6 to 12 years and (v)12 to 18 years:
    A. 10 to 15 kgs
    B. 20 to 40 kgs
    C. 15 to 20 kgs
    D. 5 to 10 kgs
    E. 40 to 70 kgs

25. **Please match the following mean weights to drug doses:**

(i) 5 to 10kgs, (ii) 10 to 15 kgs, (iii) 15 to 20 kgs, (iv)20 to 40 kgs and (v) 40 to 70 kgs.
A. ¾ to Total Adult Dose.
B. 2/5ᵗʰ to ½ Adult Dose.
C. ¼ of Adult Dose.
D. 1/3ʳᵈ Adult Dose
E. ½ to ¾ Adult Dose

26. **Aspirin is not:**
   A. An Antipyretic Anti-Inflammatory Analgesic
   B. An Analgesic Antihistamine
   C. An Antiplatelet antithrombotic preventive medication.
   D. To be used in children under 12, but from 12 to 16 years of age Aspirin is safe.
   E. To be used in anyone under the age of 16 due to Reye's Syndrome.

27. **Paracetomol is not:**
   A. A controlled substance.
   B. Anti-inflammatory.
   C. Moderately antipyretic and analgesic.
   D. Any of the above.
   E. Associated with hepatoxicity.

28. **Antidepressants are among the most widely prescribed of all medications and in dentistry they can be used for:**
   A. Tooth ache.
   B. Ear ache
   C. Atypical Facial Pain
   D. Tempero-mandibular joint pain dysfunction syndrome.
   E. Anxiety for nervous patients before undergoing conscious sedation.

29. **In the doses used in dentistry midazolam will have the following properties:**
    A. Anxiolytic, hypnotic and sedative for routine dentistry.
    B. Analgesic sedative for nervous patients who are needle phobic.
    C. Anaesthetic for dental outpatient general anaesthesia.
    D. Anxiolytic hypnotic sedative and can be used in an emergency as an anticonvulsant.
    E. An oral premedication drug when prescribed by a medically qualified practitioner.

30. **Midazolam is a water soluble benzodiazepine that binds to GABA $_A$ receptors on the cell surfaces in the Central and Peripheral Nervous System, the effect of such benzodiazepine binding is:**
    A. Sodium ions flow out of the cell
    B. Chloride ions flow into the cell
    C. There is hyperpolarization of the cell membrane with inhibition.
    D. There is hypopolarization of the cell membrane with inhibition.
    E. There is a conformative change in the GABA $_A$ receptor site resulting in adjacent receptors closing down and midazolam can no longer bind to them.

31. **What proportion of our dental patients over 55 years old will be taking prescribed medication?**
    A. One in eight of them.
    B. One in four of them.
    C. One in two of them.
    D. Three quarters of them.
    E. All of them.

32. **Pharmacokinetics are what our patients bodies will do to the drugs we give them, which of the following are not pharmacokinetic factors:**
    A. Introduction.
    B. Excretion

C. Agonism

D. Antagonism

E. Metabolism

33. **Which of the following drugs cannot be topically applied to exert their influence?**

A. Methylxanthines

B. Benzocaine

C. Eutectic mix of local anaesthetic.

D. Triamcinolone acetonide and dimethylchlortetracycline.

E. Glyceryl trinitrate

34. **A drug that is injected will have a 100% bioavailability, but which of the following factors govern bioavailability for intravenous and other routes of drug administration?**

A. The physical and chemical properties of a drug.

B. The functioning of the patient's gastro-intestinal tract.

C. The health and age of the patient.

D. Interaction with other drugs.

E. All of the above can influence the bioavailability of a drug.

35. **Drugs will bind to plasma proteins such as albumin, which of the following conditions may increase drug binding and reduce the available free drug?**

A. A drug that is more basic than acidic will result in higher levels of circulating plasma free drug.

B. A drug that is more acidic or neutral rather than basic will result in higher levels of the drug in plasma.

C. Liver and kidney disease can reduce plasma protein levels increasing the availability of free drugs.

D. The pH of the drug has no bearing on its level of plasma protein binding.

E. Liver and kidney disease can increase plasma protein levels reducing the availability of free drugs.

36. **A patient who is dehydrated will be at risk of:**
    A. Hyperalbuminaemia.
    B. Hypoalbuminaemia.
    C. Increased effects from reduced binding to plasma proteins.
    D. Decreased drug effects from a relative increase in plasma protein binding.
    E. Dehydration has limited if any effect on the actions of drugs.

37. **With respect to our patients who are either young or very young:**
    A. Drug metabolism is faster in the younger child than it is in the adolescent.
    B. The activity of metabolic enzymes in children is 1/5th to 3/4 of an adult's with drug elimination also being far slower
    C. The glomerular filtration rate (GFR) in neonates is 2 X to 3 X faster than the adult level.
    D. The GFR increases rapidly during the first 2 weeks of life, due to an increase in renal blood flow combined with a postnatal drop in renal vascular resistance. The GFR then rises rapidly until the adult values are reached at only 8 to 12 months of age.
    E. All of the above are correct

38. **With respect to our patients who are either old or very old:**
    A. Lean muscle mass decreases but adipose layers increase. Thus, the distribution, relative concentration and half-life of lipophilic drugs will increase, while the same parameters will correspondingly decrease for aqueous drugs in the elderly patient.
    B. Between the older patient and the younger patient, there is no difference in pharmacokinetics.
    C. In older patients hepatic drug clearance of some drugs can be increased by up to 3 X in the elderly and renal drug excretion can rise by a factor of 2 X in the majority of our elderly patients.

D. Hepatic drug clearance of some drugs can be reduced by up to $1/3^{rd}$ in the elderly and renal drug excretion can fall by ½ in the majority of our elderly patients.

E. None of the above answers are correct.

39. When administering a drug by any route but especially when injecting local anaesthetics into our patient we must:

A. Go as fast as possible getting as much of the drug into the patient before they know what is happening to them, this way the optimum dose reaches the target tissues rapidly and the risk of a needle phobic patient fainting or grabbing the syringe is reduced.

B. With any dose, with any rate and with any route of drug administration the axiom is: Start Low and Go Slow.

C. Whenever we inject, we need to use the longest needle with the largest bore to ensure we follow answer A.

D. Whenever we inject, we need to use the least invasive technique with the most appropriate needle gauge ensuring the bevel is towards the bone to reduce the risk of neuro-vascular trauma and advance the needle steadily, then aspirate before we slowly inject.

E. Both the technique and speed of administration are irrelevant; as the dose has been calculated we only have to wait long enough and the effects of a drug will become clinically evident.

40. Some 1% of the UK population and 8% of those older than 80 are taking Warfarin, which of the following conditions is Warfarin useful in controlling or preventing?

A. Atrial fibrillation and ischaemic heart disease.

B. Heart valve incompetence, defects or replacements.

C. Coagulation defects.

D. Deep vein thromboses with a risk of Cerebro-vascular Accidents and pulmonary embolisms.

E. Hypertension.

41. **Drugs such as aspirin compete with binding sites normally occupied by warfarin. If this occurs, we will be presented with a haematological risk to the patient as their INR rapidly rises and there is a risk of uncontrollable bleeding. An indication of such a risk is the drug's TI or Therapeutic index, the TI of warfarin is:**
    A. Very high
    B. Very Low
    C. Neither high nor low.
    D. Overall warfarin is a poorly controlled drug with a very low or narrow TI that requires constant monitoring.
    E. Concomittant drug use with warfarin is irrelevant as it is a safe drug with a good safety margin and a low TI.

42. **Following an extraction of a tooth a patient continues to bleed from the socket, you might consider using the following measures to achieve haemostasis:**
    A. Pressure with a swab soaked in saline then suturing after the bleeding slows down and stops.
    B. Use of proprietary cellulose gel inserted into the socket and suturing.
    C. Tranexamic acid although this is not a widely used measure and while being undertaken by specialists and not being widely adopted, it is nevertheless an option.
    D. All of the above.
    E. None of the above, you can send the patient to the local Accident and Emergency Department, you've done your work and you don't get paid any more on the NHS to stop bleeding, clinico-legally: It isn't your responsibility anymore!

43. **Which of the following are true?**
    A. Warfarin exerts an immediate effect while heparin takes several days to reach a therapeutically effective dose.
    B. Warfarin takes several days to reach a therapeutic steady state and an effective anticoagulation bridge can be achieved with heparin.

C. Warfarin acts to reduce clotting factor **IIX** by inhibiting the Vitamin K dependent enzyme: epoxide reductase.

D. Warfarin inhibits epoxide reductase the enzyme is responsible for recycling and reducing Vitamin K, after becoming oxidized, it carboxylates the glutamic acid residues on the precursors of the Calcium dependent clotting factors: **II, VII, IX** and **IX**, together with the regulatory proteins **C S** and **Z**.

E. Heparin can be given orally while warfarin is injected.

44. **In our patients their kidneys are:**
   A. A pair of extremely important organs responsible for everything from drug metabolism and excretion to maintaining the patient's blood pressure and we do need to know at least something of how they work.
   B. Organs excreting drugs either by active <u>glomerular filtration</u> or by passive <u>tubular secretion</u>.
   C. Organs in which glomerular filtration only removes unbound drugs (the plasma free drugs). While those bound to protein and drugs present as organic acids will be actively secreted.
   D. Organs, where following filtration, passive <u>reabsorption</u> can return a drug to plasma then into circulation once more.
   E. A complete irrelevance to us and we can conveniently forget about what we learned in 2nd year BDS physiology, nothing we do has anything to do with the renal system.

45. **First-order pharmacokinetics applies to nearly 95% of all orally administered drugs, there is an exponential pattern of drug elimination that is proportional to the drug concentration. Which of the following statements is correct?**
   A. With first order pharmacokinetics, the half-life is variable, being dependent on drug concentration.
   B. With first order pharmacokinetics, the half-life is constant, being independent of drug concentration.
   C. The elimination process does not actually end, but tends towards zero with exponential reduction.

D. The elimination process does end, as it tends towards zero with linear reduction.

E. With first-order elimination, a plasma concentration of the drug will be reached that is no longer pharmacologically effective, at this point, the drug ceases to exert a clinical effect

46. **Certain foods eaten at the same time as the administration of a drug can increase or decrease the absorption of that drug, this is an example of a pharmacodynamic interaction, which of the following are not pharmacodynamic interactions?**
A. Agonism
B. Antagonism
C. Synergism
D. Glomarization
E. Summation

47. **Drug potentiation is a useful property for medical treatments, which of the following can be a source of troublesome potentiation interactions:**
A. Caffeine and NSAIDs.
B. Midazolam and Alcohol.
C. Acetyl salicylic acid and Ibuprofen.
D. Ketoconazole and Warfarin.
E. The oral contraceptive pill and broad spectrum antibacterial drugs.

48. **In the UK, the EU and the USA, diuretics form part of a peculiarly effective medical response to the high prevalence of diet and lifestyle induced cardiovascular disease, please match the following to their site of action:** (i) Carbonic Anhydrase Inhibitors, (ii) Osmotic Diuretics, (iii) Loop Diuretics, (iv) Thiazides and (v)Potassium Sparing Diuretics:
A. The proximal tubules and descending limb of Henle.
B. The thick ascending limb of Henle.
C. The distal convoluted tubule.

D. No site specificity but they do enhance the cortical collecting ducts.

E. The proximal convoluted tubules

49. **Having successfully matched the drug to their site of action, please now match them to their mode of action:** (i) Carbonic Anhydrase Inhibitors, (ii) Osmotic Diuretics, (iii) Loop Diuretics, (iv) Thiazides and (v)Potassium Sparing Diuretics:

A. Improve thiazides and the inhibitor action of aldosterone.

B. Inhibit Na^+ reabsorption

C. Simple osmotic pressure effects

D. Inhibit the Na^+ Cl^- symporter

E. Decrease Na^+ absorption and increase bicarbonate and H^+ excretion.

50. **Adverse Drug Interactions (ADI) of NSAIDs with diuretics should be borne in mind for the following reasons:**

A. There is a risk of an allergic reaction.

B. The patient may complain of stomach upset, diarrhoea and headaches.

C. The patient's renal function can be altered by COX 1 pathway block that disrupts blood flow and filtration in the nephron.

D. There can be a block in the COX 2 pathway that will impact on the regulation of Na^+ and CL^- ion excretion.

E. Both C and D are correct.

51. **More than 5 days use of an NSAID may reduce the ability of a diuretic to lower or control hypertension, this statement is:**

A. True

B. False

C. Only applies to those patients who are cardiovascularly compromised.

D. Is most likely to apply to those patients taking Angiotensin Converting Enzyme (ACE) Inhibitors to lower their blood pressure, either in the advent of, or the wake of a cardiac event.

E. Is of theoretical importance only with no practical safety importance in clinical practice.

52. **In addition to minerals binding to antibiotics, nutrients can bind to other drugs preventing their absorption which of the following may affect our dental prescribing?**
    A. Insoluble dietary fibres bind to and reduce the uptake of cardiac glycosides such as digoxin.
    B. Soluble dietary fibres can bind to and reduce the uptake of antibiotics such as Penicillin.
    C. In addition to answer B the absorption of drugs such as paracetomol, statins, lithium and carbamazapine can also be affected by soluble dietary fibres.
    D. All of the above can affect dental drug prescribing.
    E. None of the above answers are correct.

53. **The possible interactions of the oral contraceptive pill and antibiotics are important with respect to their effect on GI tract flora. Which of the following antimicrobials are bacteriostatic and which are bacteriocidal?**
    A. Amoxycillin
    B. Metronidazole
    C. Erythromycin
    D. Tetracycline
    E. Rifampicin.

54. **Of the following drugs which could demonstrate an increase in action if the patient is taking the OCP?**
    A. Bronchodilators
    B. Anti-epileptics
    C. Diuretics
    D. Anxiolytics
    E. All of the above can have increased clinical effects when the oral contraceptive pill is being used at the same time.

55. **Taking combinations of over the counter NSAIDS and prescribed NSAIDs is:**
   A. Careless and to be discouraged.
   B. Not acceptable if an NSAID such as ibuprofen is taken before aspirin.
   C. Acceptable if the aspirin is taken before the ibuprofen as taking the ibuprofen first can result in a potentially significant decrease in the efficacy of the aspirin.
   D. All of the above answers are correct.
   E. None of the above answers are correct.

56. **The maximum safe dose of acetaminophen (paracetomol) is:**
   A. 200–250 mg/kg body weight, equivalent to 7 grams total ingestion within a 24-hour period.
   B. 4 g/day in adults and 50-75 mg/kg/day in children.
   C. Both of the above can be used.
   D. There is no upper limit as paracetomol is freely available from any pharmacist it is perfectly safe and harmless.
   E. Answer B, but a dose reduction must be considered if the patient has a compromised renal or hepatic function from any cause and is malnourished.

57. **Combining paracetomol with an NSAID either as a prescription or by our patients:**
   A. Can improve the efficacy of both paracetomol and an NSAID, while reducing the risk of hepato-toxicity.
   B. Can reduce the efficacy of both paracetomol and an NSAID while doing little if anything to lower the risk of hepatotoxicity.
   C. Is generally useless and nothing more than a placebo or a marketing initiative.
   D. Such drug combinations are both theoretically and practically questionable and our patients are to be discouraged from combining OCMs and POMs
   E. May be thought of as being useful and hepatocyte sparing due to different drugs being metabolized by different enzymes.

58. **Opioids act on the μ or mu receptors, which of the following is _not_ true following medication with opioids?**
   A. There is depression in GI tract motility and respiratory functioning.
   B. There is excitation in GI tract motility and respiratory functioning.
   C. The pupillary and oro-pharyngeal reflexes are decreased but the gag reflex is spared with no risk to the patient's airway.
   D. The pupillary and oro-pharyngeal reflexes are decreased and gag reflex is affected with a risk to patient's airway.
   E. Opioid dependence is a very real risk with even the shortest dosing regimen such as those used in dentistry.

59. **In addition to your correctly identifying the above effects, the opioid: tramadol can interact with MAOIs and SSRIs to cause:**
   A. Dry mouth and or excessive sweating.
   B. Spontaneous or inducible excessive or inappropriate muscle twitching especially of the facial muscles.
   C. A rapid rise in body temperature above 38 °C
   D. All of the above in a serotonin toxicity syndrome due to tramadol's inhibition of serotonin re-uptake.
   E. None of the above, tramadol is a very safe drug which we can prescribe.

60. **In combination, the antidepressants such as MAOIs and TCAs:**
   A. Are harmless with no risk of a drug interaction between MAOIs and TCAs.
   B. Combinations of TCA and MAOIs will have a marked cardiotonic potential, the use of any sympathomimetic drug with these two antidepressants carries the further risk of additional cardiac excitation.
   C. There is no risk of rapidly increasing blood pressure from any theoretical or actual interaction between MAOIs TCAs and exogenous adrenaline.

D. With patients taking MAOIS and TCAs, the total number of adrenaline containing local anaesthetics could be limited to not more than two cartridges of 2.2ml lidocaine with a concentration of 1/80,000 adrenaline.

E. Reducing the numbers of anaesthetic cartridges is of no clinical benefit to the patient, pain control is more important than pharmacodynamic considerations and giving more anaesthetics gives more anaesthesia.

61. **The differences between adrenergic receptor beta blockers: propranolol and atenolol are:**

A. Propranolol non-selectively blocks activation of all types of β-adrenergic receptors, while the cardio-selective atenolol only acts on the β_1 receptor.

B. Atenolol non-selectively blocks activation of all types of β-adrenergic receptors, while the cardio-selective propranolol only acts on the β_1 receptor.

C. Propranolol has proven to be an indispensable treatment for hypertension and the management of angina pectoris

D. Propranolol cannot be used to treat hypertension and the management of angina pectoris but atenolol can be.

E. There are no differences between propranolol and atenolol.

62. **With respect to Beta adrenergic receptors:**

A. β_1-adrenergic receptors increase heart rate and output.

B. As a result, β1- stimulation, renin will be released, causing arterial vasoconstriction and an increase in renal perfusion pressure. Na+ and H20 will be resorbed from the renal tubules to maintain or raise systemic blood pressure.

C. B2-adrenergic receptors cause smooth muscle relaxation but can cause an unwanted tremor in skeletal muscles.

D. With β_1 and β_2 stimulation, glycogenolysis from both the liver and skeletal muscles will result in increased levels of blood glucose.

E. All of the above can follow from the stimulation of beta adrenergic receptors.

63. **With respect to beta blockers, adverse reactions can be seen such as:**

    A. Bronchospasm leading to breathlessness and bradycardia leading to hypotension.

    B. A reduction in the distal systemic circulation, which could be of critical importance for our patients who have Raynaud's phenomenon.

    C. An alteration in both glucose and lipid metabolisms but this is less common with the β_1-cardio-selective drugs.

    D. Non selective beta blockers such as propranolol can easily cross the blood–brain barrier and can cause psychological disturbances, such as aberrant or inappropriate dream states, or indeed a complete loss of sleep.

    E. Should a complete block of the renal β_1 receptors in the macula densa occur, then renin release will be lowered, and aldosterone secretion drops. The end-point is that a critical state of hyponatremia and hyperkalemia can quickly follow.

64. **When treating patients taking non cardio-selective beta-blockers we must exercise caution when using local anaesthetics containing adrenaline due to the risk from the following physiological actions and reactions:**

    A. If our patient is taking a non cardio-selective beta-blocker, the effect of adrenaline on their vasculature will be different from the patient who has not been medicated with beta-blockers.

    B. If our patient is taking a non cardio-selective beta-blocker, the effect of adrenaline on their vasculature will be the same as the patient who has not been medicated with beta-blockers.

    C. If we inject a dental local anaesthetic containing adrenaline and some of the solution inadvertently enters an artery, the resulting arterial dilation can initiate a rapid but transient drop in diastolic blood pressure, but this effect is dose dependent.

    D. In the medicated patient: β-2 receptors on systemic arteries will be non-functional and so adrenaline will now activate the remaining α-1 receptors leading to vasoconstriction and an increase in diastolic blood pressure.

E. In the medicated patient: β-2 receptors on systemic arteries will be functional and so adrenaline cannot activate the remaining α-1 receptors there is no further vasoconstriction and diastolic blood pressure remains constant.

65. **Taking the physiological considerations of the interaction of beta-blockers and adrenaline one stage further: If there is an increase in diastolic blood pressure following the accidental intravascular injection of a local anaesthetic containing adrenaline:**

A. To counter an increase in resistance, the myocardium responds with a greater contraction force and the systolic blood pressure will also rise.

B. The mean arterial pressure will rise, however a sudden spike in arterial pressure will be picked up by the carotid sinus baro receptors and a paradoxical cardiac reflex will then initiate a sudden and striking bradycardic response.

C. The effects in A and B above can be increased further because the SAN β-1 receptors have already been blocked in patients taking cardio-selective or non-cardioselective beta blockers.

D. All of the above is total nonsense and is of theoretical consideration only

E. While answers A, B and C may be theoretical, the theory behind these answers is sound and we should bear this in mind when treating patients taking beta-blockers.

66. **Which of the following are correct for adrenaline contained in local anaesthetics?**

A. Adrenaline activates β-1 receptors in the Sino Atrial Node (SAN) to increase the heart rate and β-1 receptors on myocardial cells will also be stimulated increasing their force of contraction.

B. Adrenaline stimulates the α1 receptors in capillary vessel walls closing them down and stimulates the β-2 receptors in blood vessel walls opening them up.

C. The capillaries in the oral mucosa contain only α1 receptors and adrenaline will constrict them.

D. The walls of the larger systemic arteries contain both α1 and β -2 receptors, the latter being more numerous and stimulation of these will dilate arteries.

E. All of the above are correct.

67. **Which of the following apply to the use of dental local anaesthetics?**

A. There is no upper limit for the use of dental local anaesthetics, you can use as many as you want or the patient needs.

B. The maximum safe limit we can use is defined by the manufacturer.

C. The maximum limit is defined by the patient's medical health and issues such as cardiovascular pathology, hepatic and renal disease can reduce the maximum safe dose from the manufacturer's safe limits.

D. Every anaesthetic should aim to use the minimum dose to achieve the maximum effect but do so with the longest period of drug administration.

E. Empirically the safe dose of local anaesthetics can in theory be calculated from the patient's age and body weight.

68. **If incorrectly positioned, the Inferior Alveolar Nerve Block (IANB) can:**

A. Do no harm as it has a very high rate of success and will achieve anaesthesia almost all of the time.

B. Can transect either the Maxillary Artery and/or several of its branches, including the Inferior Alveolar Artery with the risk of a serious haematoma following from this.

C. Not result in an intravascular injection as there are no major arteries in either the pterygo-maxillary or pterygo-mandibular spaces.

D. Can encroach on the branches of the CN VII (Facial Nerve) resulting in a clinical presentation similar to a Bell's <u>like</u> Palsy.

E. Not affect the CN VII as it is a motor nerve and as such it is not susceptible to the effects of a local anaesthetic which only work on sensory nerves.

69. Should an anaesthetic injection-accident impact on the CN III (Third Cranial or Oculomotor Nerve), the clinical signs differentiating this from a Horner's Syndrome are:

A. The injection-accident will cause pupillary dilation (mydriasis) while one of the classic signs of Horner's Syndrome is pupillary constriction (miosis).

B. The injection accident will cause pupillary constriction (miosis) while one of the classic signs of Horner's Syndrome is pupillary dilation (mydriasis).

C. There is no difference in pupil sizes between an injection-accident and Horner's syndrome, the clinical differences are seen in the musculature, with an injection accident the patient's eyeball on the affected side will be displaced downwards and outwards and with Horner's syndrome only drooping of the eyelid (ptosis) is seen.

D. There will be a difference in pupil sizes between an injection-accident and Horner's syndrome, however with both an injection accident and Horner's syndrome the patient's eyeball on the affected side will be displaced upwards and inwards together with drooping of the eyelid (ptosis).

E. Answer A is correct, however with an injection-accident different groups of extra-ocular muscles could be affected or different muscles could be affected individually, including the intra-ocular ciliary muscles, so the clinical presentation could be quite variable, with the patient's vision being affected too. In contrast to this, in Horner's syndrome it is the sympathetic innervation that is disrupted, causing the classic clinical picture of: <u>Miosis</u> (a constricted pupil), <u>Ptosis</u> (a weak or drooping eyelid) and <u>Anhidrosis</u> (decreased sweating) on the affected side.

70. **An IANB injection accident that spares the pupil but affects the extra-ocular muscles is a result of:**
    A. Haematoma and haemorrhage only: Also known as a surgical 3rd
    B. Pharmacological effects of the anaesthetic diffusing into the nerve supply of muscles. Also known as a medical 3rd.
    C. Both haematoma, haemorrhage and the pharmacological effects of the anaesthetic.
    D. The mechanical trauma of the injection itself.
    E. None of the above.

71. **By which of the following routes can a misplaced dental local anaesthetic reach the Inferior Orbital Fissure to cause direct anaesthesia of the CN III, CN IV or CN VI?**
    A. Through passive tissue diffusion, venous absorption, or arterial intravascular injection.
    B. Through the Pterygoid Venous Plexus onto and into the Inferior Ophthalmic Vein, either directly or through communicating branches.
    C. Through the Cavernous sinus through the Infratemporal Fossa and the Pterygoid Plexus and the connecting Emissary Veins as they pass through the Foramen Ovale and Foramen Lacerum.
    D. Through all of the above means and routes.
    E. None of the above means or routes.

72. **In terms of anatomical location which of the following Cranial Nerves is most at risk from a misplaced posterior <u>maxillary</u> dental local anaesthetic?**
    A. CN II The Optic Nerve.
    B. CNIII The Oculomotor Nerve.

C. CNIV The Trochlear Nerve.

D. CN V The Trigeminal Nerve.

E. CNVI The Abducens Nerve.

73. **With a rushed or badly placed local anaesthetic which of the following clinical signs might be seen:**

A. Blanching of the skin in CN V $_1$ (Ophthalmic Division) and CN V$_2$ (Maxillary Division).

B. Ocular Complications: Loss of muscle control, Palpebral Ptosis and the Down and Out Orbit.

C. Ophthalmic Complications: Mydriasis, Presbyopia, Blurred Vision, Diplopia or Loss of Vision.

D. Agitation, drowsiness and possibly: loss of consciousness.

E. All of the above.

74. **Following the delivery of a local anaesthetic, if complications arise, what must be done?**

A. Nothing as the symptoms will be transient and will soon pass.

B. The symptoms of diplopia and blurred vision must be documented in the clinical notes, together with the type and dose of LA used; the affected eye must be examined for signs of muscular paralysis and pupillary involvement.

C. The patient must be reassured that their symptoms are temporary, with the affected eye being protected.

D. If necessary, the patient should be escorted home and not allowed to drive, recall for review is essential.

E. If the ocular or ophthalmic complications last longer than six hours then referral to a hospital for a specialist assessment is mandatory.

75. **Which of the following statements is correct?**

A. With maxillary infiltrations, pulpal anaesthesia is normally achieved in 10 to 15 minutes and with an IANB, pulpal anaesthesia is normally achieved in 2 to 5 minutes.

B. With maxillary infiltrations, pulpal anaesthesia is achieved in 2 to 5 minutes and with an IANB, pulpal anaesthesia is achieved in 5 to 20 minutes.

C. With maxillary infiltrations, pulpal anaesthesia is achieved in 2 to 5 minutes and with an IANB pulpal anaesthesia is also achieved in 2 to 5 minutes

D. With maxillary infiltrations, pulpal anaesthesia is achieved in 10 to 15 minutes and with an IANB pulpal anaesthesia is also achieved in 10 to 15 minutes.

E. All of the above are correct.

76. **The nerve fibres that will respond more quickly to the effects of a local anaesthetic are:**

A. Those fibres that are smaller diameter and unmyelinated rather than the larger diameter myelinated fibres.

B. Those fibres that are larger diameter and myelinated rather than the smaller diameter unmyelinated fibres.

C. Those nerve fibres with rapid firing rates rather than nerve fibres with slower firing rates.

D. Those nerve fibres with slower firing rates rather than nerve fibres with more rapid firing rates.

E. All nerve fibres will respond at the same rate regardless of their diameter or the extent of their myelination.

77. **You will know that with higher protein binding the duration of a local anaesthetic will be greater, but which of the following anaesthetic drugs also cause vaso-dilation?**

A. Mepivicaine.

B. Bupivicaine.

C. Lidocaine.

D. All of the above.

E. None of the above.

78. **While it is safer to over-estimate rather than under-estimate all drug doses, ideally a working knowledge of units and**

concentrations must be used, please match the following to their SI concentrations: (i) 0.5%, (ii) 1.0%, (iii) 2.0%, (iv) 1/100,000 and (v) 1/80,000:
A. 12.5 µgms/ml
B. 5mgs/ml
C. 20mgs/ml
D. 10mgs/ml
E. 10 µgms/ml

79. The safety critical factors associated with the accidental intravascular injections of dental local anaesthetics leading to systemic complications are:
A. The rate or speed at which the injection is given.
B. The dose or concentration of the injection that is given
C. The total volume of the injection.
D. All of the above
E. None of the above.

80. With which of the following conditions would we consider using an alternative local anaesthetic other than lidocaine with epinephrine?
A. Cardiac conduction defects, from partial to complete blocks, syndromes and artificial pacemakers.
B. Any cardiovascular condition, especially if anti-arrythmic drugs are needed or are being used
C. Impaired liver function.
D. Diabetes Types 1, 11 and gestational diabetes.
E. All of the above

81. An alternative to a dental local anaesthetic containing epinephrine is to use one containing octapressin; a vasopressin analogue, however this might cause problems with which of the following conditions?
A. Patients with impaired hepatic and renal functions.

B. Patients with breathing difficulties or allergies to drugs, medicines or local anaesthetics.

C. Patients who are either pregnant or are breast feeding.

D. Blood disorders such as anaemias, dyscrasias or coagulopathies.

E. All of the above.

82. **Both the Inferior Alveolar Nerve (IAN) and the Lingual nerve are at risk from local anaesthetic injury, but which of the following reasons are the correct explanations for the vulnerability?**

A. The IAN within a bony mandibular canal is more at risk than the lingual nerve from the primary toxic and the secondary ischaemic effects following an injection.

B. The lingual nerve, located on the mesial mandibular border, within a soft tissue sheath is more at risk from the direct physical and secondary patho-physiological damage from an accidentally placed IAN block.

C. The structure of the lingual nerve proximal to the lingula with far fewer nerve fibres and bundles than the IAN means it is at an increased risk of trauma from an injection.

D. All of the above reasons are correct.

E. None of the above reasons are correct.

83. **In comparing articaine with lidocaine which of the following statements are true?**

A. The benzene ring in lidocaine is one reason it is less neurotoxic than articaine which has a thiopentone ring.

B. With respect to neurotoxicity, both lidocaine and articaine are on parity, it is the dose that determines neurotoxocity, the benzene and thiopentone rings only confer a difference in lipid solubility.

C. Both A and B are correct.

D. Both A and B are incorrect.

E. On best accepted practice and clinical evidence, both articaine and lidocaine can be useful and are used for IAN blocks with no risk of nerve damage.

84. **Articaine is metabolized by esterase enzymes in plasma, whereas lidocaine and prilocaine are metabolized by de-alkylating enzymes in the liver, which of the following are true?**

A. Plasma esterases show no significant age related decline, however in patients over 65 years old, the levels of hepatic de-alkylating enzymes will have fallen by half.

B. Plasma esterases show a significant age related decline falling by half in patients over 65 years old, however the levels of hepatic de-alkylating enzymes will remain constant showing no age related decline

C. Many older patients will have been prescribed medication that can either directly or indirectly interact with the vasoconstrictors in our local anaesthetics.

D. Many older patients are never prescribed medication that can either directly interact with the vasoconstrictors in our local anaesthetics.

E. Any medication that decreases renal and hepatic blood flow could also reduce the ability of the patient's innate drug handling enzymes to excrete the metabolic products of local anaesthetics.

85. **The difficulty in achieving anaesthesia if tissue are inflamed or infected, but not yet abscessed can be explained by:**

A. An increase in pH of infected tissues higher than 7.4 which favours the water soluble but not the lipid soluble phase of the local anaesthetic.

B. An increase in pH of infected tissues higher than 7.4 which favours the lipid soluble but not the water soluble phase of the local anaesthetic.

C. A decrease in pH of infected tissues lower than 7.4 which favours the water soluble but not the lipid soluble phase of the local anaesthetic.

D. A decrease in pH of infected tissues lower than 7.4 which favours the lipid soluble but not the water soluble phase of the local anaesthetic.

E. All of the above factors.

The third group of 30 questions deal with the neuro-anatomy of the mouth and those injection techniques used in clinical dentistry.

In addition to gaining Enhanced CPD, reading the text and answering these test questions should provide a useful form of revision for those of you studying for clinical examinations:

86. **In comparison to the mandible the maxilla is generally:**
    A. More dense but less vascularised with fewer neuro-anastamoses.
    B. Less dense and less vascularised but has greater neuro-anastamoses.
    C. Less dense but more vascularised with greater neuro-anastamoses.
    D. More dense and more vascularised and with greater neuro-anastamoses.
    E. None of the above are correct, bone density in the maxilla and mandible are the same and the neurovasculature is identical.

87. **Which of the following can impact on the success of either maxillary or mandibular local anaesthesia:**
    A. The location of the tooth in the arch eg: incisors being easier to anaesthetise than molars.
    B. The position of the root apices with respect to their distance from the periosteum, teeth with roots closer to the bone surface being easier to anesthetise.
    C. Whether the tooth is multi rooted or single rooted.
    D. Developmental, Metabolic, Dysplastic, Neoplastic or Infective changes in bone could alter the direction and duration of local anaesthesia.

E. None of the above factors, they are all irrelevant to the success or failure of dental local anaesthesia.

88. **Using needles with a gauge of 30 or narrower...**
   A. Are beneficial causing less pain for the patient on injection than a needle with a bore of 25 to 27.
   B. Are easier to aspirate than needles of 25 to 27 gauge.
   C. Will be less prone to needle breakage than wider bore needles.
   D. Are easier to deposit local anaesthetic solutions than wider bore needles.
   E. All of the above are incorrect, it is preferable to use needles of 27 gauge or wider.

89. **Which of the following are correct for CNV$_2$?**
   A. The Maxillary Nerve is the Second Division of the Fifth Cranial Nerve or CNV$_2$ it arises from Mendlessohn's ganglion, located in Fingal's Cave in Staffa's part of the temporal bone.
   B. The CNV$_2$ is the sensory maxillary division of the Trigeminal Nerve. It leaves the middle cranial fossa through the foramen rotundum to enter the pterygopalatine fossa with combined branches of the greater petrosal nerve with preganglionic parasympathetic fibres and the deep petrosal nerve with its postganglionic sympathetic fibres.
   C. CNV$_2$ is the sensory-motor mandibular division of the Trigeminal Nerve. It leaves the middle cranial fossa through the foramen ovale in greater wing of the sphenoid bone to enter the infra-temporal fossa.
   D. A Pterygopalatine ganglion can be found suspended from the CNV$_2$. From the pterygopalatine fossa, the CNV$_2$ passes laterally on the anterior aspect of the mandible and then enters the orbit via the Superior Orbital Fissure.
   E. All of the above are incorrect for the CNV$_2$

90. **The Pterygopalatine Fossa is a cone-shaped depression deep to the** Infratemporal Fossa, **lying on the posterior aspect of the**

maxilla, with which of the following structures does it directly communicate?

A. The nasal and oral cavities.

B. The Infratemporal Fossa.

C. The Orbit, the Pharynx, and the Middle Cranial Fossa.

D. All of the above.

E. None of the above.

91. **Within the pterygopalatine fossa, the CNV$_2$ is closely associated with:**

A. Nothing whatsoever, CNV$_2$ is not in any way anatomically involved with any arteries or veins.

B. The pterygopalatine ganglion only.

C. The infraorbital branches of the terminal third of the maxillary artery and the maxillary vein are intimately involved with CNV$_2$ in the pterygopalatine ganglion.

D. The CNV$_1$ the ophthalmic division and CNV$_3$ the mandibular division of the Trigeminal nerve are intimately involved with CNV$_2$ in the pterygopalatine ganglion.

E. The CNVII the Facial Nerve is also found in the pterygopalatine ganglion.

92. **The Anterior Superior Alveolar (ASA) infiltration in one side of the maxilla will anaesthetize:**

A. Everything in the upper arch including some contra-lateral teeth due to cross over innervations.

B. Only the central and lateral incisors on one side.

C. The upper central and lateral incisors extending to the lateral aspect of the canine too, their periodontal ligaments, alveolar bone, supporting periosteum and surrounding buccal soft tissues.

D. Only the periodontal ligaments, alveolar bone, supporting periosteum and surrounding buccal soft tissues of the upper central and lateral incisors.

E. Any of the above can be seen due to the highly variable nature of the upper arch CNV$_2$ innervation.

93. **In some patients, the Middle Superior Alveolar (MSA) nerve is absent, this nerve supplies sensations to the distal aspect of the maxillary canines and premolars. In such patients to avoid pain in these teeth when working on them we can:**
   A. Use an ASA or PSA (Anterior and Posterior Superior Alveolar) nerve infiltrations which will effectively cover the missing MSA territory. One LA cartridge divided equally; anteriorly and posteriorly will then achieve anaesthesia.
   B. Refer the patient for a specialist sedation or general anaesthetic as local anaesthetics will never work on these teeth.
   C. Keep injecting into the MSA area and eventually after as many local anaesthetic cartridges as it takes the patient will go numb so you can carry on.
   D. All of the above are appropriate.
   E. None of the above are appropriate, the solution is to use a different local anaesthetic.

94. **The Posterior Superior Alveolar (PSA) infiltration will anaesthetize:**
   A. The maxillary molars.
   B. The maxillary molars but rarely the mesio-buccal aspect of the first molar, which will be supplied by the MSA and extended branches of the ASA and infrequently some branches of the PSA.
   C. All of the above and the periodontal ligament, alveolar bone, supporting periosteum, and surrounding buccal soft tissue adjacent to those teeth innervated by the PSA nerve territories.
   D. None of the above.
   E. The PSA infiltration will only anaesthetise the hard palate and area around the maxillary tuberosity.

95. **The Nasopalatine Block (NPB) will anaesthetize:**
   A. The palatal soft tissues of the premaxilla.
   B. The upper central incisors and the lateral incisors.
   C. The canines.

D. All of the above dependent on the precise location of the roots of these teeth relative to the nasopalatine foramen.

E. None of the above.

96. **The Greater Palatine Block (GPB) anaesthetizes all the** maxillary **teeth, their periodontal tissues, the hard and the soft palate to the midline septum, the sinuses. Which of the following are correct for the greater palatine nerve?**

A. The Greater Palatine nerve carries motor fibres from the Pterygopalatine ganglion and sympathetic fibres from both the Greater and the Deep Petrosal nerves.

B. The Greater Palatine nerve carries sensory fibres from the Otic ganglion and parasympathetic fibres from both Lesser and Superficial Palatal nerves.

C. The Greater Palatine nerve carries sensory fibres from the Pterygopalatine ganglion and parasympathetic fibres from both the Greater and the Deep Petrosal nerves, additionally its highly variable path is often intimately associated with the Maxillary artery.

D. The Greater Palatine nerve carries sensory and motor fibres from the Semilunar ganglion and sympathetic fibres from both Greater and Deep Palatine nerves.

E. All of the above are incorrect.

97. **Complete the missing bone parts (i) to (v), using all 5 answers: A to E in the following description of the CNV$_3$:**

A. Foramen Ovale

B. Foramen Rotundum

C. Foramen Spinosum

D. Petrous part of Temporal Bone

E. Greater Wing of Sphenoid Bone

"The Ophthalmic Division: CNV$_1$, the Maxillary Division: CNV$_2$ and the Mandibular Division: CNV$_3$ all arise from the Trigeminal Ganglion located in Meckel's Cave, near to the apex of the (i).......... The CNV$_3$ departs from the skull via the (ii)..........., located in the (iii).......... . This can be found to the outside and just behind the (iv).......... .from where CNV$_2$ emerges, but to the inside and just in front of the (v).........., from where the *Middle Meningeal Artery*, the *Middle Meningeal Vein*, and the *Meningeal Branch of the CNV$_2$* re-enter the cranium".

98. Despite being skeletal muscles, one neurological difference between the masticatory muscles and those of facial expression is:

    A. Facial muscles and purely voluntary, while those of mastication are involuntary or under autonomic control.

    B. There is no difference between the masticatory muscles and the facial muscles, both are under the control of the same cranial nerves.

    C. The masticatory muscles are controlled by the CNV$_3$ while those of facial expression are controlled by the CNVII.

    D. The masticatory muscles are controlled by the CNVII while those of facial expression are controlled by the CNV$_3$.

    E. All of the above are incorrect.

99. In the following section place the muscles (i) to (v) in the correct order using all 5 answers: A to E.

Passing inferiorly between the (i)........... and the (ii).........., the CNV$_3$ divides into two trunks, a small one to the front and a large one to the rear. Both of these trunks are mixed sensory-motor nerves. Firstly the small anterior trunk provides sensory input from the Long Buccal Nerve supplying the cheek and the first and second mandibular molars. There is a motor output to the four masticatory muscles: the (iii).........., the (iv)........... (with Sphenomandiularis) and the (v)........... .

    A. Masseter

    B. Lateral Pterygoid

    C. Temporalis

D. Tensor Veli Palatini

E. Medial and Lateral Pterygoids

100. **The CNV$_3$ posterior trunk is interesting in that one branch the Auriculo-temporal nerve:**

A. Carries fibres from the Facial Nerve.

B. Forms the eye of a needle through which the Middle Meningeal Artery passes like a thread before the nerve reunites.

C. Also carries fibres for the submandibular salivary gland.

D. Is also known as the nerve of Jefferies in that it: Goes Nowhere and Does Nothing (GNDN).

E. All of the above are incorrect.

101. **The ganglion through which sensory fibres of the CNV$_3$ pass without synapsing, but parasympathetic fibres that originate from the Glossopharyngeal Nerve (CN IX) synapse, which are then transported into the CNV$_3$ via the Tympanic Nerve is the:**

A. Otic Ganglion

B. The Pterygopalatine Ganglion.

C. The Submandibular Ganglion.

D. The ganglion of Gideon or Heister's Ganglion.

E. None of the above.

102. **Even though the Auriculotemporal nerve is not the target for dental anaesthesia, it is worth knowing something about the anatomy; the origins, destinations and connections of this nerve, because:**

A. The Auriculotemporal nerve is the main nerve supply to the TMJ.

B. Parotid gland injury, pathology and surgery can also give rise to complications should Auriculotemporal nerve fibres become incorrectly reattached. Given the complex input to this nerve, Frey's Syndrome is an unfortunate but thankfully a rare occurrence.

C. The Pleomorphic Salivary Adenoma (PSA) is one of the most common oral neoplasias and this most frequently occurs in the Parotid Gland. Considering the current increase in use of mobile phones with the attendant risks to sensitive neural tissues from radiation we need to be aware of these issues.

D. All of the above.

E. None of the above.

103. In the following text, fill in the spaces from (i) to (v) using the correct answers from A to E:

The (i)......... provides a sensory secreto-motor supply, achieving this by carrying fibres from The (ii).........These relay taste sensations via the (iii).........from the anterior 2/3rd of the tongue, while the posterior 1/3rd of the tongue is supplied by the (iv)........... The Lingual nerve lies beneath the <u>Lateral Pterygoid muscle</u>, medial to and in front of the <u>Inferior Alveolar Nerve</u> and is joined to this nerve by a branch which may cross over the <u>Internal Maxillary Artery</u>. The above noted <u>Chorda Tympani</u> also carries parasympathetic fibres to the (v)........., which is suspended from the Lingual Nerve by two very fine twig-like nerves.

A. Submandibular Ganglion.

B. Lingual Nerve

C. Facial Nerve (CNVII)

D. Chorda Tympani

E. Glossopharyngeal Nerve (CN IX)

104. Lingual Nerve injuries are caused most frequently either by surgery or local anaesthetic (Articaine) use. Overall, these risks have been quantified by the Royal College Surgeons (England) as:

A. 20% Temporary Injury and 2% Permanent Injury.

B. 2% Temporary Injury and 0.2% Permanent Injury

C. 0.2% Temporary Injury and 2% Permanent Injury.

D. All of the above.

E. None of the above.

105. **In common with the Lingual Nerve, there is a risk of injury to the Inferior Alveolar nerve too, but this is most likely to be from.**

   A. Procedures such as root canal treatment, extractions, or an implant placement encroaching upon or compromising the Mandibular Canal or its contents.

   B. Such problems are direct and immediate through technical error.

   C. Such problems are indirect as a result of a haematoma, or an infection.

   D. All of the above.

   E. None of the above.

106. **A good working knowledge of the whereabouts of the lingual nerve is important, please complete the following text (i) to (v) with the correct answers A to E.**

   Passing lateral to the (i).......... and positioned against the medial aspect of the (ii).........., the Lingual Nerve crosses over both the (iii).......... and the (iv).......... to run along the inferio-lateral margin of the tongue. Between the (v).......... and the Submandibular Salivary Gland, the Lingual Nerve runs towards the mandibular midline crossing over Wharton's duct of the Submandibular Salivary Gland. Located just below the tongue and just below the surface of the oral mucosa, the Lingual Nerve eventually terminates as the Sub-Lingual Nerve.

   A. Styloglossus

   B. Medial Pteryogoid

   C. Hyoglossus

   D. Superior Pharyngeal Constrictor

   E. Mandibular Ramus.

107. **The Inferior Alveolar Nerve (IAN) travels down a groove on the medial surface of the mandibular ramus, just behind the lateral pterygoid muscle where it gives off a motor branch to:**

Mylohyoid and then another motor branch to the: Anterior Belly of the Digastric in addition:

A. Both the nerves to Mylohyoid and the Anterior Belly of the Digastric also have a sensory element.

B. The mesial root of the mandibular first molar and the chin can be innervated by branches from the nerve to Mylohyoid.

C. There is an incredible range of variation not only with the IAN but throughout the entire path of the CNV_3. Communications have been noted between the Auriculotemporal nerve and the IAN and between the Mylohyoid nerve and the Lingual nerve

D. Further communications between the IAN and the Lateral Pterygoid have also been documented and the presence of these anatomical variations could provide one explanation for the failure rate in IANB being recorded as 20 to 25%.

E. All of the above are correct answers.

108. **The IANB will anaesthetize the mandibular teeth from the wisdom teeth to the central incisors, the intra-oral connective and soft tissues from the premolars anteriorly including the gingiva and periodontium will be covered. The extra-oral tissues around the chin and lower lip will be involved when an IANB is used and numbness in these areas is a good indication of successfully delivery. Which of the following needle sizes should be used?**

A. 27 Gauge 32 mm

B. 25 Gauge 32 mm

C. 30 Gauge 21 mm

D. 30 Gauge 25mm

E. All of the above are perfectly fine and acceptable.

109. **In the following description of an IANB place the answers (A to (E) in their correct places (i) to (v) in the text:**

For the IANB, the point of entry can be defined as (i)...... ......mm above the occlusal plane, between the tendon of the Temporalis muscle anteriorly and the Pterygomandibular raphe posteriorly. After a clear aspiration is demonstrated, up to (ii).......... mL of local anaesthetic can be safely and slowly injected into the area around and above the lingula, where both the IAN and the Lingual Nerve are located. Should you choose to specifically target the Lingual nerve, then following deposition of (iii).........mL, the remaining contents of the anaesthetic cartridge (iv).......... mL can be administered at a depth (v)..........cm superficial to that depth; just above the periosteum around the Lingula, where the IANB was previously placed.

A. 1.5

B. 10 to 15

C. 1 to 1.5

D. 0.5 to 0.7

E. 1

110. **In addition to the Halsead-Hall technique that you have correctly defined above, the Gow-Gates and the Vazirani-Akinosi methods can be used to deliver an IANB. With these two techniques, the main difference is:**

A. The Gow-Gates is a closed mouth technique.

B. The Vazirani-Akinosis is an open mouth technique.

C. The Gow-Gates is an open mouth technique.

D. The Vazirani-Akinosi is a closed mouth technique.

E. The Gow-Gates needs patient consent and compliance, while the Vazirani Akinosi should be used on a patient who will not consent to having an injection in their mouth.

111. **Between open and closed mouth techniques the Gow Gates will differ from the Vazirani-Akinosis in that:**

A. Gow-Gates will capture the: Inferior Alveolar Nerve (IAN), Auriculotemporal Nerve, Lingual Nerve, Buccal Nerve and Mylohyoid Nerve.

B. Akinosi will capture: The IAN, the Lingual Nerve, the Long Buccal and the Mylohyoid nerves but not the Auriculotemporal Nerve.

C. Gow-Gates will capture the: Inferior Alveolar Nerve (IAN), Lingual Nerve, Buccal Nerve and Mylohyoid Nerve but not the Auriculotemporal Nerve.

D. Akinosi will capture: The IAN, the Lingual Nerve, the Long Buccal and the Mylohyoid nerves and the Auriculotemporal Nerve.

E. There is no difference between these two techniques with nerves being covered

112. The Long Buccal Nerve can be anaesthetized with:

A. Not less than 2 cartridges of Lidocaine and/or Articaine as the nerve is so deeply buried.

B. This nerve is so superficial, a ¼ cartridge injected to a depth of 2mm to 3mm is sufficient.

C. A deep injection penetrating the maxillary periosteum is needed for this nerve

D. A deep injection penetrating the mandibular periosteum is needed for this nerve.

E. Topical anaesthetic is all that is needed for the Long Buccal Nerve.

113. The mental nerve provides a sensory supply to the:

A. The lower lip.

B. The chin.

C. The bucco-labial mucosa around the incisors.

D. The canines and the pre-molars.

E. All of the above.

114. Which of the following are correct?

A. There is cross over innovation in the midline of the mandible.

B. The Incisive nerve will also have some communication with sensory branches of the Facial nerve.

C. The buccal soft tissues will not be anaesthetized with an Inferior Alveolar Nerve Block, and the lingual soft tissues will not be covered by a Mental Nerve Block.

D. All of the above are correct.

E. All of the above are incorrect.

115. If after giving three cartridges of local anaesthetic and no effect is reported or observed you might then:

A. Carry on giving more local anaesthetic until the patient goes numb at some point they will, you can use up to 10 cartridges without any real safety concerns.

B. Stop to reassess the situation both you and your patient are now in and if necessary consider another approach including openly discussing the problem with your patient and your colleagues, waiting assessing and reassessing, referring if necessary are the safest options you should take.

C. Refer the patient for conscious sedation.

D. Try using a different local anaesthetic.

E. All of the above are incorrect if you wait long enough and give enough local anaesthetic, everyone will go numb....very numb at some point.

The fourth group of 15 questions deal with the consenting process for dental treatment and conscious sedation:

116. When referring a patient to a colleague for conscious sedation which of the following should be usefully included in your referral letter?

A. The reasons and justification for the use of conscious sedation with an outline of the dental treatment being requested, including treatment attempted and failed with reasons.

B. An up to date and complete medical dental and social history with ease and likelihood of attendance.

C. The scope and extent of sedation treatment with the total number of visits estimated.

D. All of the above.

E. Nothing, just complete the referral with the data set as requested by the health authority.

117. With respect to consent which of the following apply?

A. The patient must have capacity being both able and capable of making the decision to receive, or undertake or undergo treatment.

B. The patient must be informed_receiving <u>all relevant data</u> to reach the decision that the treatment option they have chosen is the most appropriate for them.

C. The patient doesn't need to have capacity as long as they sign a consent form.

D. The decision to receive dental treatment once obtained cannot be changed at any time.

E. The decision to receive treatment is voluntary and can be withdrawn at any time.

118. In the following famous legal dictum from Lord Denning in 1969, (which cleared the way forward for the rights of children), at what age does the legal right of a parent cease?

*"The legal right of a parent to custody of a child ends at the: ....
and even up till then, it is a dwindling right which the courts will
hesitate to enforce against the wishes of a child, and the more so the
older he is. It starts with a right of control and ends with little more
than advice".*

A. 12th birthday

B. 13th birthday

C. 16th birthday

D. 18th birthday

E. 21st birthday

119. **From the cases of Hewer v Bryant in 1969 and Gillick in the House of Lords 1985 which of the following should we now consider when dealing with the child patient?**
   A. The concept of the limitations in the rights and the responsibilities of children, the essence being judgment is based more on the facts surrounding the individuals at the time of the events in question and less on applying the law as it stood at the time of the events in question.
   B. The concept of the limitations in the rights and the responsibilities of parents, the essence being judgment is based more on the law surrounding the individuals at the time of the events in question and less on applying the facts as they stood at the time of the events in question.
   C. The concept of the limitations in the rights and the responsibilities of parents, the essence being judgment is based more on the facts surrounding the individuals at the time of the events in question and less on applying the law as it stood at the time of the events in question.
   D. The concept of the absolute rights and the responsibilities of parents, the essence being judgment is based more on the law surrounding the individuals at the time of the events in question and less on applying the facts as they stood at the time of the events in question.
   E. The concept of the absolute rights of children, the essence being judgment is based more on the law surrounding the individuals before and not after the events in question and less on applying the facts as they stood at the time of the events in question.

120. **For the patient younger than 18 years old, place the following options: (i) to (v) in their correct order from highest to lowest precedence for parental responsibility and legal guardianship:**
   i.   Birth father if the child was born after 1st December 2003.
   ii. Surrogate mother unless a parental or court order removes this.
   iii. Birth mother unless an adoption order has removed this.

iv. If the father is neither biological nor married to the mother, the father does not have parental responsibility; however joint responsibility can be applied for.

v. Biological father if married to the birth mother either at the time of birth or subsequently.

    A.....B.....C.....D.....E.....

121. **Following from immediate family members place the following options for legal guardianship in their correct order of precedence from highest to lowest:**

i. Local authorities with arrangement orders also having parental responsibilities.

ii. Special guardians consenting for a child but the birth parents do maintain some rights.

iii. Foster carers.

iv. Adoptive parents with an adoption order.

v. Guardians with responsibility following the death of a parent or other responsible person.

    A.....B.....C.....D.....E.....

122. **With respect to gaining consent for treating a child which of the following is correct?**

A. Only one person can have responsibility and should any doubt arise it is important that consent has been obtained from the correct person, normally a Social Worker who will tell you they are in charge.

B. Only one person can have responsibility and that person holds an Adult Protection Order and you must see this document.

C. It is possible that more than one person can have responsibility and should any doubt arise it is important that consent has been obtained from the correct person, the persons or individual officer within an organisation, such as a local authority who is authorised to hold a Child Arrangement Order.

D. It is possible that more than one person can have responsibility and in such cases all those involved will be Specialist Social Workers with Adult Protection Orders.

E. It is possible that more than one person can have responsibility and should any doubt arise you can all sit down and discuss what you think is best inviting the Social Workers along for a practice meeting to meet the staff for tea, biscuits and cake.

123. Which of the following apply to the 2005 Mental Capacity Act for adults?

A. There is no presumption of capacity, individuals are not to be supported to make their own decisions, unwise decisions cannot be made, decisions must not be made in the patient's best interests and the most restrictive option is to be made.

B. There is a presumption of capacity, individuals are supported to make their own decisions, unwise decisions cannot be made, decisions must be made in the patient's best interests and the most restrictive option is to be made.

C. There is a presumption of capacity, individuals are supported to make their own decisions, unwise decisions can be made, decisions must be made in the patient's best interests and the least restrictive option is to be made.

D. There is a presumption of capacity, individuals are supported to make their own decisions, unwise decisions cannot be made, decisions must be made even if they are in the patient's worst interests and the most restrictive option is to be made if you think it might be best for the patient.

E. All of the above are incorrect.

124. Mental capacity is the ability to make a decision. Which of the following can be applied to determine if capacity is present?

A. Does your patient have an impairment or disturbance in the functioning of their mind at the time of your consultation, if so, then what is the diagnosis and how will this affect the person? If an impairment or disturbance of the mind can be documented, does this mean the person is unable to make the decision for treatment required of them at this time?

B. If your patient has an impairment or disturbance in the functioning of their mind at the time of your consultation, you don't need to know either the diagnosis or the medication the patient is taking as these are irrelevant. However if an impairment or disturbance of the mind can be subsequently documented, you will have obtained consent in the form of a patient's signature and this will have been sufficient to go ahead and treat the patient.

C. You are certain your patient has no impairment or disturbance in the functioning of their mind at the time of your consultation. However if they have an impairment or disturbance of the mind you can make the decision for their treatment and even if consent wasn't valid you will have acted in the patient's best interests anyway.

D. You are certain your patient has an impairment or disturbance in the functioning of their mind at the time of your consultation. However as you are a dental professional you can make the decision for their treatment.

E. One answer you can rely on is that the 2005 MCA applies to a patient's mental needs and not their dental needs.

125. A functional test of capacity can be assessed by:
A. Understanding information relevant to the decision and retaining information to make a decision.
B. Balancing information to reach a decision and understanding the risks and benefits in making or not making the decision.
C. Communicating the decision.
D. All of the above: A, B and C.
E. None of the above.

126. In the process of gaining consent you have a clear duty to disclose those material risks that may give rise to adverse outcomes. From the 2004 judgment of Lords: Steyn, Hope

and Walker, in Chester v Afshar, which of the following statements is correct?

A. *"It is a basic principle of good medical practice that adults should consent on a fully informed basis to surgery, so they are aware of the risks you as a professional person with your clinical knowledge think might apply to them".*

B. *"Good medical practice should not be dependent on the decisions of the Lords; adults are old enough to know what is good and what is not good for them without interference from the law".*

C. *"Good medical practice is just that and adults undergoing dental procedures do not need to follow the onerous rules that apply to medicine, we will be telling hairdressers and manicurists what to do next if this nanny-state meddling is allowed to continue".*

D. *"It is a basic principle of good medical practice that adults should consent on a fully informed basis to surgery, so they are aware of all the risks."*

E. *"It is a basic principle of good dental practice that adults should only hear about the risks that a dental professional thinks will help them to undergo treatment and not those which, if they knew about would stop them from undergoing treatment."*

127. **With the ascendency of Scarman which of the following statements is the most correct?**

A. A failure to warn a patient of any and all risks is irrelevant to whether consent is valid or not.

B. A failure to warn a patient of a risk inherent in an operation that is recommended constitutes a breach in the patient's rights, but nevertheless consent is still valid.

C. A failure to warn a patient of the risks inherent in an operation which is recommended constitutes a failure to respect the patient's right to make their decision and if the risk materializes and injury follows, the patient can make a claim for compensation and damages in law.

D. A failure to warn a patient of the risks inherent in an operation which is recommended constitutes a failure to respect the patient's right to make their decision, however even if such a risk materializes and injury then follows, the patient cannot make a claim for compensation as they have consented for the procedure and are restricted by the legal documents they will have signed before the operation.

E. All of the above are incorrect.

128. **The judgment in the 2015 Supreme Court Appeal of Nadine Montgomery is:**

A. Only prospective from 2015 onwards

B. Absolutely and clearly both retrospective from 2015 and prospective from 2015.

C. Still unsettled as a further appeal is planned from the Lanarkshire Health Board and Scottish Courts.

D. A legal decision that the clinical indemnity providers in the UK are concerned about.

E. Due to the retrospective nature of Montgomery consent, answers B and D are correct.

129. **Today patients are increasingly accessing information from wider sources such as the internet and patient support groups, therefore patients should be thought of as:**

A. Seeking solutions to their problems with litigation rather than medication.

B. Persons holding active rights, rather than as being the passive recipients of our care.

C. Persons holding passive rights rather than being the active recipients of our care.

D. Persons who must accept what is told to them in the clinic no matter how paternalistic, the doctor and dentist will always know what is best for them.

E. None of the above are relevant to patient care.

130. **The move away from paternalism does come with the caveat of therapeutic exception. Therapeutic exception is:**
   A. Information which may compromise the decision of the patient to undergo treatment or information that if revealed would be detrimental to the patient's health and as such it can be withheld.
   B. An extremely narrow concept and it should not be use to subvert the principle of consent.
   C. Useful in those circumstances where the patient is liable to make a choice which may be contrary to their best interests and therapeutic exception must not be used to influence a decision that favours the practitioner rather than the patient *eg*: Extractions rather root treatment in a molar tooth.
   D. Defined by all of the above.
   E. Not defined by A to D above.

The fifth group of 35 questions will deal with conscious sedation.

To begin with; the questions will revise Relative Analgesia or Inhalation Sedation and after this; Intravenous Sedation will be revised. The level at which these questions are set will help you to revise your physiology and pharmacology for both E- CPD and your clinical examinations.

131. **With nitrous oxide relative analgesia, the lowest concentration of oxygen that can be delivered is:**
   A. 15%
   B. 20%
   C. 25%
   D. 30%
   E. 40%

132. **When considering the use of Relative Analgesia (RA) which of the following are important?**

A. The patient needs to be treated in a supportive understanding manner and within a clinical environment that is calming.

B. The patient doesn't need to be treated in a calm manner and the environment in which treatment is carried out has no effect on the treatment outcome.

C. The pharmacological effect of nitrous oxide is sufficient to achieve the desired effect on its own without the need to be supportive to the patient in any way.

D. Communication with the patient is not needed as they will be asleep throughout the procedure.

E. The patient must be told they will remember nothing and they must let the dentist get on with the work to be done, if necessary this message must be given clearly and if necessary emphatically and quite forcefully as the patient may be nervous and anxious patients respond well to threats.

133. **RA with N_2O and O_2 is inherently safe with a 100% safety record, however there are certain patients for whom the use of RA could potentially lead to clinical and legal complications, from the following options, please choose the patients for whom you would exercise caution before treating them with N_2O:**

A. Patients with upper obstructive airways diseases such as COPD.

B. Patients who are being medicated for behavioural or psychiatric illnesses and the input of their medical specialist will be needed.

C. Patients who are pregnant especially those in the first trimester of pregnancy.

D. Patients with bowel obstructions, strictures or those having recent surgery such as colostomy or ileostomy and for whom Vitamin B12 absorption is compromised.

E. Patients undergoing any or all forms of eye surgery especially vitreo-retinal procedures.

134. For COPD which of the following are true?

   A. COPD is a common condition mapped out across the UK in a North-South socio-economic divide.

   B. 5% of the world's population affected to a lesser or a greater degree.

   C. Those over 40 years, smokers, or those with industrial, occupational or recreational exposure to pollutants, irritants or tobacco smoke are affected by COPD.

   D. Non-smokers can suffer from COPD.

   E. The condition is invariably incurable and patients can die with it and from it.

135. Patients with Type 1 Respiratory Failure will:

   A. Have normal blood CO_2, but lowered levels of O_2 this is a result of a V/Q mismatch.

   B. Have elevated blood CO_2 and lowered levels of O_2 this is a result of a V/Q mismatch.

   C. Have lowered blood CO_2 and elevated levels of O_2 this is a result of a V/Q mismatch.

   D. Have normal blood CO_2, but lowered levels of O_2 there is no V/Q mismatch.

   E. All of the above can apply to a Type 1 Respiratory Failure.

136. Patients with a Type 2 Respiratory Failure will:

   A. Have decreased blood CO_2, together with increased levels of O_2

   B. Have increased blood CO_2, together with increased levels of O_2

   C. Have increased blood CO_2, together with lowered levels of O_2

   D. Have decreased blood CO_2, together with lowered levels of O_2

   E. Have neither increased or decrease CO_2, nor lowered or increased levels of O_2

137. Which of the following can cause a Type 1 Respiratory Failure?

   A. Insufficient O_2 in the air resulting in a V/Q mismatch

   B. Pulmonary embolism, pneumonia or Acute Respiratory Distress Syndrome so O_2 cannot diffuse into the blood stream.

C. Arterio-Venous shunting with oxygenated blood mixing with non-oxygenated blood.

D. Alveolar hypoventilation from respiratory muscle weakness.

E. All of the answers above can cause a Type 1 Respiratory Failure.

138. Which of the following can cause a Type 2 Respiratory Failure?

A. Increased airway resistance from COPD Asthma or suffocation.

B. A reduced ability to breathe effectively due to medication, TIA, CVA or morbid obesity.

C. Decrease in alveolar area due to chronic bronchitis, asthma or pulmonary tuberculosis.

D. An inability to use the muscles of respiration due to paralysis, medication or other neuromuscular condition or skeletal deformity such as extreme kyphosis or a malformed chest cavity.

E. All of the answers above are recognized causes of Type 2 Respiratory Failure.

139. There are definite risks from chronic exposure to N_2O with the doses and durations used for GA procedures being capable of inducing megaloblastic changes in bone marrow cells after 24 hours, however the actual risk from the concentrations used in a dental environment are very low, which of the following options are appropriate safety measures to take?

A. Active scavenging with suction systems and external gas exhaust are now mandated.

B. Passive scavenging is adequate.

C. Any concerns are based on theoretical extrapolation rather than practical consideration; in so far as work in the dental clinic is concerned and so no scavenging measures are needed.

D. No scavenging is needed but you might consider working with the doors and windows open.

E. Opening the doors and windows will only work if there is a breeze, to ensure there is a draft blowing from behind your back towards the patient a fan is necessary to blow the gas away and this much more effective than active scavenging (and cheaper too).

140. The rate of a patient's respiration is finely controlled by very small increases or decreases in:

A. The partial pressure of CO_2 dissolved in blood.

B. The partial pressure of O_2 dissolved in blood.

C. The partial pressure of both CO_2 and O_2 dissolved in blood.

D. The amount of CO_2 carried by Haemoglobin.

E. The amount of O_2 carried by Haemoglobin.

141. In the following text place the answers A to E in their correct places (i) to (v):

With (i) .... of the diaphragm and accessory muscles of respiration: the Pectorales Major and Minor, the Sternocleidomastoids and Platysma, negative pressure develops in the patient's lungs and air will be drawn in. Of note in COPD, the involvement of the accessory muscles of respiration become critically important to aid breathing. While (ii).......... is an active event, (iii).......... is in the main a passive event, as the muscles of respiration are in a state of (iv).......... However with coughing and in asthma, it is the rapid contraction of the internal intercostal muscles that are responsible for creating the (v).......... associated with forceful expiration.

A. Relaxation

B. Positive pressure.

C. Contraction

D. Inspiration

E. Expiration

142. The three physiological mechanisms of Ventilation, Perfusion and Diffusion occur in the lungs with the V/Q ratio being an important factor in the concentrations of Alveolar (PA) levels of O_2 and CO_2 and arterial (Pa) levels of O_2 and CO_2, which of the following statements are correct?

A. An increase in the V/Q ratio can come from either lowered ventilation or raised perfusion, the effect is that both PA O_2 and Pa O_2 will decrease, while PA CO_2 and Pa CO_2 will increase.

B. A decrease in the V/Q ratio results in an increase in PA O_2 and Pa O_2 with a decrease in PA CO_2 and Pa CO_2

C. A decrease in the V/Q ratio can come from either lowered ventilation or raised perfusion, the effect is both PA O_2 and Pa O_2 decrease and PA CO_2 and Pa CO_2 increase.

D. An increase in the V/Q ratio results in an increase in PA O_2 and Pa O_2 with a decrease in PA CO_2 and Pa CO_2

E. All of the above are correct.

143. **With a low V/Q ratio, which of the following physiological compensatory mechanisms might occur to allow a rise in Pa O_2 and a fall in Pa CO_2 ?**

A. Hypoxic vasoconstriction to decrease perfusion to allow normalization of the V/Q ratio.

B. Hypoxic vasodilation to decrease perfusion to allow normalization of the V/Q ratio.

C. Hypoxic vasodilation to increase perfusion to allow normalization of the V/Q ratio.

D. Hyperoxic vasoconstriction to decrease perfusion to allow normalization of the V/Q ratio.

E. Hyperoxic vasoconstriction to increase perfusion to allow normalization of the V/Q ratio.

144. **With a high V/Q ratio which of the following physiological mechanisms might occur?**

A. Broncho-constriction can reduce the ventilation to match the compromised perfusion.

B. Broncho-constriction can increase the ventilation to match the compromised perfusion.

C. Broncho-dilation can reduce the ventilation to match the compromised perfusion.

D. Broncho-dilation can increase the ventilation further to match the compromised perfusion.

E. Neither Broncho-dilation nor broncho-constriction can match the compromised perfusion.

145. N_2O is a simple molecule, with a low blood; gas partition co-efficient its solubility is low and its absorption is the highest of all anaesthetic agents, N_2O achieves its effect by:

A. A pressure gradient of Oxygen in the tissues, plasma and blood being responsible for actively forcing O_2 out of blood so hypoxia is responsible for the relative analgesia that is seen.

B. Active absorption and distribution through specific receptors and channels.

C. A pressure gradient of N_2O in the tissues, plasma and blood being responsible for driving N_2O across the blood brain barrier to the CNS.

D. Passive absorption and distribution through specific cell membrane receptors and channels.

E. All of the above mechanisms have a part to play in N_2O conscious sedation.

146. All inhalation sedative agents exert some physiological effects on a patient's respiratory function, while not altering blood pressure or heart rate, N_2O will cause a decrease in tidal volume, in response to this mechanism...which of the following statements is correct?

A. Due to the CNS sedation of all skeletal muscle function, a decrease in respiratory rate will be observed in your patient being sedated with N_2O and O_2.

B. The overall effect is that net ventilation will increase, in common with other inhalation anaesthetics; N_2O lowers the intrinsic tone of skeletal muscles.

C. Due to the CNS sedation of all skeletal muscle function, a compensatory increase in respiratory rate will be observed in your patient being sedated with N_2O and O_2.

D. The overall effect is that net ventilation remains unaltered. Unlike other inhalation anaesthetics, N_2O does not lower the intrinsic tone of skeletal muscles.

E. All of the above are correct.

147. **N2O has a MAC of 104%, which of the following statements apply to N2O?**
A. MAC decreases with extremes of age, with the use of recreational drugs such as cannabis, and an excess of alcohol consumption.
B. MAC increases in the young healthy athletically fit, with the use of recreational drugs such as cocaine or other CNS stimulants.
C. MAC increases in the chronic alcoholic whose CNS and hepatic metabolic pathways have developed a high tolerance to exogenous sedatives
D. N_2O could (but not in all cases) have almost has almost no effect on an athletically fit male using anabolic steroids.
E. All of the above are correct.

148. **On cessation of N_2O relative analgesia there is a risk of:**
A. The patient becoming uncontrollably aggressive as the disinhibition effect is always maximal just before the end of any procedure.
B. The patient falling asleep as the concentration of N_2O after a few minutes has accumulated to a MAC level sufficient to induce general anaesthesia.
C. The patient demanding more gas as N_2O is highly addictive.
D. Post procedural diffusion hypoxia due to a relatively high volume of O_2 leaving the blood stream to enter the alveoli together with the outflow of N_2O due to the pressure differential ceasing.
E. Heightened awareness of pain and surroundings due to the disinhibition effect being minimal at the end of the procedure.

149. **Please place the correct answers from A to E in the text from (i) to (v):**

N_2O will not cause (i).......... in respiratory activity; however the patient taking opioids will show a pronounced circulatory and respiratory (i).........from the combination of N_2O and opioids resulting in an unmasking of the pharmacological actions of N_2O. This effect on the patient's circulatory ability must be borne in mind in those opioid medicated patients who are cardiovascularly compromised. Against this potential for (ii)......... of N_2O to depress the hypoxic O_2 dependent drive, the venous return will show an (iii)........ due to an (iv)......... in the contractility of venous smooth muscles due to an (iv).......... in sympathetic tone from (v)......... of N_2O. The net effect is arterial blood pressure will therefore remain unaffected by the concentrations of N_2O used for dental RA.

A. Depression
B. Increase
C. Elevation
D. Lower doses
E. Higher doses

150. When considering intravenous sedation which of the following might we use as part of our patient assessment?

A. Body weight of the patient
B. The height of the patient
C. The Body Mass Index (BMI) of the patient, together with their heart rate, their systolic and their diastolic blood pressure.
D. The ASA, Mallampati and SARI index.
E. All of the above are useful if not mandatory measurements to take.

151. When midazolam is injected intravenously the bioavailability is:

A. 100%:
B. 75%
C. 50%
D. 25%
E. Zero

152. Which of the following must we follow when using IV Midazolam for Conscious Sedation?

A. The NICE and SIGN Guidelines defining the rapid and safe use of midazolam for IV conscious sedation.

B. The pharmacodynamics for patients in various states of either health or disease needs to be understood, together with the pharmacokinetics (I ADD ME) and any drug Interactions for midazolam.

C. The patient's response to local anaesthesia, anxiolysis and analgesia must be continuously and accurately assessed.

D. The need for drug reversal with flumazenil, together with an understanding of the doses and pharmacology of this reversal agent.

E. All of the above need to be followed.

153. **The intravenous administration of midazolam produces a predictable curve. The changes in plasma concentration versus time can be plotted and the shape of the curve produced will be dependent on the drug redistribution in the anatomical compartments of the patient. The area under the curve or AUC is an indication of:**

A. The pharmacokinetic properties and the bioavailability of a drug

B. The AUC represents the *total drug exposure over time.*

C. The the average concentration over a time interval: AUC/t.

D. The rate of drug <u>elimination</u> or clearance. Clearance (volume/time) * AUC (mass*time/volume).

E. All of the above.

154. **Which of the following are correct for Midazolam?**

A. Midazolam has anxiolytic, amnesic and sedative properties.

B. Midazolam has sedative properties but it is neither anxiolytic nor amnesic.

C. Paradoxical stimulation with agitation, hallucinations and euphoria could occur in children.

D. Paradoxical stimulation with agitation, hallucinations and euphoria never occur.

E. Vasodilation and a depression in myocardial function can occur together with skeletal muscle relaxation.

155. **Flumazenil can be used to antagonise midazolam and we know the half life of midazolam is longer than that of flumazenil (the elimination half life of flumazenil at 40 to 80 minutes is far less than that of midazalom at 90 minutes to 2.5 hours, with a peak effect at 13 minutes). However which of the following drugs can induce the metabolism of midazolam?**
   A. Omeprazole
   B. Rifampicin
   C. Phenytoin
   D. Carbamazapine
   E. Diltiazem

156. **Fentanyl is a potent synthetic opioid with incredibly small doses being sufficient and these are in the range of: 0.25 – 0.50 μgm/Kg body weight of the patient. Please place the correct answers A to E in (i) to (v) for the pharmacokinetics of fentanyl:**

While (i)..... will be available intravenously, remarkably over (ii)...... will be available transdermally and orally around (iii)...... of fentanyl will become metabolically active. Some (iv)....... of fentanyl will become protein bound with a very rapid elimination half life of some 10 to 20 minutes. The metabolism of fentanyl is decreased by with concomitant use of the antifungal azole drugs such as fluconazole. A similar inhibitory effect could be seen with the antiviral drug ritonavir. Renal elimination is seen with some (v).......of fentanyl being excreted in an unchanged state.
   A. 100%
   B. 90%
   C. 33%
   D. 10%
   E. 80%

157. Which of the following could occur with the use of fentanyl?

A. Bradycardia.

B. Tachycardia

C. Apnoea and decreased tidal volume with rigidity in the respiratory muscles.

D. Reduction in blood gas responses and lowering in effectiveness of the gag reflex.

E. Hyperventilation.

158. Which of the following effects are seen with naloxone?

A. A rapid reversal of the physiological effects of pain control, leading to intense pain and distress, this is especially relevant to those patients in palliative care being given opioids.

B. Stimulation of the sympathetic nervous system can be increased from a dramatic rise in cytokine levels and an acute opioid withdrawal crisis rapidly develops.

C. Hypertension, cardiac arrhythmias, pulmonary oedema and cardiac arrest may result from the inappropriate use of naloxone.

D. All of the above can be seen with naloxone.

E. None of the above effects are seen, these effects are only seen with Flumazenil.

159. With respect to the use of propofol which of the following are correct?

A. Propofol is an anaesthetic and hypnotic drug with amnesic properties.

B. The above are correct but of note: Propofol has no analgesic properties

C. The metabolism of midazolam can be significantly reduced by the concurrent administration of propofol.

D. Propofol is an extremely fast acting sedative with a maximal effect noted in only 1 to 3 minutes from administration.

E. None of the above effects are seen with propofol.

160. **Which safety critical concerns apply to the use of propofol?**

    A. The use of propofol can induce vasodilation, blocking the cardiovascular mechanisms physiologically compensating for this and the net result could be a lowering of the patient's myocardial output.

    B. If the above answer is correct, then an inhibition of the sympathetic neural output by propofol can result in blood pressure decreasing by up to 30%.

    C. The use of propofol can induce vasoconstriction and will also block the cardiovascular mechanisms physiologically compensating for this; the net result is the patient's myocardial output will be increased.

    D. If the above answer is correct, then an excitation of sympathetic neural outputs by propofol can result in blood pressure increasing by up to 30%.

    E. Propofol injections are noted to be less painful than injections with other sedative drugs so the patient could be unaware of how much has been administered if they are self medicating with propofol.

161. **Ketamine is a versatile drug with many recreational users. When used in dentistry which of the following are correct?**

    A. Ketamine is an anaesthetic hypnotic drug with sedative, analgesic and amnesic properties.

    B. On administration: A trance like state can be rapidly induced, with no loss of consciousness

    C. Despite being conscious profound relief from pain has been observed in patients given ketamine.

    D. Ketamine agonises both mu and kappa receptors while inhibiting the uptake of serotonin.

    E. The pharmacological action of ketamine is still poorly understood and there are safety concerns with its use.

162. **Given that a considerable number of our patients may have experimentally or recreationally taken ketamine which of the following could be <u>problematic</u>?**
   A. In contrast to the other sedative agents we have considered, ketamine can elevate both the blood pressure and the heart rate in a patient.
   B. There will be a noticeable increase or stabilization in cardiac output when ketamine has been administered.
   C. Ketamine can maintain or increase the drive to ventilate and usefully from a safety point, airway reflexes are maintained as the bronchioles are dilated with ketamine use.
   D. In contrast to midazolam but in common with fentanyl and propofol, ketamine can induce nausea and vomiting.
   E. Ketamine causes increased salivation.

163. **Which of the following are correct?**
   A. Midazolam: Can be antagonised with Flumazenil
   B. Fentanyl: Can be antagonised with Naloxone
   C. Propofol: Has no Antagonist
   D. Ketamine: Has no Antagonist
   E. All of these are correct.

164. **Which of the following are correct?**
   A. The potential pharmacokinetic competitive drug interactions we commonly see have a minimal effect.
   B. The pharmacodynamic additive drug interactions we rarely see will have a maximal effect.
   C. The potential pharmacokinetic competitive drug interactions we commonly see have a maximal effect.
   D. The pharmacodynamic additive drug interactions we rarely see will have a minimal effect.
   E. From the clinical evidence: Answers A and B are more correct than C and D. However, to be safety critical: The risk of any drug interaction whether competitive or additive, maximal or

minimal must be borne in mind when not only sedating be treating any patient!

165. James Badenoch QC (who successfully led the 2015 appeal for Montgomery consent) as a patient advised his anaesthetist to be sure if he was putting him to sleep to make sure he woke up when he was finished. For all of your patients you would:

A. Ensure that any medication you gave would follow the safety maxim that a good sedative should not be a strong analgesic and a strong analgesic should be a weak sedative.
B. Ensure your consenting process is up to date.
C. Ensure your medical and medication histories were complete and up to date.
D. <u>All of the above should, would and now must apply.</u>
E. None of the above would apply.

Answers to Questions on Medicine and Drug Safety

1. Answers to questions on prescribing drugs:

1. D	4. E	11. C D E	14. E True
2. E	5. A C D	12. D	15. C E
3. A: 1	6. E	13. A B C	16. B C D
3. B: 3	7. E	14. A: False	17. A C D E
3. C: 5	8. C D E	14. B: False	18. A C
3. D: 4	9. E	14. C: False	19. D
3. E: 2	10. C D E	14. D: False	20. B C

2. Answers to questions on drug safety and pharmacology:

21. B C D E	25. (i): C	29. D E	37. B D
22. B	25. (ii): D	30. B C	38. A D
23. A B C E	25. (iii): B	31. D	39. B D
24. (i): D	25. (iv): E	32. C D	40. A B D
24. (ii): A	25. (v): A	33. A	41. C E
24. (iii): C	26. B E	34. E	42. A B C D
24. (iv): B	27. A B	35. C	43. B D
24. (v): E	28. C D	36. A D	44. A C D

45. B D E	49. (i): E	53. A: Bactericidal	57. B C D
46. D	49. (ii): B	53. B: Bactericidal	58. A D
47. B	49. (iii): C	53. C: Bacteristatic	59. D
48. (i): E	49. (iv): D	53. D: Bacteristatic	60. B D
48. (ii): A	49. (v): A	53. E: Bactericidal	61. A C
48. (iii): B	50. E	54. A D	62. E
48. (iv): C	51. D	55. D	63. A B C D E
48. (v): D	52. D	56. E	64. A C D

65. E	73. E	78. (iv) E	85. C
66. E	74. B C D E	78. (v) A	
67. C D E	75. B	79. A B	
68. B D	76. A	80. E	
69. E	77. C	81. E	
70. B	78. (i) B	82. D	
71. D	78. (ii) D	83. A	
72. E	78. (iii) C	84. A C E	

3. Answers to questions on neuro- anatomy and local anaesthesia:

86. C	98. C	106. (i): B	114. D
87. A B C D	99. (i): D	106. (ii): E	115. B
88. E	99. (ii): B	106. (iii): D	
89. B	99. (iii): A	106. (iv):A	
90. D	99. (iv): C	106. (v): C	
91. C	99. (v): E	107. E	
92. C	100. B	108. A	
93. A	101: A	109. (i): B	
94. C	102: D	109. (ii): A	
95. D	103. (i): B	109. (iii): C	
96. C	103. (ii): C	109. (iv): D	
97. (i): D	103. (iii): D	109. (v): E	
97. (ii): A	103. (iv): E	110. C	
97. (iii): E	103. (v): A	111. A	
97. (iv): B	104. B	112. B	
97. (v): C	105. D	113. E	

4. Answers to questions on the process of consent:

116. D	120. (iv): E	122. C	129. B
117. A B E	120. (v): C	123. C	130. D
118. D	121. (i): D	124. A	
119. C	121. (ii): C	125. D	
120. (i): D	121. (iii): E	126. D	
120. (ii): B	121. (iv): A	127. C	
120. (iii): A	121. (v): B	128. E	

5. Answers to questions on conscious sedation:

131. D	141. (iii): E	149. (iii): C	156. (iv): E
132. A	141. (iv): A	149. (iv): B	156. (v): D
133. A B D E	141. (v): B	149. (v): E	157. A C D
134. A B C D E	142. C D	150. E	158. D
135. A	143. A	151. A	159. A B C D
136. C	144. A	152. E	160. A B
137. E	145. C	153. E	161. A B C D E
138. E	146. C D	154. A C E	162. D E
139. A	147. E	155. B C D	163. E
140. A	148. D	156. (i): A	164. E
141. (i): C	149. (i): A	156. (ii): B	165. D
141. (ii) D	149. (ii): D	156. (iii): C	

Certificate of Enhanced CPD in
Medicine and Drug Safety

C U S P I D
Clinically Useful Safety Procedures In Dentistry

| CPD Topic: | Medicine and Drug Safety |
| Focussed subject: | |

Enhanced CPD Record and Certificate for:

Name:	
GDC Number:	
Professional Role:	

Pages accessed:	
For the CPD Period:	
MCQ Questions answered:	
Enhanced CPD hours claimed:	

Signed: Date:	
Counter signed: Date:	
Name + GDC number:	

Please copy to add further focussed subject areas as required.

CUSPID Log sheet for Enhanced CPD
in Medicine and Drug Safety

Date and venue	Method eg: self study or training sessions	Topic(s) Covered	Pages studied:	MCQs used:	Reflection and areas for improvement? If so what?	CPD Hours	Signed

(Copy as necessary to add further CPD).

Total hours this page:

Evaluation and Self Satisfaction Survey

CUSPID - CPD in Medicine and Drug Safety

Name:	
Date:	
Venue:	

Section A. Please consider the following statements and decide if they reflect your views.

Please score each statement from: 1 - Strongly Disagree to: 5 - Strongly Agree

1	This CPD has improved my knowledge of the subject.	1 2 3 4 5
2	This CPD has confirmed my perception of current best practise.	1 2 3 4 5
3	As a result of this CPD, I plan to make changes to my practice.	1 2 3 4 5
4	The learning aims and objectives for this CPD were appropriate.	1 2 3 4 5
5	The learning aims and objectives for this CPD were met.	1 2 3 4 5
6	I was given enough background information about this CPD.	1 2 3 4 5
7	I was satisfied with the educational standard of this chapter.	1 2 3 4 5
8	The CPD organisation and delivery was excellent.	1 2 3 4 5
9	The venue was appropriate and conducive to learning.	1 2 3 4 5
10	I would recommend this CPD to my colleagues.	1 2 3 4 5

Section B. Please answer each of the following questions:

1.	Is there any part of the CPD activity that you felt was particularly successful?
2.	Is there any part of the CPD activity that you felt needed improvement?
3.	If so, how would you like to see it improved?
4.	Do you have any other comments or suggestions relating to this CPD?

(For CPD to be verifiable the GDC state the opportunity to give feedback should be provided.)

Section C.
Please add your further notes and updates

Professional and Personal Development
in Medicine and Drug Safety

CUSPID – Medicine and Drug Safety Reflective Notes

Name:	
Date:	
Topic:	Medicine and Drug Safety
Subject:	

The Main Points I have learned from this CPD activity:

1.	
2.	
3.	

Do these points have a relevance to my work?

Yes	
Possibly	
No	

The possible changes to improve safety for my patients and my profession:

1.	
2.	
3.	

On review the actual changes to my practise of dentistry were:

1.	
2.	
3.	

Verifiable Enhanced CPD Hours claimed for:

Preparation	
Activity	
Reflection	
Review	
Total hours:	

Name, GDC Number Signed.	
Dated.	
Name, GDC Number Countersigned.	
Dated.	

Index List of Terms
CUSPID Volume 1

A

alveolar:

of the lungs:

dead spaces 592–5

ventilation 68, 586, 595; *see also in lung function and physiology*

amalgam, dental amalgam, *see volume 2, chapters 3, 4, and 5*

amaurosis 300; *see intravascular injection accidents; see also blindness caused by local anaesthetic injections*

amides, local anaesthetics 458, 464, 470, 472–5, 478, 493

amoxycillin 303, 375–6

AMT (applied muscle tension technique in fainting) 63, 443–4, 561

anaesthesia:

consent 504, 559, 562

general 112, 241–2, 582, 609

local 82, 295, 361, 445, 448–9, 461, 467, 471, 487, 493, 509, 514, 525, 537, 539–40

analgesia 381, 394, 398, 400, 562, 581, 600, 611, 618

pain management 43, 277–8, 296, 316, 408

anaphylaxis 31, 95–100, 102–3; *see also* ACE inhibitors; aspirin; ibuprofen; penicillin

clinical presentation 98

management 98, 102

angina pectoris:

clinical presentation 143

differential diagnosis and Prinzmetal angina 147

management 143, 145

stable 139, 141–2, 144–5

unstable 139, 141–2, 144–5

angioedema, *see* anaphylaxis

angiotensin 364

angular stomatitis 97, 123

ANP (atrial natriuretic peptide) 107

antagonists 280, 304, 352–3, 404–5, 609, 624

anti-inflammatory drugs 278, 333, 380

antibacterial drugs 251, 283

interaction 312–13

antibiotic 135, 263, 266–7, 270, 330, 345, 375, 419–20

allergies 83, 97, 103, 278

breast feeding 330–1

interaction with oral contraceptive pills 283, 303, 375

resistance 266

stewardship 110, 262, 270–1, 282, 313, 343, 369

synergy 354–5

antibodies 108, 587; *see under specific diseases*

anticoagulants, *see* aspirin; heparin; *see under* warfarin

anticoagulants, interactions 369–70, 383–4

antidepressants 279, 355, 409–10; *see also* atypical facial pain; TCA
(tricyclic antidepressants); MAOIs (monoamine oxidase inhibitors)

antifungal drugs 135, 258, 263, 282, 313, 368, 618

antigens 301

antihypertensive medication 415; *see under specific drugs*

antimicrobials, *see* antibiotic

anxiolytics and beta blocker use 280–1, 304, 325, 412–16, 615

aphthous ulcer 278

APTT (activated partial thromboplastin time), *see* heparin

AR (applied relaxation in hyperventilation) 63

arrhythmias 163, 178, 240, 360–1, 412, 478, 480, 498

arterio-venous shunting 586

articaine 474, 486, 488–9, 491–3, 497, 510, 518

ASA (American Society of Anaesthesiologists) 40; *see also* ASA grading

ASA in medical assessment of patients and emergencies:

ASA DS 44–5

ASA PARS 43–4

ASA PS 40, 42–3

see NEWS (National Early Warning Score); Karnofsky

ASA grading 42, 164

ASA (anterior superior alveolar nerve) 451, 475, 507–10

aspiration 86–7, 505, 508–9, 523, 526; *see also* FBAO (foreign body airway
obstruction)

aspirin 98, 146–8, 151–2, 277–8, 286, 297, 309, 330, 333, 363–4, 369–70,
382–4, 387, 408

asthma:

deaths from 81; *see NRAD report*

emergency management of 80, 361

spacer use 79

see also LABA (Long Acting Beta Agonists); PAAP (Personal Asthma
Action Plan)

atheroma, atheromatous plaques 60, 139–40, 147; *see clots*

atrial fibrillation 311, 411

atypical facial pain 279, 409

AUC (area under the curve) 332, 613

auditing xxvii–xxviii, 12, 246, 476, 554, 560

autonomy 576; *see also* Dworkin, autonomy and consent to treatment; Steyn

AVPU, level of responsiveness 33–4, 51, 119, 129, 139, 146, 151–2, 173

B

B, breathing 14, 25, 27–8, 59–60, 99, 119, 131, 143, 155

bacteria:
    acute (infections caused by), *see volume 2, chapter 3, infection control*
    aerobic 367
    anaerobic 368
    antibiotic resistant 266–8, 270
    associated with oral cancer, *see volume 2, chapter 5, oral cancer*
    hospital acquired, *see volume 2, chapter 3, infection control*
    synergism with viruses and oral cancer, *see volume 2, chapter 5, oral cancer*
    see specific infections and types

Badenoch, James QC 566, 627; *see chapter 2, consent for treatment and Montgomery*

BADN (British Association of Dental Nurses) 245–6

bag, bag valve mask 29, 80, 90, 99–100, 102, 130–1, 146, 152, 176, 605

BDIA (British Dental Industry Association) 87, 343

behaviour, professional standards of, *see volume 2, chapters 3, 4, and 5*

Bell's palsy 453

benzocaine 295, 444, 474, 504, 511

benzodiazepines 83, 131, 280–2, 325, 354, 356, 358, 411, 445
    mechanism of action of 324, 353, 357

beta adrenoreceptor agonists, *see* salbutamol; *see under* asthma

beta blockers 353, 414, 492, 499

betamethasone, *see under* steroid

bioavailability:
    age 306–7, 323
    factors 298
    protein binding 304, 609

biotransformation 370–1, 597

bisphosphonates, *see volume 2, chapter 4, radiation safety; the justification for radiography*

bladder 277

bleeding:

  disorders 32, 278, 309, 316, 320, 370, 384–6, 394, 408, 451–2, 482, 587

  management 320

  medical history 31

  post-operative 317, 323

blindness:

  following intravascular injection accident 451

  permanent 300, 458

  temporary 451–2

  see also amaurosis

blood:

  analysis 596

  coagulation 251, 309, 363, 385–6

  pressure 31, 56, 61, 99, 108, 111–12, 142, 242, 323, 361, 389, 393–4, 405, 412–13, 442–3

  transmission (risks from) 576, 590; *see under specific pathogens and viruses*

blue:

  card, steroid treatment 109

  inhaler, salbutamol, and asthma relief from 77, 79

BMI (Body Mass Index) 265, 269

BNF (British National Formulary) 22, 246, 260–1, 272–4, 286, 294, 351, 424; *see also* DPF (Dental Practitioners' Formulary)

bradycardia 61, 414, 618

brain (the protection of), *see under* consent

breast feeding, *see under* drugs

breathing:

  sounds 27–8, 155, 174

  stridor 28

  wheeze 28, 78, 89, 98, 100, 149

bronchodilators 378

  beta-adrenoreceptor agonists and COPD treatment 585

brown, inhaler steroid and asthma prevention 77

bupivicaine, *see under* local anaesthetics

buprenorphine, *see under* smoking

burning mouth syndrome, *see* glossodynia

C

C, circulation 25, 29, 60, 99, 119, 143, 155

CAD (coronary artery disease) 139, 141

caffeine 297, 356, 362

calcium, *see* calcium channel blockers

calcium channel blockers 308, 325, 353, 361, 368, 389, 414

calories, *see volume 2, chapter 5, oral cancer*

cancer 41, 44, 356–7, 390; *see under specific forms, lesions, and types but especially refer to volume 2, chapter 5*

candidosis, *see volume 2, chapter 5, premalignant presentations*
    AIDS/HIV infection, *see volume 2, chapter 3*
    candidal leukoplakia, *see volume 2, chapter 5*
    iron deficiency, *see volume 2, chapter 5*

cannabis 598

capacity, *see* competence; *see under* consent

carbohydrate 124

carbon dioxide, *see under* COPD (chronic obstructive pulmonary disease); medical emergencies

carcinogens, *see volume 2, chapter 5, oral cancer*

cardiac arrest 15, 26, 29, 98, 152–3, 155, 157–8, 161–5, 170–1, 178, 241, 403, 477, 621

cardiovascular disease:
    cigarettes, *see volume 2, chapter 5, oral cancer*
    local anaesthetics and 497–8
    obesity 586
    smoking 585

carotid 59–60, 451, 457, 591; *see also under* medical emergencies

catecholamines 142, 410

cavernous sinus 399, 456–7

CD4 cells, *see volume 2, chapter 3, HIV and AIDS*

CD8 cells, *see volume 2, chapter 3, HIV and AIDS*

CDC (Centre for Disease Control) 399

cell mediated immunity, *see volume 2, chapter 5, oncogenesis*

cellulitis, *see volume 2, chapter 3, infection control*

cephalosporins 421

cerebral palsy 579

chain of survival 25, 164, 166

cheese, tyramine reaction with 410

cheilitis, *see* angular stomatitis

chemicals, *see under RIDDOR and workplace or occupational hazards in volume 2*

chemokines, *see volume 2, chapter 5, oral cancer*

chemotherapy 314–15

chest 27, 70, 73, 90, 155–6, 174, 176–7, 180, 256

    pain 22, 138–9, 141–3, 147–8

chickenpox, *see volume 2, chapter 3, infection control*

child, *see under algorithms for medical emergencies involving children*

children:

    consent to treatment 568–9

    drugs 99, 254, 260, 274, 278, 306, 331, 344

    puberty 569

chlorhexidine, *see volume 2, chapters 3 and 5*

chloride channels, *see* GABA (gamma amino butyric acid), $GABA_A$

    receptors; *see under* benzodiazepines

choking, *see* FBAO (foreign body airway obstruction)

cholesterol 140

CHORE (Conjugation, Hydrolysis, Oxidation, Reduction, Excretion), *see*

    biotransformation

chromosomes, *see volume 2, chapter 5, oral cancer*

    abnormalities

chronic, *see under specific diseases and condition, but of importance:*

    asthma 75, 78

    bronchitis 587, 595

    drug abuse, use, and treatment 133, 390, 406–8, 424

    emphysema 595

    hepatitis B 257, 301

    pain and its management 43, 277, 363, 401, 408

    periodontal disease 123, 368

cigarette smoking, *see volume 2, chapter 5, oral cancer*

    nicotine

    see also tobacco

circumoral:

    pallor 459

    paraesthesia 407, 488, 517

cirrhosis:

alcohol abuse 305

non viral and viral hepatitis 305, 390

clinical examination:

cervical lymph nodes, *see volume 2, chapter 5, oral cancer*

cranial nerves 123, 453

face 56, 65, 96, 98

head and neck 35, 56–7

clinical record keeping 52, 90, 245

CNS (central nervous system) 61, 135, 277, 280, 296, 352, 354, 364, 398, 401, 477, 591, 597–8, 617, 620

coagulation:

cascade 251, 309, 319

defects 393, 531–2

cocaine 127, 355, 415, 500, 533, 598

COCP (combined oral contraceptive pill) 303, 421

codeine 277, 354, 399

cognitive behavioural therapy 562

cold, the common cold virus 78

collapse:

adrenal crisis 109

airway obstruction 89

anaphylaxis 95, 98

asthma 78

cardiac arrest 154

diabetes 115, 117–18, 120–1, 124–5

epilepsy 127

fainting 57, 61

hyperventilation 65

see chapter 1 medical emergencies; see under the specific medical emergencies

communication 147, 151; *see communicating medical emergencies to first responders*

competence 566–9, 571–6, 580

compressions of chest; in cardiac arrest 155–8, 176–7

conscious sedation:

blood pressure monitoring 616

chaperone 281

drugs 602–3, 608–9, 611–26

counterfeit medicines 343, 345; *see also* BDIA (British Dental Industry Association); MHRA (Medicines and Healthcare Products Regulatory Authority or Agency); SSFFC (substandard, spurious, falsely-labelled, falsified, or counterfeit)

COX 1 and COX 2:
  actions of 363–4, 386
  inhibitors 366, 384, 394

Coxsackie virus, *see volume 2, chapter 3, infection control*

CPR (cardiopulmonary resuscitation) 9–10, 12, 25, 155–6, 158–9, 161–2, 164–6, 170, 173, 178, 181–4, 408
  management in a medical emergency 159, 172–3, 178, 181–2

cranial nerves:
  I (olfactory), *see volume 2, chapter 5, oral cancer*
  II (optic) 452
  III (oculomotor) 454–7
  IV (trochlear) 454–7
  V (trigeminal), *see under* mandibular; maxillary
  VI (abducens) 454–7
  VII (facial) 453, 490, 515, 517, 521, 536
  VIII (auditory), *see volume 2, chapter 5, oral cancer*
  IX (glossopharyngeal) 516, 518
  X (vagus) 59–61, 76
  XII (hypoglossal), *see volume 2, chapter 5, oral cancer*

Crohn's disease 587

CRT (capillary refill time) 30

Cushing's disease 115; *see also* corticosteroids; hyperglycaemia

Cushing's syndrome 115

CVA (cerebro-vascular accidents) 41, 44, 308, 586; *see also* stroke; TIA (transient ischaemic attack)

cyclo oxygenase, *see* COX 1 and COX 2

cytochrome 372; *see also* P450

cytokines 621

cytotoxic 357; *see CD8 cells in volume 2, chapter 3*

D

D, disability 25, 32; *see under ABCDE in chapter 1, management of medical emergencies*

DDD (defined daily dose of drugs) 263, 271–2

medical history 12, 17, 19, 22, 97, 255, 305, 325, 354, 402, 406, 486, 498, 500, 582

metabolism 306, 322–3, 325–6, 342, 370, 374, 379

older patients 282, 306–7, 323–5, 384, 423, 492

oral ulceration 278, 295

overdose 281, 285, 313, 350, 395, 401, 404, 406–7, 415, 619–21; *see also* paracetomol; Rumack-Mathews nomogram for paracetomol overdose

pigmentation, *see volume 2, chapter 5, oral cancer*

reactions 243, 349, 372, 414

urine 107, 307, 329–30, 480, 625

xerostomia, *see volume 2, chapter 5, oral cancer*

DVT (deep vein thromboses) 308; *see also under* coagulation

Dworkin, autonomy and consent to treatment 576

E

E, examination and exposure (ABCDEF in medical emergencies) 25, 37

eating disorder, bulaemia 305

ECDC (European Centre for Disease Prevention and Control) 262

eczema 77

Eisenmenger syndrome 593; *see also* Down's syndrome; *see under* lungs

elderly 260, 282, 306–7, 323–4, 382, 384–5, 493, 598, 621; *see also under* old/older

embolism, pulmonary 27, 83, 148–9, 304, 308, 586, 592–5, 621

emergencies and emergency:

emergency drugs 22, 286

medical emergencies, *see chapter 1*

EMLA (eutectic mix of local anaesthetic) 296, 444, 474, 504, 511

emphysema, *see* COPD (chronic obstructive pulmonary disease)

endocarditis 20, 237

endocrine glands 20, 106, 108, 115, 365, 487

endorphins 621

environment vii, 16, 29, 38, 62, 132, 166, 170, 180, 236, 245, 284, 347–8, 411, 444

epilepsy:

classification 134

drugs 130–1, 134–5

emergency management 128, 130–1

medical emergencies 130
SUDEP death 132
epinephrine:
adrenaline 99, 102, 475, 480–1, 486–7, 492, 496–9, 502, 513
allergy to 447
anaesthesia, local 481, 486–7, 496, 498–9, 502, 513
anaphylaxis use in medical emergency 99–100, 102
neurotransmitter 106, 410
Epipen 99, 102–3
erythromycin 313, 375, 421–3
ethanol 280, 296–7, 354, 362, 393; *see also* alcohol abuse, alcoholism
ethmoid bone 457
exercise 72–3, 76, 123, 148
exposure in medical emergencies 25, 37
extractions:
bleeding 316–17, 323
teeth 30, 66, 314, 504, 518–19, 535
extrinsic:
asthma 75–6, 83
clotting and coagulation cascade 309, 319
eyes:
amaurosis 300
anaesthetic intravascular accidents 453–5
blindness 300, 451–3, 458, 584
cranial nerves (II, III, IV, and VI.) 454
examination 453
ophthalmitis, herpetic, *see volume 2, chapter 3, infection control*
pupil 453, 455

F

F, follow up (ABCDEF in medical emergencies) 24, 37
face, facial:
bones 457–8, 501, 503, 506, 511, 514, 524, 526, 529–30, 536
pain, atypical 279, 409
palsy 453
paralysis 453
facial:
nerve, *see under* cranial nerves

G

gases

    medical emergencies 27, 68, 586, 592–3, 595–6

    see under conscious sedation

gastrointestinal tract 297, 375, 385, 616, 619, 624, 626

    aspirin and 384

    disorders of 298, 363, 381, 384, 388, 398

    flora in 313, 368, 375–6, 421

GCS (Glasgow Coma Scale) 33–4, 40, 51

GDC (General Dental Council): vii–viii, x, xix–xx, xxii–xxvii, xxix–xxx, 9, 11, 85, 235–6, 239–43, 258–60, 349, 408, 520, 557

    AED 157–9, 162, 178, 181, 183, 408

    CPD x–xi, xix–xx, xxii–xxviii, 9, 235, 239–40, 520, 557–8

    Principle 1.54 245

    Standard 1: Putting patients first 245

general anaesthesia:

    complications 83, 112, 609

    contraindications 83, 445–6, 582

    morbidity 445, 504

    mortality 242, 445, 504

genes 322, 372, 379

genital, *see volume 2, chapter 3, infection control*

    herpes

    infections

genito-urinary tract, *see* medical history; *see under* infections

gestational diabetes 116

GFR (glomerular filtration rate) 306

Gillick competence 568–9

gingival, *see volume 2, chapter 3, infection control*

    hyperplasia

    swelling

gingivitis, *see volume 2, chapter 5, oral cancer*

glossitis, *see volume 2, chapter 5, premalignant presentations*

glossodynia 123

glossopharyngeal nerve

    neuralgia 370

    see under cranial nerves

glucagon 22, 37, 119–21, 286, 299, 414

glucose 22, 117, 119, 414

glucose 6 phosphate dehydrogenase pathway 484

glycogen, *see volume 2, chapter 5, non-odontogenic tumours: the Ewing's Sarcoma*

GMC (General Medical Council) xxiv, 240–1

Gow-Gates, *see* mandibular: local anaesthetic techniques; *see also Vazirani Akinosi and Halsted techniques*

GPB (greater palatine block), maxillary local anaesthesia 512–13

grand mal, epilepsy 128, 130

granuloma, *see volume 2, chapter 5, non-odontogenic tumours*

grapefruit juice and drug interactions 379

GTN (glyceryl trinitrate) 22, 138, 141–2, 146–8, 150–2, 286, 296, 367

guardianship 570; *see also* precedence, the legal order of

H

HAART (highly active anti retro-viral treatment) 312
    HIV and AIDS medication 312
    see PEP (post-exposure prophylaxis)

haematoma 450–1, 455, 510, 513

haemoglobin 296, 394, 482–5, 589–90, 597

haemoglobinopathy 484

haemophilia 315

haemorrhage 30–2, 112, 316–17, 450–1, 455

haemostasis:
    blood 386
    disorders 386
    factors 124, 386

hairy leukoplakia, *see volume 2, chapter 3, infection control*

half life, *see under drugs, especially refer to chapter 2*

hallucinations 354, 407, 615, 623

Halsted 528, 532–3; *see inferior alveolar nerve block techniques*

hand, foot, and mouth disease, *see volume 2, chapter 3, infection control*

hands, *see volume 2, chapter 3, hand hygiene*
    cleaning
    contamination
    washing

hay fever 77

HBc antigen, HBe antigen, HBs antigen, *see volume 2, chapter 3, infection control*

disease progression, *see volume 2, chapter 3, infection control*

epidemiology, *see volume 2, chapter 3, infection control*

incidence 162

mortality from, *see volume 2, chapter 3, infection control*

neoplasms associated with, *see* Kaposi's sarcoma; *see volume 2, chapter 3, infection control*

opportunistic infections, *see volume 2, chapter 3, infection control*

post-exposure prophylaxis, *see volume 2, chapter 3, infection control*

prevalence, *see volume 2, chapter 3, infection control*

society, *see volume 2, chapter 3, infection control*

transmission from needle stick injuries, *see volume 2, chapter 3, infection control*

see AIDS (acquired immunodeficiency syndrome)

hoarseness 98, 278

homeostasis, *see* RAAS (Renin Angiotensin Aldosterone System); ACE (angiotensin converting enzyme) (inhibitor drug)

Hope (law lord in consent) 575

hormones 115, 251, 304, 352

Horner's syndrome 453–4; *see also* medical third and surgical third

hospitals, referral to 38, 121, 452, 459, 560, 565

HPV (human papilloma virus), *see volume 2, chapters 3 and 5 for:*

epidemiology

lesions

method of infection

oral cancer

vaccination

vaccines

HRT (hormone replacement therapy), *see volume 2, chapter 5, oral cancer*

HSV (herpes simplex virus) 283, 285

human factors 403; *see also* PROUD (Pilot Recognition for Operational Up-skilling and Development from CAA and comparison with GDC ECPD for dental registrants)

hyperadrenocorticism 115

hyperalbuminaemia 304–6

hypercapnia 28, 32, 594, 598

hyperglycaemia:

coma 117, 121

diabetes 115–17, 121–2, 124

minerals 368–9

miosis, *see under* pupils; *see also comparison with mydriasis*

MODY (maturity onset diabetes in the young) 116–17, 121

monitoring:

cardiac 26, 146, 151

conscious sedation 564, 608–9, 616

medical emergency ix, 26, 33, 45, 49, 51, 124, 271

mono amine oxidase inhibitors 401, 409

monoclonal, *see volume 2, chapter 5, oral cancer*

antibodies

tumour origin in neoplasia

Montgomery consent 518, 520, 578, 580; *see also* Badenoch, James QC

morbidity viii, 16, 31, 86, 91, 253, 267, 342, 387, 396, 407, 423, 445, 504

morphine 277, 352, 354, 399, 404, 533, 600, 617; *see also section on N_2O for equivalence and doses*

mortality viii, 16, 86, 91, 103, 132–3, 164, 267, 342, 387, 396, 407, 422–3, 445, 504

motor, branches of the cranial nerve VII 453, 515

mouth:

examination of 524, 526

pain 44, 143, 278

ulcers 278, 295

MOVE, *see under* medical emergencies

MRSA (methicillin-resistant Staphylococcus aureus) 367

MSA (middle superior alveolar) 451, 475, 507–10

mucocutaneous candidosis 108

mucosa 250, 295, 367, 371, 375, 384–5, 416, 448, 461, 471, 487–8, 496–7, 508–10, 529–30, 535–6

mucosal lesions 283–4

multidrug resistant infections 268

multiple myeloma 344

muscles:

affected by local anaesthetics 455–6

orbital muscles 454–6

mycobacterium, *see volume 2, chapter 3, infection control*

mycobacterium tuberculosis, *see volume 2, chapter 3, infection control*

mydriasis, *see under* pupils

myeloma, *see* multiple myeloma

myocardial infarct:
>   cardiac arrest 152–3, 155, 157–8, 161–5
>   chest pain 138–9, 141–3, 147–8, 150
>   clinical presentation 149–50
>   depression 387, 615
>   diagnosis 149–50, 153
>   immediate treatment 150–2
>   Killip classification 163–4
>   management 148, 151–3
>   mortality from 164
>   ventricular fibrillation 161, 181
>   *see under* heart

myocardium 139–40, 149, 417
>   effects of anaesthetic on 416

N

NAC (n-acetylcysteine), *see* Rumack-Mathews nomogram for paracetomol
>   overdose

naloxone 404–5, 600, 619–20, 626

NAPQI (n-acetyl-p-benzoquinone imine paracetomol metabolic toxicity)
>   391–3

NASH (non-alcoholic steato-hepatitis) 390–1

nasopalatine block 510–11

nausea 108, 143, 277, 331, 406, 626

neonates 306, 482, 484

nephron, *see* kidneys

neuralgia 370

NEWS (national early warning score) 40–2, 45–7, 50, 52
>   observation charts 46, 59, 80
>   weighting score 46

NICE, also NIHCE (National Institute for Health and Care Excellence)
>   51, 237–8, 260, 279, 555, 611

nicotine, *see volume 2, chapter 5, smoking and oral cancer*

nitrous oxide (N_2O), *see* conscious sedation: relative analgesia

non-adrenaline (containing local anaesthetics) 43, 142, 408

non-alcoholic steato-hepatitis 390

non-opioid analgesics 380, 398, 400

NOSID (non-insulin dependent steroid induced diabetes) 116

respiratory depression 401, 404, 621

opportunistic infections:

    HIV 108, 133, 162, 257

    immunocompromised 256, 282

optic nerve, *see under* cranial nerves

oral health 561, 563

oral hygiene 43, 583

oral infections 44

oral lesions, *see volume 2, chapter 5, oral cancer*

    drug related lesions and pigmentations

    HIV AIDS and oral lesions

    lichenoid reactions

    see specific lesion types

oral route of drug administration 285, 299, 301, 331

oral ulcers, drug related 278, 295

orofacial, *see volume 2, chapters 3, 4, and 5 for the following:*

    lesions

    leukaemias

    lymphomas

    pain

orofacial infections, *see volume 2, chapter 3, infection control*

    bacterial

    fungal

    HIV

    viral

oropharyngeal, lesions, *see volume 2, chapter 5, oral cancer*

orthodontics/orthodontists 88, 519, 531

osteoblasts, *see volume 2, chapter 5, oral cancer*

osteoclasts 363

osteoma, *see volume 2, chapter 5, oral cancer*

otitis media 584

oxycodone, *see under* hillbilly heroin

oxygen:

    cardiac arrest 29, 157, 176, 182

    cardiac failure 413

    CD (cylinder sizes) 22–3, 286–7

    conscious sedation 83, 581

    COPD 29, 590

panic attacks 66, 69, 127, 134, 407

papillomavirus, *see specific virus types in volume 2*

paracetomol 277, 312–13, 364, 370, 384, 386, 390–7, 400, 408
    overdose 243, 391, 393, 395, 399–400, 404, 407–8

paracetomol dose toxicity 277, 313, 354, 384, 389–93, 395–6, 400–1

paracetomol metabolic toxicity 396

paraesthesia 407, 488, 517

parasitic infections, *see specific types and species in volume 2, particularly in chapter 3*

Parkinson's disease 411

parotid, salivary gland 515–17, 521, 528; *see also volume 2, chapter 5, tumours of the parotid*

penicillin:
    allergy to 83, 97, 103
    probenicid use and penicillin 330

PEP (post-exposure prophylaxis), *see volume 2, chapter 3, HIV and sharp injuries*

periapical 441, 535

periodontal:
    abscess 110, 263, 419
    disease 123, 368

pernicious anaemia 587; *see also under* vitamins

pharmacodynamics:
    definition 342
    drug reactions 303, 313, 322, 355, 383, 389, 609, 611, 615, 618, 623, 625–6

pharmacokinetics 295, 611
    definition 295, 342
    drug reactions and 297, 319, 321, 334, 342, 355, 367, 371, 609, 611–12, 615, 618, 622, 625
    first-order 320, 332–3
    zero-order 333–4

pharynx 87, 97, 506, 584

phenytoin 334, 615
    adverse effects 135

phobia 16, 28, 63, 69, 73, 141, 162, 165, 259, 281, 398, 440–3, 504, 558, 561
    fainting 62–3, 442

progesterone 375, 420

prognosis 45, 163–4, 182

prophylactic, antibiotic prescribing 237–8

propofol 358–61, 404–5, 603, 617, 621–4, 626; *see also* PIS (propofol infusion syndrome)

prostaglandins 76, 363, 389

PROUD (Pilot Recognition for Operational Up-skilling and Development), from UK CAA 349

PSA (posterior superior alveolar nerve) 451, 475, 507, 509–10

psychoactive, drugs 127, 355, 415, 500, 533, 598

pterygomandibular space 450, 526, 532

pterygopalatine fossa 457, 506–7

PTLBW (preterm low birth weight babies), *see volume 2, chapter 5, effects of smoking*

ptosis 453, 455, 459

puberty 569

pulmonary, *see* embolism, pulmonary

pupils:
    constriction 453–4
    dilation 56, 121, 453–4, 459

P>WHEAT, *see under* pharmacokinetics

Q

quality assurance, *see auditing and volume 2, chapter 3, standards of radiographic images*

quality of life, *see end of life care in volume 2*

R

RAAS (renin angiotensin aldosterone system) 364–6, 414

rabies 301

radiation and radiography, *see volume 2, chapter 4, radiation safety*

radiotherapy, *see volume 2, chapter 5, cancer care*
    dental effects of
    mucosal effects of

RAS (recurrent aphthous stomatitis) 278

Raynaud's phenomenon 414; *see also* beta blockers

RCP (Royal College of Physicians) 45, 47, 50–1; *see NEWS in management of medical emergencies*

RCS (Royal College of Surgeons) vii, 236, 555

recovery position in medical emergencies 37, 131, 155, 174, 176

red blood cells, *see volume 2, chapter 5, oral cancer*

renal function 307, 323, 363, 623

rescue breaths 156–8, 161, 176, 178

respiratory:

    COPD and 586, 589–90, 594

    distress 26, 28, 100

    failure 586, 589, 596

    infections 76, 78, 584

    muscles of 27–8, 78, 587, 590

    obstruction 97; *see also* FBAO (foreign body airway obstruction)

    see also aspiration

Reye's syndrome 278, 297

rheumatic fever 20

rheumatoid arthritis 388

rifampicin 375, 421, 615

risk assessment 24, 39–40, 486

rubella, *see volume 2, chapter 3, infection control*

Rumack-Mathews nomogram for paracetomol overdose 277, 313, 354, 384, 389–93, 395–7, 400–1

S

salbutamol 77, 79–80, 100, 361, 415

saline 255

saliva 128, 130, 334, 536

salivary glands:

    minor 512

    palate 512

    parotid 515–17, 521, 528

    sublingual, *see volume 2, chapter 5, oral cancer*

    submandibular 518

salivation 128, 517, 626

    excessive 128, 130, 626

    xerostomia, *see volume 2, chapter 5, oral cancer*

SARI (simplified airway risk index) 606

Scarman (the ascendency of and the demise of Diplock in rulings on consent) 568–9, 577

SDCEP (Scottish Dental Clinical Effectiveness Program), *see under* conscious sedation

secondary, *see specific conditions*

sedatives:
alcohol abuse and use 354, 356, 598
conscious sedation uses for 582–3, 602

seizures:
epilepsy 127–9, 132–5, 378
medical emergencies 128–31

serotonin 385, 401–2, 625
serotonin syndrome 354–5, 402–4, 408
SSRI (serotonin specific reuptake inhibitors) 279, 312, 355, 385–8, 401, 408–10
see also 5HT (5 hydroxytryptamine)

serum, serous, and sero 304, 375, 388, 477–8, 587
hepatitis 301
see specific diseases

SILENT (syndrome of irreversible lithium-effected neuro-toxicity) 388

simplified airway risk index 606

sinus, cavernous 399, 456–7

Sjogren's syndrome, *see volume 2, chapter 5, oral cancer*

skin cancer, *see volume 2, chapter 5, oral cancer*

skull, *see under this volume, mandibular and maxillary for anaesthesia; see also volume 2, radiography*

sleep, lack of, *62; see also causes of fainting in medical emergencies*

smoking 42, 139, 325, 585
cessation 352, 355
see also tobacco; nicotine; *see volume 2, chapter 5, cancer*

sodium:
biochemistry in blood 469, 472
hypochlorite 252–3

spasms:
carpo-pedal 68
laryngeal 65, 68

sphenoid 457, 506, 514

spine, spinal cord, or spinal column 173, 591
head and neck support in medical emergencies, *see chapter 1*

SSFFC (substandard, spurious, falsely-labelled, falsified, or counterfeit) 345

SSRI (serotonin specific reuptake inhibitors) 279, 312, 355, 385–8, 401, 408–10

staphylococcal, bacterial infection, *see volume 2, chapter 3, infection control*

statins 370, 422–3

status epilepticus 130–1

STD (sexually transmitted diseases), *see volume 2, chapter 3, infection control*

steroid:
    anti-inflammatory effects of 278
    betamethasone 278
    hydrocortisone 111–12
    prednisolone 112, 278
    triamcinolone acetonide 278
    see specific types of steroids and treatments

Steyn 575–6

stomach 67, 72, 278, 363, 367

stomatitis:
    angular 123
    recurrent aphthous 278

stroke 22, 41, 43–4, 133, 140, 156, 366, 387; *see also* CVA (cerebrovascular accidents); TIA (transient ischaemic attack)

substance abuse:
    analgesics 391, 393, 395, 398–400, 404, 406–7, 619–21
    drugs 133, 243, 270, 354, 399–400, 404, 407–8, 415
    emergency care (in cases of) 402, 406
    opioids 398–9, 404, 406–7, 619–21
    oxycodone *see under hillbilly heroine*
    paracetomol 243, 391, 393, 395, 399–400, 404, 407–8
    see specific drugs

SUDEP (sudden unexpected death in epilepsy) 132–3

suicide 395; *see mechanisms of and paracetomol overdose*

summation 280, 304, 352, 356–7

sun exposure, *see volume 2, chapter 5, risk factors for cancer and oral cancer*

supportive care, end of life care, *see volume 2, chapter 5, end of life care*

surgery, *see volume 2, chapter 5, oral cancer*
    in cancer
    compared to medical care

surgical third 455

syncope 14, 127, 442, 504–5, 513

synergism, drugs 280, 304, 352–3, 355–7, 391

syphilis, *see volume 2, chapter 3, infection control*

T

T cells, *see volume 2, chapter 5, oral cancer with relevance to:*
    AIDS
    APC (antigen presenting cells)
    CD4 cells
    CD8 cells
    HIV

tachycardia 70, 78, 181, 354, 414

taste:
    cranial nerves involved in 517–18
    disorders of, *see volume 2, chapter 5, oral cancer*
    facial nerve CN VII 517
    glossopharyngeal nerve CN IX 518
    loss of, *see volume 2, chapter 5, oral cancer*

TCA (tricyclic antidepressants) 355, 369, 400, 409–10, 499

teeth 503
    abrasion, *see volume 2, chapters 3 and 5*
    discoloration, *see volume 2, chapter 3*
    erosion, *see volume 2, chapter 5*

temporal bone 457, 506, 514

tetanus 448

thalidomide 344–5

thiamine, *see volume 2, chapter 5, end of life care*

thrombin 319

thyroid 378
    function 325

TIA (transient ischaemic attack) 127, 586

TMJ (tempero-mandibular joint) 279, 516–17
    pain dysfunction 279

tobacco 325, 379, 585
    cessation advice, *see volume 2, chapter 5, oral cancer*

tongue 22, 128, 131, 146, 152, 517–18, 521, 534; *see also* hypoglossal nerve

tonic clonic, seizure in epilepsy medical emergency 128, 130 topical anaesthetic, *see* benzocaine; EMLA (eutectic mix of local anaesthetic)

tranexamic acid 316–17, 320

transplants 109, 395–6

trauma:

accidents 296, 531

haemorrhage 31

triamcinolone acetonide (steroid) 278; *see also* di-methyl chlortetracycline (antimicrobial)

trigeminal nerve (cranial nerve CN V):

branches of 457, 459, 470, 502, 506–8, 513–17, 519–21, 523, 525–6, 533

neuralgia 370

trismus 527

trypanophobia, *see under* phobia, *specifically needle phobia*

tuberculosis 108

BCG vaccine 448

drug resistance, *see volume 2, chapter 3, infection control*

drug treatment 375, 420

tumours 108, 133, 379

tympanic membrane 584; *see also* otitis media; *see under* conscious sedation

U

UK DOH (Department of Health) 164, 240, 403

UK GDC (General Dental Council):

CPD x–xi, xix–xx, xxii–xxviii, 9, 235, 239–40, 520, 557–8; *see ECPD from 2018 onwards*

guidelines xxiii, 11, 235, 243

standards 10, 245, 260

UK GMC (General Medical Council) xxiv, 240–1

UK NMC (Nursing and Midwifery Council) xxiv

ulcers and ulceration 278, 295, 316, 363, 369, 384–5, 388, 395; *see also* oral ulcers

unstable angina 139, 141–2, 144–5

urine 107, 121, 307, 329–30, 360, 479–80, 625; *see also under* kidneys

URTI (upper respiratory tract infection) 78, 584

V

vaccination, *see volume 2, chapter 3, infection control*

vaccine 301; *see also under* hepatitis

vagus, cranial nerve X (CN X), *see under* cranial nerves; medical
    emergencies: vasovagal syncope

vancomycin 369; *see also vancomycin resistant species of bacteria in volume 2,
    chapter 3*
    enterococci
    staphylococcus aureus species

varicella, *see volume 2, chapter 3, infection control*
    chickenpox
    virus

vascular:
    accidents from local anaesthetic injections 457, 459, 487, 496, 499, 530,
        532–3
    strokes 41, 44

vasoconstrictors, local anaesthetics 416, 465, 467, 476, 478, 487, 492, 496

vasodilators 415

vasovagal attack, *see syncope and fainting in chapter 1, medical emergencies*

Vazirani-Akinosi inferior alveolar neve (IAN) block technique, *see*
    mandibular: local anaesthetic techniques

vegetables, *see fruit and vegetables diet 5 a day in volume 2, chapter 5, oral cancer*

veins 30, 299, 405, 450, 456–7, 501, 608

ventricular fibrillation 161, 181

viral:
    hepatitis 305, 390
    immunisation, *see volume 2, chapter 3, infection control*
    infections 76, 265
    see specific types

vitamins:
    A (retinol), *see volume 2, chapter 5, oral cancer*
    B_1 (thiamine), *see volume 2, chapter 5, oral cancer*
    B_{12} (cobalamin or folate) 368, 587
    C (ascorbic acid) 484
    D and bones, *see volume 2, chapter 5, oral cancer*
    E, *see volume 2, chapter 5, oral cancer*
    K and clotting 308–9, 313, 393, 421

W

Walker (law lord in consent) 575
warfarin:

X

Y

young / younger patients:

Z

Lightning Source UK Ltd.
Milton Keynes UK
UKHW012310070223
416610UK00001B/29